D0866251

MRI of the Eye and Orbit

MRI of the Eye and Orbit

EDITED BY

PATRICK DE POTTER, M.D.
Assistant Surgeon
Oncology Service
Wills Eye Hospital
Assistant Professor
Thomas Jefferson University
Philadelphia, Pennsylvania

JERRY A. SHIELDS, M.D.
Director
Oncology Service
Wills Eye Hospital
Professor of Ophthalmology
Thomas Jefferson University
Philadelphia, Pennsylvania

CAROL L. SHIELDS, M.D.
Associate Surgeon
Oncology Service
Wills Eye Hospital
Associate Professor of Ophthalmology
Thomas Jefferson University
Philadelphia, Pennsylvania

With 3 Additional Contributors

J. B. LIPPINCOTT COMPANY Philadelphia

Assistant Editor: Eileen Wolfberg
Production Editor: Virginia Barishek
Indexer: Roger Layne Wall
Interior Designer: Arlene Putterman
Cover Designer: Thomas M. Jackson
Production: P. M. Gordon Associates, Inc.
Compositor: Circle Graphics, Inc.
Prepress: Jay's Publishers Services, Inc.
Printer/Binder: Quebecor/Kingsport

Copyright © 1995, by J. B. Lippincott Company. All rights
reserved. No part of this book may be used or reproduced in
any manner whatsoever without written permission except for
brief quotations embodied in critical articles and reviews.
Printed in the United States of America. For information write
J. B. Lippincott Company, 227 East Washington Square,
Philadelphia, Pennsylvania 19106.

6 5 4 3 2 1

Library of Congress Cataloging-in-Publication Data

MRI of the eye and orbit / edited by Patrick De Potter, Jerry A.
   Shields, Carol L. Shields ; with 3 additional contributors.
      p.   cm.
   Includes bibliographical references and index.
   ISBN 0–397–51382–8
    1. Eye—Magnetic resonance imaging—Atlases. 2. Eye-
sockets—Magnetic resonance imaging—Atlases. I. De
Potter, Patrick. II. Shields, Jerry A. III. Shields, Carol L.
  [DNLM: 1. Orbital Neoplasms—diagnosis—atlases.
2. Orbit—pathology—atlases. 3. Eye Neoplasms—
diagnosis—atlases. 4. Eye—pathology—atlases.
5. Magnetic Resonance Imaging—atlases. WW
17 M939 1995]
RF79.M33M75   1995
617.7'1548—dc20
DNLM/DLC
for Library of Congress   94–41374
                                      CIP

The authors and publisher have exerted every effort to ensure
that drug selection and dosage set forth in this text are in
accord with current recommendations and practice at the
time of publication. However, in view of ongoing research,
changes in government regulations, and the constant flow of
information relating to drug therapy and drug reactions, the
reader is urged to check the package insert for each drug for
any change in indications and dosage and for added warnings
and precautions. This is particularly important when the
recommended agent is a new or infrequently employed drug.

To my parents who dedicate their lives for their children, to my brothers and sister as well as my close relatives that I love, to my dear friends who bring sunshine to my life and work, to each patient whom I respect for teaching me the meaning of life, and to you whom I cherish.

A mes chers parents qui ont dédié leur vie pour leurs enfants, à mes frères et soeur ainsi qu'à ma proche famille que j'aime, à mes amis qui m'apportent joie dans ma vie, à mes patients que je respecte pour m'avoir appris le vrai sens de la vie, et à toi que je chéris.

Patrick De Potter

To our wonderful children: Jerry, Patrick, Billy Bob, Maggie Mae, and John Fendell.

Jerry A. Shields
Carol L. Shields

Contributors

PATRICK DE POTTER, M.D.

Assistant Surgeon
Oncology Service
Wills Eye Hospital
Assistant Professor
Thomas Jefferson University
Philadelphia, Pennsylvania

CAROL A. DOLINSKAS, M.D.

Clinical Director, MRI
Radiology Department
Pennsylvania Hospital
Clinical Associate Professor
University of Pennsylvania
Philadelphia, Pennsylvania

WILLIAM S. MILLAR, M.D.

Neuroradiology Fellow
Radiology Department
Thomas Jefferson University Hospital
Philadelphia, Pennsylvania

JERRY A. SHIELDS, M.D.

Director
Oncology Service
Wills Eye Hospital
Professor of Ophthalmology
Thomas Jefferson University
Philadelphia, Pennsylvania

CAROL L. SHIELDS, M.D.
Associate Surgeon
Oncology Service
Wills Eye Hospital
Associate Professor of Ophthalmology
Thomas Jefferson University
Philadelphia, Pennsylvania

ROBERT A. ZIMMERMAN, M.D.
Professor of Radiology
University of Pennsylvania School of Medicine
Chief, Pediatric Neuroradiology and MRI
The Children's Hospital of Philadelphia
Philadelphia, Pennsylvania

Preface

The Ocular Oncology Service at Wills Eye Hospital has evaluated over 12,000 patients with ocular tumors and simulating lesions over the past twenty years under the direction of Dr. Jerry A. Shields. A world-reknowned practice has developed and a respected reputation evolved. Dr. Carol L. Shields, trained at Wills Eye Hospital, joined the practice in 1989 and is dedicated to full-time ocular oncology. In 1992, Dr. Patrick De Potter from Belgium became the junior associate.

Dr. De Potter's interest in imaging techniques of the eye and orbit began while he was a fellow in the Oncology Department at the University Eye Hospital in Lausanne, Switzerland. He brought his expertise in MR techniques to the Ocular Oncology Service at Wills Eye Hospital, and as a two-year fellow he shared his enthusiasm for MRI with Drs. Jerry A. Shields and Carol L. Shields. Many manuscripts, chapters of books, presentations, and research projects have resulted from this team effort. This atlas is a compilation of many years of investigating and imaging patients with ocular tumors.

This atlas is the first book dedicated exclusively to MRI of the eye and orbit. Many clinico-pathologic correlations are used to facilitate understanding of the MR features of intraocular and orbital lesions and provide a more complete understanding of the disease. A large spectrum of ocular lesions, from the most common to the most rare, is documented.

Why write an atlas specifically focused on MRI of the eye and orbit? First, several books and manuscripts have been written on the subject of computed tomography and ultrasonography of the eye and orbit and few have focused in detail on MRI of ocular diseases. Second, MRI has revolutionized the ability to image the human body and has recently become one of the most useful diagnostic tools for the clinician. However, there is still some confusion among ophthalmologists and others in ordering and interpreting imaging studies. For these reasons we chose to write a concise atlas illustrating the MR features of intraocular and orbital lesions. Hopefully, this book will help physicians in their diagnostic and therapeutic approach to ocular lesions.

Chapter 1 covers pertinent basic principles of MRI, emphasizing its application for orbital imaging as well as the requirement for the orbital protocol. Chapter 2 illustrates with great detail the anatomy of the normal eye and orbit. Chapters 3 through 7 provide a detailed review of intraocular lesions. MR features of congenital anomalies, retinal detachments, and inflammatory conditions simulating intraocular tumors are reviewed. Chapters 6 and 7 illustrate the MR features of tumors of the uvea and retina. Chapters 8 through 19 provide a review of orbital lesions. Chapter 20 contains pertinent MR information on the anophthalmic socket, with emphasis on the recently introduced hydroxyapatite implant. Finally, Chapter 21 reviews the role of MRI in orbital trauma.

We have attempted to make each chapter clear and easy to read. Tables scattered throughout the chapters help organize the diagnostic approach and interpretation of MR features. However, we realize that new imaging protocols such as fast spin-echo techniques may further improve the MR resolution of orbital imaging. Because of these recent developments, not all the intraocular and orbital lesions presented in this atlas have been imaged by these new techniques. We hope that this atlas will provide the clinician with a solid basis for the differential evaluation of the majority of ocular and orbital lesions.

Patrick De Potter, M.D.
Jerry A. Shields, M.D.
Carol L. Shields, M.D.

Acknowledgments

Many people have contributed to the preparation of this atlas, and a few words of thanks need to be expressed. First and foremost we must give special thanks and recognition to Roger Barone, photographer in the Audio-Visual Department at Wills Eye Hospital. He devoted an enormous amount of time and expertise in the preparation of the photographs used in this book. We also thank Robert Curtin and Jack Scully for their generous ongoing photography collaboration with the Oncology Service team.

We wish to give special recognition to our own staff of the Ocular Oncology Service who have dedicated years of their time to the development of our facility. Special thanks go to Kathy Smallenburg, Queen Warrick, Sandra Dailey, Jeanine Ligon, Ruth Humm, Barbara Mace, Brenda Hall, Leslie Botti, and Patricia Schultz, R.N. The Oncology Service fellows were instrumental in assisting in the care of our patients with ocular tumors, many of whom are illustrated in this book. In this regard, we acknowledge the assistance of Drs. Arun D. Singh and Hayyam Kiratli.

Special recognition goes to Dr. Ralph C. Eagle, Jr., Department of Pathology, who provides ongoing histopathological advice on most of our oncological cases. He also contributed the superb histopathologic slides that illustrate this atlas. The expert opinions of Drs. Adam E. Flanders, Vijay M. Rao, and Carlos F. Gonzalez from the Department of Neuroradiology at Thomas Jefferson University Hospital in Philadelphia are appreciated. They offered critical analysis of our own MR interpretations. Similarly, we appreciate the technical assistance of Peter M. Natale, BSRT, and co-workers in the Department of Neuroradiology, Thomas Jefferson University Hospital, who were involved in many imaging studies of our patients. Dr. Robert I. Grossman from the Department of Radiology at the Hospital of the University of Pennsylvania in Philadelphia gave his tremendous expertise in reviewing Chapters 10, 13, 14, and 19. Dr. Jonathan J. Dutton, Oculoplastic Service, Duke University Medical Center in Durham, kindly reviewed Chapter 2 on normal anatomy of the eye and orbit. Many physicians have contributed individual cases, and they are acknowledged specifically throughout the book. We also appreciate the continued support of the Ocular Oncology Service from many members of the staff at Wills Eye Hospital and from many ophthalmologists throughout the United States as well as other countries.

Finally, we would like to recognize the support of the staff of J.B. Lippincott Company, and would especially like to thank Stuart Freeman and Eileen Wolfberg for their assistance.

Contents

MRI of the Eye and Orbit

Part One | General Considerations

MRI of the Eye and Orbit,
by Patrick De Potter, Jerry A. Shields, and Carol L. Shields.
J. B. Lippincott Company, Philadelphia © 1995.

1

Basic Principles

WILLIAM S. MILLAR

The goals of this chapter are to discuss the physical basis for magnetic resonance (MR) imaging at the atomic level and then to provide insight into how electromagnetic signals are produced, acquired, and subsequently transformed into MR images. The physics of tissue contrast is then discussed and applied to basic MR image analysis of the orbit. A basic MR imaging protocol for the orbits is presented. The chapter concludes with a discussion of the physics of image artifacts.

A detailed discussion of the complexities of MR physics is beyond the scope of this chapter. However, a basic understanding of MR physics is useful to produce technically acceptable images, to maximize diagnostic information, and to avoid or reduce artifacts. Exposure to college-level physics is helpful in this endeavor, but not essential. The interested reader is referred to the Bibliography at the end of this chapter, which includes several excellent MR physics texts that have been written at different levels of technical sophistication.

BASICS OF MR IMAGE PRODUCTION

The basis for MR image production begins at the atomic level with the concept of *nuclear spin* (angular momentum). Only the nuclei of atoms with an odd number of protons, neutrons, or protons and neutrons have nuclear spin. Atoms with nuclear spin include ^1H, ^{13}C, ^{14}N, ^{23}Na, and ^{31}P. An important consequence of nuclear spin, and the foundation of MR imaging, is that each positively charged, spinning ^1H nucleus produces a miniature magnetic field (similar to the way an electrical current in a coil of wire induces a magnetic field). This miniature magnetic field can be likened to a tiny bar magnet which has both a north and south pole. Because the magnetic field has both magnitude (strength) and direction (north/south), it can be represented by a vector (usually depicted by an arrow). The miniature nuclear magnetic field vector is called the *magnetic dipole moment* (MDM). In medicine, MR images of patients are obtained by inducing electromagnetic signals from the MDMs of ^1H nuclei within living tissues and then converting these signals into diagnostic cross-sectional images. Hydrogen is chosen over other atomic elements with nuclear spin owing to its relative abundance in body tissues and its efficient MR signal production.

In MR imaging, radio frequency (RF) energy is transmitted via an antenna located around the patient (called a body coil). It is then transferred to ^1H nuclei within the body's tissue and temporarily stored in a coherent, in-phase arrangement of MDM motion. During and after the RF pulse, special electromagnetic coils (called *gradient coils*) produce small electromagnetic field variations (called *gradi-*

ents). These gradients are used to encode frequency and phase information in the ^{1}H MDMs in order to mark and later determine the location of their signal information. When the RF pulse is terminated, the MDMs of the ^{1}H nuclei begin to relax and decay to their original equilibrium energy levels. During this relaxation process, a complex RF electromagnetic signal is produced by the MDMs that reflects their progressive loss of energy and decreasing coherence. These complex RF signals are then detected by a receiver antenna (a body, head, or surface coil), analyzed by specialized computer hardware and software, and converted from frequency- and phase-encoded signal intensity information into image data via a mathematical algorithm called a *2D Fourier transformation* (2DFT). These data can then be transferred to a computer monitor or onto photographic film to produce useful MR images.

THE RF PULSE AND NUCLEAR MAGNETIC RESONANCE

When the ^{1}H nuclei are placed in a strong magnetic field, their MDMs begin to precess (or revolve) about the axis of the magnetic field. The precessional motion of the MDMs and the nuclear spin can be likened to a spinning top, where the slower wobbling motion of the top is the MDM precession and the faster rotating axis of the top is the nuclear spin. The precessional frequency (in revolutions per second) of the MDMs is known as the *Larmor frequency* and is proportional to the strength of the external magnetic field. When the precessional frequency of the MDMs matches the frequency of the RF input pulse, transfer of energy occurs by a process called *nuclear magnetic resonance* (NMR). An analogy is useful to make this important point: the transfer of energy at resonance frequency is similar to a tuning fork transferring sound (vibrational) energy to other neighboring tuning forks that have the same pitch; those tuning forks with a different pitch will not sympathetically vibrate. For ^{1}H MDMs, the frequency at which this resonant transfer of energy occurs is approximately 42.5 MHz/T of external magnetic field strength.

COILS FOR MR IMAGING

There are four functionally distinct types of coils used in MR imaging: (1) the X, Y, and Z axis gradient coils, (2) the RF transmit/receive coils, (3) the main magnetic field coil, and (4) the shim coils. The gradient coils are used to induce small linear magnetic field variations upon the much stronger constant external magnetic field to produce the slice-select, frequency (readout), and phase-encoding gradients that are necessary to locate the origin of MDM signals. The transmit/receive coils are radio antennae which are used to transmit the input RF pulse, which transfers energy to the ^{1}H MDMs via resonance, and to receive the complex output RF wave. In 1.5-T MRI units, the main external magnetic field is produced by a large cylindrical superconducting coil that is bathed and cooled in liquid helium. The superconducting magnet produces a very strong, slightly inhomogeneous magnetic field. Nonsuperconducting magnets (electromagnets, and permanent and resistive magnets) that are used at lower field strengths (0.4 T, 0.3 T, and 0.15 T, respectively) have greater magnetic field inhomogeneities. Shim coils make the external magnetic field more uniform by reducing the larger magnetic field inhomogeneities.

RF TRANSMITTER AND RECEIVER COILS

The *body coil* is contained within the MRI unit and may be used both as an RF transmitter and receiver antenna. However, other specialized antennas, such as *head coils* or *orbit coils*, may be used in place of the body coil as a receiver antenna. This approach combines the advantage of the uniform excitation produced by the body (transmitter) coil with the higher sensitivity of the head or orbit (receiver) coils.

When placed close to the body surface, the receiver coils are known as *surface coils*. By locating the receiver coil directly over the region of interest, a much stronger NMR signal is obtained. In addition, the relative contribution to the overall background noise signal from the nonimaged portions of the body is reduced. This results in an increased *signal-to-noise ratio* (SNR). Owing to the increased SNRs obtained with surface coils, images with thinner sections, better resolution, and shorter acquisition times can be obtained.

One type of orbit coil is the 3-inch surface coil, which is a circular coil with a 3-inch diameter. As a rule of thumb, the maximum depth of tissue that can be imaged by a circular coil is equal to the radius of the coil. Therefore, in orbital imaging, the 3-inch coil is best used for examination of the anterior orbit and globe. A limitation of the 3-inch surface coil is a drop-off in signal intensity with increasing distances from the coil. This drop-off in signal intensity (shading artifact) limits evaluation of the posterior orbit from the retrobulbar region to the orbital apex (see the later section on Shading Artifacts). Another limitation of the orbit coil is that the signal intensity from orbital fat may be so strong that it overwhelms the lesser signal intensity of adjacent intraorbital structures. This may require the use of one of the fat-suppression techniques (detailed in a later section).

A pair of 3-inch surface coils can be modified to obtain information simultaneously from both orbits (Fig. 1–1). The limitations of dual-orbit coils are coil size, geometric configuration, and the placement skill of the MR technologist. Asymmetric coil placement can produce asymmetric fat suppression (see the section entitled Asymmetry Artifacts). One solution to asymmetric placement is the butterfly coil, which is a soft, pliable mask that is molded to the patient's facial contour. However, this configuration has the disadvantages of slightly decreased SNRs compared with 3-inch coils, and the increased cost of a specialty coil. Although there are exceptions, surface coils should not generally touch the patient for reasons of safety, motion artifact, and tuning ability.

If disease of the orbital apex is suspected, or if there is possible extension of disease into the optic chiasm or other, more posterior structures, a head coil should be used (Fig. 1–2). This coil receives a uniform RF signal from the head tissue and does not suffer from the shading artifact of the surface coils. Problems related to motion artifact and positioning are also decreased compared to the surface coil. However, the tradeoffs are decreased resolution, thicker sections, and increased imaging time. The newer quadrature head coils have better signal-to-

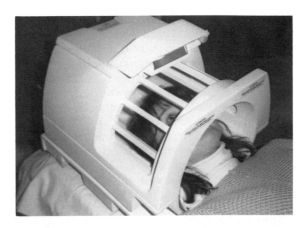

FIGURE 1–2 *Quadrature Head Coil*
The head coil produces a more uniform signal and is less physically confining than orbit coils. However, because of decreased signal-to-noise ratios, scan times are longer than with surface coils.

noise characteristics than standard linear head coils by a factor of approximately 30%. Images similar to those acquired in a linear head coil may be obtained in about half the time with a quadrature head coil.

MR BASIS FOR TISSUE CONTRAST

When a patient is placed in an MR imaging unit, the MDMs in body tissues align themselves along the longitudinal axis of the patient (the Z axis of the external magnetic field) and begin to precess at the Larmor frequency. A strong RF pulse at resonance frequency is then transmitted by the body coil, which tilts (flips) the MDMs 90 degrees into the transverse X–Y plane. At the conclusion of the RF pulse, the MDMs begin to return to their original low-energy (unflipped) position from the higher-energy (flipped) position. The magnitude and direction of all of the ^1H MDMs may be represented by a net vector (M). This M vector can be broken down into two perpendicular vector components: (1) a longitudinal M_z component parallel to the Z axis, and (2) a transverse $M_{x,y}$ component in the X–Y plane. Immediately after the 90-degree RF input pulse, the M vector consists almost entirely of the $M_{x,y}$ component. However, with increasing time, the M_z component will increase in size by a process called *T1 relaxation*, and the $M_{x,y}$ component will decrease in size by a process called *T2 decay*.

Both T1 relaxation and T2 decay occur exponentially at rates determined by tissue-specific T1 and T2 constants. This situation is analogous to radio-

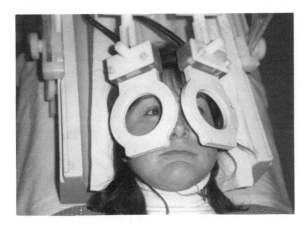

FIGURE 1–1 *Dual Modified Orbit Coils*
A cushioned plastic frame holds a pair of 3-inch surface coils in place. These are symmetrically positioned as close as possible to the orbits without touching the skin.

active decay curves, whereby constants called half-lives determine rates of decay for various radioactive nuclei. The *T1 constant* is the time required for the longitudinal M_z vector to exponentially return (relax) to 63% of its original value. Similarly, the *T2 constant* is the time it takes for the transverse $M_{x,y}$ vector to decay to 37% of its initial value at the end of the RF pulse. Because different tissues have different T1 (and T2) constants, their respective M_z (and $M_{x,y}$) vectors vary in relative magnitude during the relaxation (and decay) process. The relative difference in magnitudes between the different M_z (and $M_{x,y}$) vectors at any point in time is the basis for T1 (and T2) tissue contrast. An MR image that predominantly reflects the T1 relaxation signal information from each tissue type is referred to as a *T1-weighted* (T1W) image. Similarly, an MR image that predominantly consists of T2 decay signal information from each tissue type is called a *T2-weighted* (T2W) image.

SPIN ECHO PULSE SEQUENCES AND MEASUREMENT OF TISSUE CONTRAST

Central to the understanding of tissue contrast is the RF pulse sequence. A pulse sequence consists of an initial RF pulse, which is usually, but not always, followed by one or more secondary RF pulses. The time delay between initial RF pulses is known as the *TR* (time to repeat). The initial RF pulse can flip the M vector less than 90 degrees (as in gradient echo [GRE] imaging), 90 degrees (as in spin echo [SE] imaging), or 180 degrees (as in inversion recovery [IR] imaging). The strength and duration of the RF pulse determines the flip angle.

The most common method of measuring T1 (and T2) contrast uses the *spin echo pulse sequence*. Shortly after the initial 90-degree RF pulse, a second input RF pulse—a 180-degree refocusing pulse—is introduced. This refocusing pulse reverses the direction of precession of the dephasing MDMs, producing a refocused (in-phase) signal a short time later. The delayed signal produced by the refocusing pulse is referred to as an *echo*. The time between the initial RF pulse and the refocused echo signal is known as the *TE* (time to echo).

The T1 relaxation in the longitudinal plane (represented by M_z) releases energy in the form of heat to its surroundings. The T2 decay releases energy through progressive dephasing of MDMs in the transverse plane. An electromagnetic signal is only generated in the transverse plane.

In 1946, Felix Bloch described this "nuclear induction" process with a set of mathematical equations, now known as the *Bloch equations*. Solving these equations for the transverse signal intensity (I_s) generated by a spin echo pulse sequence yields the following equation:

$$I_s = N_h \cdot f(v) \cdot (e^{-TE/T2}) \cdot (1 - e^{-TR/T1})$$

where N_h is the local hydrogen (proton) density, $f(v)$ represents the fraction and velocity of hydrogen nuclei that are mobile, T1 and T2 are tissue parameters, and TR and TE are RF pulse variables as previously described. From the equation, it can be seen that there are two competing exponential curves, one dependent on TE/T2 and the other on TR/T1. In spin echo imaging, the tissue signal (I) can be varied from T1-weighting, to intermediate weighting (between T1 and T2), and finally to T2-weighting by adjusting the degree of competition between the two exponential functions. This is accomplished by varying the timing of the initial RF pulses (TR) and the timing of the secondary refocusing RF pulse (TE/2). The T1 and T2 constants are tissue-specific parameters that vary according to the tissue type being examined, but that are not affected by the RF pulse sequence. The clinical goal is to adjust the operator-dependent variables (TR and TE) to exploit the tissue-specific parameters (T1 and T2), thereby producing signal information and contrast between tissues of clinical concern.

A T1W image is produced with a short TR (to maximize T1 contrast) and a short TE (to minimize T2 contrast). Because the magnitudes of the M_z vector are different for different voxels (volume elements) of tissue (fat, brain, or water) at short TRs, a T1W signal difference (contrast) can be detected between these different tissue types. However, because the magnitudes of the $M_{x,y}$ vector components of all tissue types at short TEs are still nearly equal, there is little T2W tissue contrast that is contributed to the image.

A T2W image is produced with a long TR (to minimize T1 contrast) and a long TE (to increase T2 contrast). At long TRs, the M_z component of each tissue type has returned (relaxed) to near-original levels of longitudinal magnetization. As there is little difference between the magnitudes of the M_z vectors, there is little difference in T1W signal intensities between tissue types (hence, little T1 contrast contribution). However, the longer TEs permit the difference in the T2 decay constants between tissues to produce a difference in their transverse magnetization ($M_{x,y}$) vectors. The relative difference in signal intensity between each voxel of tissue results in an MR image with T2W contrast.

Intermediate-weighted (IW) images are produced by using a long TR (to minimize T1-weighting) and a short TE (to minimize T2-weighting). These are sometimes referred to as *balanced images* because the signal intensity (I_s) is balanced between the contributions of T1-weighting and T2-weighting. In the past, they have been referred to as *proton-density–weighted images* because they reflect the number of mobile ^{1}H nuclei contributed by the N_p (proton density) portion of the signal intensity equation.

FAT-SUPPRESSED MR IMAGES

The short T1 constant of fat produces a bright signal intensity on T1W images. Although fat acts as a natural contrast agent when it is located adjacent to structures with low signal intensity, it also limits MR imaging in several ways. First, *chemical shift misregistration artifact* (see section bearing same title) at fat/water interfaces produces bright and dark signal bands that can obscure detail at these interfaces. Furthermore, the extremely strong signal intensity from fat may overwhelm structures of intermediate and low signal intensity that are immediately adjacent to the fat. Finally, there may be minimal, if any, contrast between bright fat signal and adjacent bright signal from either unenhanced or contrast-enhanced abnormalities. A solution to these limitations is found in various fat suppression techniques. These techniques can be divided into four general classifications: (1) frequency-selective presaturation methods, such as chemical shift selection (CHESS), also known as "fat sat" techniques; (2) phase-dependent chemical shift methods (such as Dixon and Chopper techniques); (3) short TI inversion recovery (STIR); and (4) hybrid and experimental methods. A discussion of the technical aspects of these fat suppression techniques is beyond the scope of this chapter.

FAST MR IMAGING TECHNIQUES

Recent advances in RF pulse techniques show great promise for orbital MR imaging. These techniques are based on the RARE (rapid acquisition with relaxation enhancement) sequence. One imaging technique, known as fast spin echo (FSE) imaging (General Electric) or turbo SE imaging (Siemens), provides high-quality images in a fraction of the time of conventional SE imaging. This has two possible advantages: (1) the overall scan time can be shortened for patients with medical problems, such as positional pain, motion disorders, or claustrophobia; or (2) the overall scan time can remain more or less the same, but the number of signal excitations (NEX) can be increased. In the latter case, more signal averaging results in improved SNRs and greater image resolution.

These fast techniques are also subject to less magnetic susceptibility artifact (see later section bearing that title) from metallic foreign bodies, such as surgical clips, than is conventional SE imaging. Tradeoffs include decreased visualization of hemorrhage, brighter orbital fat on T2W images, new artifacts, and limits to motion-suppression techniques.

Fast fat suppression techniques, such as FMPIR (fast multiplanar inversion recovery), also have great potential compared to the previously discussed fat-suppression techniques, such as STIR and CHESS. The diagnostic role and clinical efficacy of these special techniques remain to be investigated.

CONTRAST-ENHANCED MR IMAGES

Owing to its excellent soft tissue contrast, MRI can diagnose many pathologic processes that might otherwise be missed by unenhanced computerized tomographic (CT) imaging. However, because contrast-enhanced CT images, under certain circumstances, can be superior to unenhanced MR imaging, a need emerged for an intravenous contrast agent that could be used for MR imaging. Although newer contrast agents are under investigation, the current standard is *gadopentetate dimeglumine*. This is a complex organic carrier molecule that carries the paramagnetic element called gadolinium. Contrast-enhanced MR imaging with this agent has been shown to be superior to contrast-enhanced CT in most orbital MR applications.

Gadolinium (Gd) is a metal ion (3 +) in the lanthanide series of the periodic chart. Like many similar elements with unpaired electrons in the outer shell, gadolinium is *paramagnetic*. When molecules with high-energy state ^{1}H MDMs closely approach a paramagnetic ion, such as gadolinium, they quickly relax their MDMs to lower-energy states. This rapid relaxation is most pronounced in molecules with long T1 constants and produces a bright signal on T1W images.

Gadolinium, however, is an extremely toxic substance in its unbound state. To reduce this toxicity, the Gd ion is covalently bound (chelated) to the center of a large carrier molecule called diethylenetriamine penta-acetic acid (DTPA). The Gd-DTPA molecule has a molecular weight and biodistribution similar to that of the iodinated contrast media used in CT scanning. Consequently, Gd-

DTPA contrast enhancement occurs in those lesions that would be expected to enhance with iodinated contrast agents. Gd-DTPA is distributed in the extracellular space, does not cross an intact blood–brain barrier, and is rapidly excreted by the kidneys. Currently, Gd-DTPA is administered as a dimeglumine salt (gadopentetate dimeglumine) and is used clinically at intravenous doses of 0.1 mmol/kg. This contrast agent has an excellent safety profile compared with that of iodinated contrast agents. Reported side effects include hypotension and transient elevation of serum levels of bilirubin and iron. Severe allergic reactions and death have been reported, but fortunately are rare.

BASICS OF ORBITAL MR IMAGE INTERPRETATION

Although skilled interpretation of MR images remains in the realm of the diagnostic radiologist, basic image analysis can be performed with knowledge of a few fundamental concepts. First, the expected signal intensities of orbital fat, optic nerve, and brain, as well as of water, vitreous, and cerebrospinal fluid (CSF) should be known for all basic pulse sequences. Awareness of "ballpark" TR and TE numbers that produce T1W and T2W images is also useful. However, overdependence on the TR and TE numbers that are provided on the image page can lead to diagnostic inaccuracy. For example, a basic T1W image and a fat-suppressed T1W sequence both have short TRs and TEs, but produce significantly different images and associated image artifacts. Therefore, knowledge of the specific RF pulse sequence used, not just the TRs and TEs, is very important in MR image analysis. As the prevalence of other specialized RF pulse sequences increases, cursory analysis of MR images will be fraught with other diagnostic pitfalls.

ANALYSIS OF T1-WEIGHTED ORBITAL MR IMAGES

On a 1.5-T magnet, a TR of 500 ms and a TE of 20 ms typically produce a T1W image. The hallmark of a T1W image (Fig. 1–3) is the bright signal intensity seen in orbital fat, subcutaneous tissues, and, to a lesser extent, bone marrow. This is attributable to the fast T1 decay constants of these tissues and consequent rapid T1 relaxation.

Intermediate signal intensity is seen in the cerebral gray matter. The cerebral white matter is

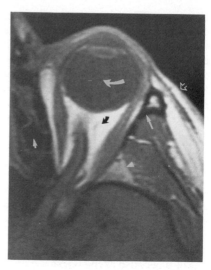

FIGURE 1–3 *Axial T1W Image of the Left Orbit* Bright signal intensity is seen in the orbital fat (*curved black arrow*), subcutaneous tissue (*open white arrow*) and bone marrow (*white arrowhead*). Intermediate signal intensity is seen in the extraocular muscles, optic nerve, and brain. Low signal intensity is seen in the vitreous (*curved white arrow*) and CSF. Very low signal intensity is seen in cortical bone (*long solid white arrow*). A signal void secondary to air is seen in the ethmoid sinus (*short solid white arrow*).

slightly brighter than the gray matter on T1W images. Optic nerve and extraocular muscles also have moderate signal intensities on T1W images.

Low signal intensity in the vitreous and in the CSF of the subarachnoid spaces is also a sign of a T1W image. This is because of the extremely long T1 relaxation constant of water. Fluid collections on T1W images that contain proteins will have variable signal intensities, depending on the amount of paramagnetic effect produced by the constituent proteins.

Very low signal intensity is found in cortical bone (the MDMs are not mobile), calcifications, and fibrous tissues. Small calcific foci may be idiosyncratically bright on T1W images. Total signal voids are seen as a result of air in the paranasal sinuses (fewer and less mobile MDMs to produce a signal) and rapidly flowing blood in vessels (owing to out-of-slice flow of the MDM signal).

In general, T1W images have inherently good anatomic detail owing to their high SNRs. (The SNR is simply a voxel's NMR signal strength divided by the background noise contribution.) Orbital fat is also a major contributor to anatomic contrast, as its bright signal demarcates the lower signal intensities of intraorbital structures, such as the optic nerve sheath, extraocular muscles, and orbital veins. However, the strong orbital fat signal can overwhelm and mask the intermediate signal intensity of small, adjacent structures. Also, there is poor contrast between brighter, intermediate signal intensity structures, such as the lacrimal gland, and the adjacent bright orbital fat. In addition, T1W images provide poor contrast between the vitreous humor and the layers of the globe, the lens, and the ciliary body owing to their similar signal intensities.

The MR signal characteristics of orbital pathology will be discussed in detail in subsequent chapters. However, some basic points should be mentioned, as they relate to the physics of MR imaging. Subacute hemorrhage (>5 days) will appear bright on T1W images because of the paramagnetic effects of methemoglobin (both intracellular and extracellular) on T1 relaxation. Melanin is also bright in signal intensity owing to similar paramagnetic effects. Excess amounts of proteins, some of which have paramagnetic effects, can be produced by the body under certain pathologic conditions. These proteins will effectively shorten the long T1 constant of water in cysts or the vitreous, thereby producing a bright signal intensity rather than the low signal intensity of water that is normally expected on T1W images. Bright signal in blood vessels may be attributable to flow-related enhancement artifact, slow flow in vascular structures after contrast enhancement, or subacute blood clot. Abnormal masses may have high, intermediate, or low signal intensities, depending on their tissue constituents and whether an intravenous contrast agent has been administered.

ANALYSIS OF T2-WEIGHTED ORBITAL MR IMAGES

On a 1.5-T magnet, a TR of 2000 ms and a TE of 80 ms typically produce a T2W image. Bright signal in the vitreous as well as the CSF are hallmarks of a T2W image (Fig. 1–4). Fat signal intensity is less bright than on T1W images. The amount of decreased fat brightness depends on the length of the TR. Heavily T2W images have longer TRs and a darker fat signal. (Fat may remain relatively bright on the newer fast SE pulse sequences.)

Intermediate signal intensity is seen in the cerebral white matter. On T2W images, cerebral gray matter now has a slightly brighter signal intensity than cerebral white matter. (Compare this to the opposite signal relationship on T1W images.)

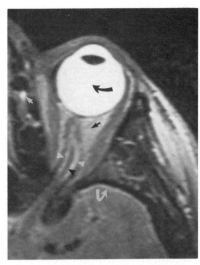

FIGURE 1–4 *Axial T2W Image of the Left Orbit*
Bright signal intensity is seen in the vitreous (*curved black arrow*), intracranial CSF (*curved white arrow*), CSF around the optic nerve (*white arrowheads*), and ethmoid sinus mucosa (*short white arrow*). Intermediate signal intensity is seen in the extraocular muscles, optic nerve (*black arrowhead*), and brain. The signal intensity in the orbital fat (*short black arrow*) and bone marrow is less bright than on T1W images. Very low signal intensity is again seen in the cortical bone.

Very low signal intensity is again seen in cortical bone and calcifications. Air in the paranasal sinuses, soft tissue gas, and rapidly flowing blood are characterized by signal voids.

In general, conventional T2W images of the orbit provide less anatomic detail than T1W images owing to inherently decreased SNRs. In addition, anatomic detail is degraded by patient motion artifact from the longer scan times of T2W images. (The scan time can be calculated by multiplying the TR by the number of phase encoding steps [N] and the NEX).

The bright signal intensity of the vitreous improves visualization of the inner surface of the globe and structures within the anterior chamber. However, the slightly decreased orbital fat signal provides less contrast relative to the optic nerve sheath and extraocular muscles than seen on T1W images. Visualization of the lacrimal gland is variable and depends upon the extent to which orbital fat decreases in signal intensity relative to the gland. On occasion, the lacrimal gland may appear artificially bright owing to its proximity to the surface coil. Depending upon the direction of the frequency-encoding gradient, the high and low signal bands of chemical shift misregistration artifact (see the section on Orbital MR Image Artifacts) may obscure the posterior portion of the globe as well as the periphery of the optic nerve and extraocular muscles. The intraorbital locations where chemical shift artifact obscures anatomic detail are visually most apparent on T2W images. Careful observation will reveal a minimal chemical shift effect on T1W images as well.

The physics of pathologic processes is also useful to discuss in terms of T2W images. Cytotoxic edema and vasogenic edema in tissue can both produce a bright signal intensity on T2W images because of their respective increased intracellular and extracellular water content. Subacute blood can be bright on T2W images, again because of its paramagnetic effect, but this is seen only with extracellular methemoglobin. Hemosiderin produces a region of extremely low signal intensity on T2W images owing to the profound T2-shortening effect of its large number of unpaired electrons, an effect referred to as *superparamagnetism*. Absence of signal secondary to *magnetic susceptibility artifact* from ferromagnetic materials also produces a signal void with a morphologically distorted periphery.

ANALYSIS OF INTERMEDIATE-WEIGHTED ORBITAL MR IMAGES

On a 1.5-T MRI unit, a TR of 2000 ms and a TE of 20 ms typically produce an intermediated-weighted (balanced) image. In these images, vitreous and CSF are less bright in signal intensity (Fig. 1–5) than in T2W images. IW images can separate the low-intensity lens from surrounding higher-intensity fluid, and can resolve the globe surface into at least two layers. However, there is poor contrast between the optic nerve and CSF, as well as between the lacrimal gland and neighboring fat. Because abnormal tissue may remain slightly bright while the adjacent vitreous or CSF signal turns intermediate to low in signal intensity, the extent of abnormal tissues may theoretically be better visualized on IW images. However, owing to their lower diagnostic yield, IW images are not frequently used for routine orbital MR imaging.

ANALYSIS OF FAT-SUPPRESSED ORBITAL MR IMAGES

Fat-suppressed T1W images can be recognized by noting the normal low signal intensity of the vitreous combined with the unexpectedly low signal

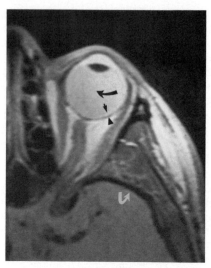

FIGURE 1–5 *Axial Intermediate-Weighted (IW) Image of the Left Orbit*
The signal intensity of the vitreous (*curved black arrow*) and CSF (*curved white arrow*) is less bright than on T2W images. Orbital fat and bone marrow are slightly brighter in signal intensity than their counterparts in T2W images. The choroid/retina (*short black arrow*) can be distinguished from the lower signal intensity fibrous sclera (*black arrowhead*).

intensity of orbital fat, subcutaneous fat, and fatty bone marrow (Fig. 1–6), as compared with a routine T1W image (Fig. 1–7). As previously indicated, there are several categories of RF pulse sequences that can produce fat suppression. The Dixon and Chopper techniques were initially available via minor software alterations to MR imaging units. For the most part, however, these phase-dependent chemical shift techniques have been replaced by the frequency-selective presaturation techniques.

Reversal of the normal signal intensity relationships between fat and intraorbital structures more accurately depicts the contour of the lacrimal gland, as well as the actual thickness of the optic nerve and extraocular muscles. A byproduct of fat suppression is the reduction or elimination of the chemical shift misregistration artifact. This permits improved anatomic delineation of the posterior portion of the globe and the optic nerve, structures previously obscured by chemical shift artifact.

Fat-suppressed images can be used to evaluate bright signal abnormalities on unenhanced T1W images. Bright signal abnormalities that remain after fat suppression of non-contrast enhanced images are usually attributable to subacute hemorrhage (methemoglobin), melanin, or fluid that contains

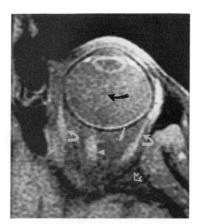

FIGURE 1-6 *Axial Fat-Suppressed T1W Image of the Left Orbit*

Orbital fat (*straight white arrow*) and fatty bone marrow (*open white arrow*) are unexpectedly low in signal intensity for a T1W image. The vitreous (*curved black arrow*) appears brighter than on routine T1W images, but is still relatively low in signal intensity. The extraocular muscles (*curved white arrows*) and optic nerve (*white arrowhead*) are normally intermediate in signal intensity, but now appear brighter owing to relative loss of normally bright fat signal. Absent fat signal reduces the signal-to-noise ratio; the resultant images now appear grainier.

paramagnetic protein. However, because of the absence of bright fat signal intensity, normal structures with low- to intermediate-signal intensity can appear artifactually bright (see Fig. 1-6). Routine T1W images should always be obtained, as fatty

masses may be obscured on fat-suppressed T1W images.

ANALYSIS OF CONTRAST-ENHANCED ORBITAL MR IMAGES

Although paramagnetic agents can theoretically produce both T1- and T2-shortening, the effects of contrast enhancement are visualized only on T1W images, not on T2W images. Because regions of contrast enhancement (lacrimal gland and extraocular muscles) can be obscured on T1W images by the adjacent bright signal fat (Fig. 1-8), contrast-enhanced MR images are best produced in conjunction with fat suppression techniques (Fig. 1-9).

Images produced with fat suppression and intravenous Gd-DTPA enhancement will show normal intense enhancement and excellent definition of the extraocular muscles and the lacrimal gland (Fig. 1-10). This should be compared with the poor visualization of the lacrimal glands on routine T1W images (Fig. 1-11). There is also enhancement of the ciliary body anteriorly, as well as a thin line of enhancement of the choroid posteriorly (see Fig. 1-9). The optic nerve does not normally enhance.

Routine (unenhanced, nonfat-suppressed) T1W images should always be obtained prior to contrast enhancement because bright signal abnormalities, such as those produced by blood or melanin, may be obscured by the bright signal from Gd-DTPA en-

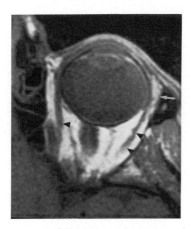

FIGURE 1-7 *Axial Routine T1W Image of the Orbit (Same Patient as in Fig. 1-6)*

Note the bright orbital fat, as well as the moderate-to-bright lacrimal gland (*white arrow*) and bone marrow. The signal intensity of the vitreous is low. The extraocular muscles (*black arrowheads*) are intermediate in signal intensity.

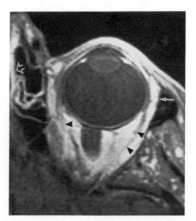

FIGURE 1-8 *Axial Contrast-Enhanced T1W Image Without Fat Suppression*

Note that the enhancing lacrimal gland (*white arrow*) and extraocular muscles (*black arrowheads*) are less well visualized adjacent to the bright orbital fat than when unenhanced (compare to Fig. 1-7). Note the contrast enhancement of the ethmoid sinus mucosa (*open white arrow*). The optic nerve does not normally enhance with contrast material.

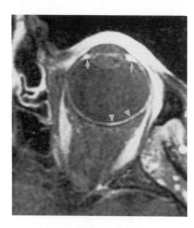

FIGURE 1-9 *Axial Contrast-Enhanced T1W Image with Fat Suppression*
Intense enhancement of the extraocular muscles and lacrimal gland is seen. There is greater conspicuity of these structures as compared with the nonfat-suppressed enhanced T1W image (compare to Fig. 1-7). The ciliary body (*white arrows*) enhances anteriorly, as does a thin line of choroid (*white arrowheads*) posteriorly. The optic nerve does not enhance and is poorly visualized against the low signal orbital fat.

hancement. Additionally, intraorbital low signal abnormalities on routine T1W images that do not enhance may be poorly visualized on fat-suppressed images owing to the lack of surrounding bright fat signal. Therefore, all routine T1W images should be carefully examined for bright signal abnormalities or potentially nonenhancing low signal abnormalities that may be missed on enhanced, fat-suppressed, T1W images. Despite careful examination, small low signal abnormalities on T1W images may

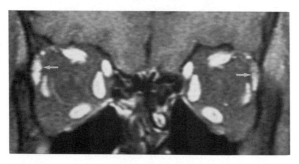

FIGURE 1-10 *Coronal Contrast-Enhanced and Fat-Suppressed T1W Image of the Orbits*
There is intense enhancement and improved definition of the lacrimal glands (*white arrows*) as compared to routine T1W images (see Fig. 1-7). Although the extraocular muscles also intensely enhance, the optic nerves do not.

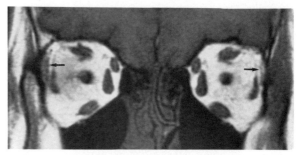

FIGURE 1-11 *Coronal Routine T1W Images (Same Patient as in Fig. 1-10)*
The lacrimal glands are slightly brighter in signal intensity than are the extraocular muscles, which have an intermediate signal intensity. Consequently, the lacrimal glands are poorly visualized adjacent to the bright orbital fat.

still be obscured by overwhelmingly bright fat signal intensity, particularly when using a surface coil or when recording the image with an inappropriate gray scale or film contrast.

Use of STIR as a fat-suppression technique in conjunction with intravenous paramagnetic contrast enhancement may have limitations compared with other fat suppression methods. Although STIR reduces fat signal, it may also reduce signal from contrast-enhancing structures as well, as a result of a phenomenon known as negative enhancement. This theoretically could reduce the conspicuity of orbital pathology.

ORBITAL MR IMAGING PROTOCOLS

A basic MR imaging orbital protocol might consist of: (1) T1W and T2W axial images through the orbits using a 14- to 16-cm field-of-view (FOV) and 3-mm thick slices with 1-mm interspaces; (2) a similar fat-suppressed axial T1W image, and (3) contrast-enhanced axial, coronal, and/or parasagittal oblique fat-suppressed T1W images with identical FOVs and slice parameters. Axial-enhanced T1W images without fat suppression are occasionally useful for the purpose of direct comparison to the pre-Gd T1W images. Fast scanning techniques, such as FSE and FMPIR, show particular promise in the evaluation of the orbit, especially the orbital apex.

ORBITAL MR IMAGE ARTIFACTS

Artifacts in image production have clinical importance because they can be mistaken for disease processes. They may also unnecessarily limit the diagnostic utility of an imaging study. With proper technique, many artifacts can be directed away from clinically important anatomic structures, reduced in spatial extent, or even eliminated entirely.

There are several sources of artifact. Some artifacts are primarily attributable to the MR imaging process itself, such as chemical shift artifact, shading artifact, asymmetric fat suppression, aliasing, and equipment malfunction. Other artifacts are directly related to the patient, as in the case of metallic foreign body artifact and patient motion artifact. Artifact may also be external to the imaging process, such as those caused by RF interference.

CHEMICAL SHIFT MISREGISTRATION ARTIFACT

Not all ^{1}H MDMs resonate at exactly the same frequency. For example, the ^{1}H MDMs in triglycerides are more shielded from the external magnetic field by orbital electrons than are the ^{1}H MDMs in water. As a result, the resonance frequency of fat is slightly lower than that of water. At 1.5 T, this frequency difference amounts to approximately 220 Hz. During signal readout (with the system frequency tuned to the water resonance frequency), the signal from fat is downshifted in location along the frequency-encoding gradient. Therefore, in the final MR image, the fat signal information will be spatially dislocated downward, along the direction of the frequency-encoding gradient, by several pixel widths. This effect produces a *chemical shift misregistration artifact* (Fig. 1–12) at fat–water interfaces,

such as parallel to the optic nerve/orbital fat interface (X-axis frequency-encoding gradient) or between the posterior globe vitreous humor and retrobulbar fat (Y-axis frequency-encoding gradient). The chemical shift misregistration artifact is located only along the frequency-encoding axis. If fat precedes water in location along an increasing frequency-encoding gradient, a black signal band (void of fat signal) is noted in the expected location of the fat pixels. Under the same conditions, if water precedes fat, a bright signal band (fat overlay) is noted at the interface overlying the expected position of water.

The effects of chemical shift are most pronounced when using strong magnetic fields, large FOVs, few phase-encoding steps, or narrow receiver bandwidth. The artifact can be reduced by using smaller pixel sizes, placing the fat–water interface parallel to the frequency-encoding direction, or instituting fat-suppression techniques. The artifact is also less pronounced when using surface coils, whereby the increased SNR permits smaller pixel sizes.

SHADING ARTIFACT

Although one advantage of surface coils is their increased SNR, the disadvantage is a decrease in signal reception with distance from the surface coil. This gradual decrease in signal intensity is known as *shading artifact* (Fig. 1–13). A more uniform

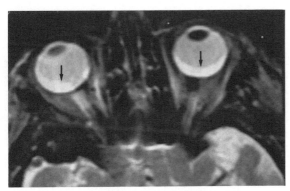

FIGURE 1–12 *Chemical Shift Artifact*
Bright curvilinear bands of abnormal signal intensity (*black arrows*) secondary to frequency down-shifted fat signal overlie and obscure the posterior wall and vitreous humor of both globes. (Here the frequency-encoding gradient is increasing from anterior to posterior in the direction of the black arrows.)

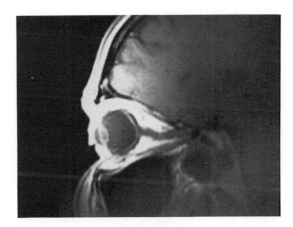

FIGURE 1–13 *Shading Artifact from Surface Coil Imaging*
The signal intensity and signal-to-noise ratio of the orbit decrease with increasing distance from the skin surface. Retro-orbital structures are poorly visualized. Extremely strong fat signal at the surface tends to obscure anterior orbital detail.

signal intensity is produced by the head coil (Fig. 1–14). Therefore, diagnostic evaluation with small surface coils should be restricted to orbital structures, preferably the globe and anterior orbit. Monocular imaging of the orbital apex can be performed with a solitary 5-inch orbit coil if there is prior knowledge of an orbital apex mass, but this technique yields SNRs that are only slightly better than those of a head coil. Retro-orbital structures, such as the optic chiasm, have much lower signal intensities than those in the orbit. Evaluation of this region with a surface coil will lead to diagnostic errors. The retro-orbital region is best imaged with a head coil.

ASYMMETRY ARTIFACT

The symmetry of anatomic structures plays an important role in MR imaging. In the appropriate setting, symmetry of shape (morphology) and signal intensity are powerful tools in making or excluding a diagnosis of pathology. Therefore, any artifact-induced asymmetry of morphology or signal intensity diminishes the diagnostic utility of an image.

Asymmetric placement of dual orbital surface coils can produce asymmetric shading artifact. When comparing signal intensities between similar right and left orbital structures, the difference in signal intensities may initially suggest a pathological process. However, awareness of this artifact should prompt recognition of right/left asymmetry

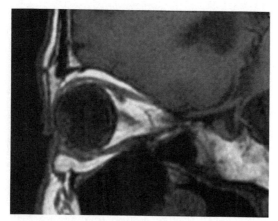

FIGURE 1–14 *Uniformity of Signal from Head Coil Imaging*
Orbital and retro-orbital structures are well visualized and uniform in signal intensity. Anterior orbital fat does not overwhelm the signal from other anterior orbital structures.

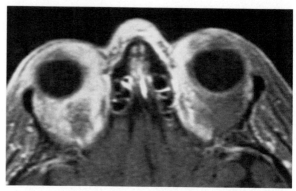

FIGURE 1–15 *Asymmetric Fat Suppression*
Partial fat suppression in the left orbit and almost absent fat suppression in the right orbit may initially suggest a retro-orbital mass or hemorrhage. Bright signal intensity that extends to the subcutaneous fat is a clue to the artifact. In T1W images, edema would be dark in signal intensity.

of signal intensity in the surrounding structures as well, thereby avoiding a misdiagnosis.

When using dual surface coils, it may occasionally be difficult to suppress completely and symmetrically the extremely strong signal from subcutaneous and orbital fat. As a result, the presence of unexpected bright fat signal may initially suggest an infiltrative process (Fig. 1–15). Incomplete fat suppression can also occur at air–fat interfaces when using frequency-selective presaturation fat-suppression techniques. Awareness of these artifacts, as well as comparison to other pulse sequences, helps to avoid this pitfall.

ALIASING

Aliasing, or wraparound artifact, occurs when a part of the body extends beyond the volume that is being imaged. For example, in axial MR images of the orbit using a head coil, aliasing might produce truncation of the tip of the nose in the anterior portion of the image, with subsequent reconstruction of the tip of the nose over the posterior portion of the image, such as over the posterior brain. Aliasing may also occur from left to right (Fig. 1–16).

Aliasing occurs when an MR signal is produced outside the imaging volume, but has a frequency higher than the predetermined sampling frequency for that volume. The frequency of an MR signal is determined by sampling it at a small number of discrete intervals rather than continuously. If the sampling pattern of the higher frequency signal

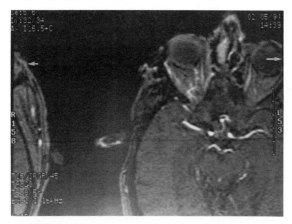

FIGURE 1–16 *Wraparound (Aliasing) Artifact*
The cut-off portion of the left orbit (*long arrow*) is reconstructed in the right portion (*short arrow*) of the image. This artifact usually occurs along the phase-encoding direction.

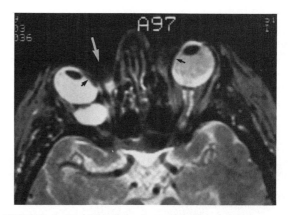

FIGURE 1–17 *Magnetic Susceptibility Artifact Secondary to Metallic Dental Work*
A large signal void (*white arrow*) is produced in the medial anterior and inferior right orbit. Magnetic susceptibility distorts the shape of both globes (*black arrows*).

from outside the imaging volume exactly matches that of a much lower MR signal frequency from within the image volume, there is frequency (and, hence, locational) ambiguity, leading to image wraparound and overlap.

Aliasing along the frequency-encoding axis can be eliminated through the use of filters that prevent the passage of frequencies above the sampling rate. However, aliasing along the phase-encoding axis cannot be eliminated so easily. Possible solutions include changing to a larger, more inclusive field of view (FOV), acquiring an image matrix that is larger than the display matrix (oversampling); and applying presaturation pulses to eliminate any contribution from the portion of the orbit that is outside of the imaging volume. The use of orbital surface coils also minimizes aliasing.

MAGNETIC SUSCEPTIBILITY ARTIFACT

The tendency and ability of any substance to become magnetized when placed in a magnetic field is known as its *magnetic susceptibility*. Most biological tissues and some paramagnetic metals (such as copper and gadolinium) have small magnetic susceptibilities. Other superparamagnetic or ferromagnetic metals (particularly iron) have magnetic susceptibilities that are thousands of times greater.

Magnetic susceptibility artifact occurs when attempts are made to image two neighboring substances of vastly differing magnetic susceptibility. This difference in susceptibility produces a local distortion of the magnetic field and leads to dephas-

ing and frequency shifts in local MDMs. Examples of magnetic susceptibility artifacts include metallic dental work (Fig. 1–17), metallic intraorbital sutures (Fig. 1–18), and iron-oxide–containing cosmetics, such as eyeliner and mascara (Fig. 1–19).

Although magnetic susceptibility artifact cannot be eliminated, its effects can be modified. Swapping frequency- and phase-encoding directions can change the shape of the distortion. SE imaging, owing to its phase-refocusing RF pulse, is less prone to magnetic susceptibility artifact than other pulse sequences, such as GRE imaging. FSE imaging is even less prone to magnetic susceptibility artifact

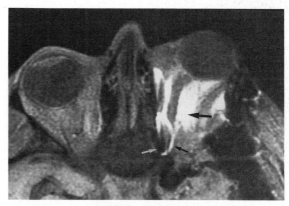

FIGURE 1–18 *Magnetic Susceptibility Artifact Secondary to a Metallic Surgical Clip*
A small signal void (*white arrow*) is produced, with an adjacent linear bright signal (*small black arrow*). This may also be producing incomplete fat suppression (*large black arrow*) within the left orbit.

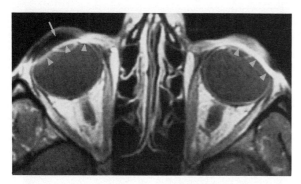

FIGURE 1–19 *Magnetic Susceptibility Artifact Secondary to an Eyelid Cosmetic Containing Iron Oxide*
Characteristic bright curvilinear signals (*white arrowheads*) are seen along the anterior periphery of both globes. Both anterior globes are mildly distorted in shape. A signal void (*large white arrow*) is also seen to obscure a portion of the anterior chamber of the right globe.

than conventional SE imaging. Using short TEs further reduces the amount of MDM dephasing that can occur. Imaging in orthogonal planes may also be useful.

PATIENT MOTION ARTIFACT

Blurred orbital MR images can result from random head/orbit motion, periodic or random globe motion, or both. The artifact that is produced can occur: (1) in the direction of the movement or (2) in the phase-encoding direction, regardless of the direction of movement.

Similar to the photographic blurring that occurs when one attempts to take a snapshot of a rapidly moving object using a camera with slow shutter speed, the first type of blurring artifact occurs when the head or globe rapidly assumes different anatomic positions during the relatively slow MR imaging process. This artifact can be reduced through education, cooperation, and mild sedation of the patient. Strategies might include administering anxiolytic medication prior to the examination, asking the patient to maintain a fixed gaze upon an imaginary point within the bore of the magnet, and emphasizing the need to restrict eye movements, blinking, and head motion. Scan times should be minimized through the use of surface coils, when appropriate, and by optimal use of tailored RF pulse sequences.

Production of the second type of motion artifact is less intuitively obvious. This artifact (Fig. 1–20) consists of multiple *phase ghosts*, which are ghostlike duplications of the moving body part along the phase-encoding gradient direction. This occurs as a result of the multiple phase-encoding gradient signal acquisitions that are required to produce an image slice. (The phase-encoding direction is within the image plane, which in axial imaging is either along the X axis (left/right) or the Y axis (anterior/posterior). Unlike the frequency-encoding step, which acquires its signal information in a matter of a few milliseconds (TE), the phase-encoding process may take seconds to minutes. (The frequency- [readout] encoding direction is always perpendicular to the phase-encoding direction within a given image plane.)

Phase ghosts secondary to eye movement may be reduced by increasing the NEX. The weaker, more random, phase ghost signals are reduced as a result of signal averaging and the increased image SNR, but the tradeoff is a doubling or tripling of examination time. Surface coils also reduce the effects of any phase ghost signals that might arise from outside of the orbit (such as from vascular pulsation). Mild sedation and restriction of head position with tape may help to reduce phase ghosting from head movements. Additionally, the swapping of phase- and frequency-encoding directions may move phase ghosts away from regions of pathology.

STRUCTURED NOISE ARTIFACT

Repetitive structured noise may occur as a result of equipment malfunction or failure. An example of structured noise secondary to gradient amplifier problems is shown in Fig. 1–21. Another type of artifact, which is gridlike in appearance, can be

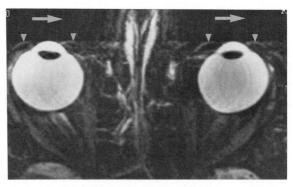

FIGURE 1–20 *Phase Ghosting Artifact*
Multiple ghosts of the cornea (*white arrowheads*) are noted along the phase-encoding direction (*large white arrows*) owing to ocular motion.

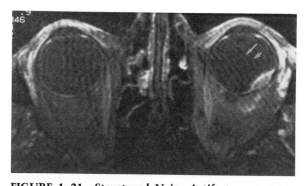

FIGURE 1-21 *Structured Noise Artifact*
Multiple thin wavy lines are produced that alternate between bright (*short arrow*) and dark (*long arrow*) signal intensity. Although they parallel each other, they do not follow anatomic structures. This artifact is frequently attributable to malfunction of electronic equipment, such as gradient amplifiers.

produced by faulty array processors or errors in computer processing of the Fourier transformation. Resolution of these artifacts usually requires a service call from the manufacturer.

RF INTERFERENCE ARTIFACT AND SHIELDING

At typical MRI field strength (1.5 T), the Larmor frequency of ^{1}H is approximately 63.87 MHz, the same frequency as VHF television (e.g., Channel 3) broadcasts. This is why MRI units are placed in a special room called a *Faraday cage*, where the MRI unit is surrounded with a grounded metallic screen to reduce interference from much stronger outside RF electromagnetic energy. This RF interference may be produced by inadvertently leaving the door to the Faraday cage open, thus allowing external RF energy to enter the room. RF interference may also occur within a closed room as a result of electromagnetic signals from patient monitoring devices, such as pulse oximeters. This RF interference artifact has a zipperlike appearance along the frequency-encoding direction.

BIBLIOGRAPHY

Anzai Y, Lufkin RB, Jabour BA, Hanafee WN. Fat-suppression failure artifacts simulating pathology on frequency-selective fat-suppression MR images of the head and neck. *AJNR*. 1992; 13:879–884.

Atlas SW, Galetta SL. The orbit and visual system. In: Atlas SW, ed. *Magnetic Resonance Imaging of the Brain and Spine*. New York: Raven Press; 1991:709–722.

De Marco JK, Bilaniuk LT. Magnetic resonance imaging: Technical aspects. In: Newton TH, Bilaniuk LT, eds. *Modern Neuroradiology*. Vol. 4. *Radiology of the Eye and Orbit*. San Anselmo, CA: Clavadel Press; 1990:1–14.

Elster AD. *Questions and Answers in Magnetic Resonance Imaging*. St. Louis: CV Mosby; 1994: 134–161.

Field SA, Wehrli FW. *Signa Applications Guide*. 5th ed. Vol. 1. Milwaukee: GE Medical Systems; 1992: 27–43.

Harms SE. The orbit. In: Edelman RR, Hesselink JR, eds. *Clinical Magnetic Resonance Imaging*. Philadelphia: WB Saunders; 1990:598–603.

Horowitz AL. *MRI Physics for Radiologists*. 2nd ed. New York: Springer-Verlag; 1992:4–54.

Lufkin RB. *The MRI Manual*. St. Louis: Mosby–Year Book; 1990:1–42.

Nelson KL, Runge VM. Basic principles. In: Runge VM, ed. *Enhanced Magnetic Resonance Imaging*. St. Louis: CV Mosby; 1989:57–73.

Prorok RJ. *Signa Applications Guide*. 4th ed. Vol. 2. Milwaukee: GE Medical Systems; 1990:21–24.

Ross JS, Ruggieri P, Tkach J, Obuchowski N, Dillenger J, Masaryk TJ, Modic MT. Lumbar degenerative disk disease: Prospective comparison of conventional T2-weighted spin-echo imaging and T2-weighted rapid acquisition relaxation-enhanced imaging. *AJNR*. 1993;14:1215–1223.

Schenck JF, Leue WM. Instrumentation: magnets, coils, and hardware. In: Atlas SW, ed. *Magnetic Imaging of the Brain and Spine*. New York: Raven Press; 1991:1–23.

Simon J, Szumowski J, Totterman S, Kido D, Ekholm S, Wicks A, Plewes D. Fat-suppression MR imaging of the orbit. *AJNR*. 1988; 9:961–968.

Sobel DF, Mills C, Char D, Norman D, Brant-Zawadski M, Kaufman L, Crooks L. NMR of the normal and pathologic eye and orbit. *AJNR*. 1984; 5:345–350.

Sze G, Kawamura Y, Negishi C, Constable RT, Merman M, Oshio K, Jolesz F. Fast spin-echo MR imaging of the cervical spine: Influence of echo train length and echo spacing on image contrast. *AJNR*. 1993;14: 1203–1213.

Tien RD, Chu PK, Hesselink JR, Szumowski J. Intra- and paraorbital lesions: value of fat-suppression MR imaging with paramagnetic contrast enhancement. *AJNR*. 1991;12:245–253.

MRI of the Eye and Orbit,
by Patrick De Potter, Jerry A. Shields, and Carol L. Shields.
J. B. Lippincott Company, Philadelphia © 1995.

2

Anatomic Considerations

PATRICK DE POTTER

The clinical history and ocular examination provide information regarding the status of the orbit, but this often needs to be supplemented by orbital imaging studies. Over the years, a variety of imaging techniques have been employed, and improvements in tissue resolution have been made. Because of its multiplanar capability and exquisite soft tissue contrast, MR provides an excellent image of the orbital tissues as well as the paraorbital structures. The signal void produced by the cortical bone of the orbital walls and the hyperintense signal of the orbital fat allow clear delineation of the orbital soft tissues. The normal anatomy of the eye and orbit is described in great detail in the illustrations of this chapter.

ANATOMY OF THE EYE

FIGURE 2-1 *Normal Right Eye*
A, Axial T1-weighted (T1W) image. *B,* Fat-suppressed axial T1W image. *C,* Axial T2-weighted (T2W) image. *D,* Axial Gd-DTPA–enhanced T1W image. *E,* Fat-suppressed axial Gd-DTPA–enhanced T1W image.

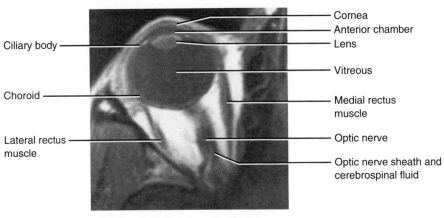

2-1A

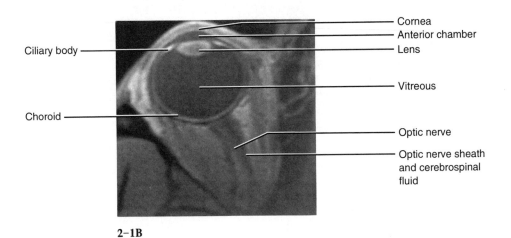

2-1B

(continued)

FIGURE 2–1 *Normal Right Eye* (continued)

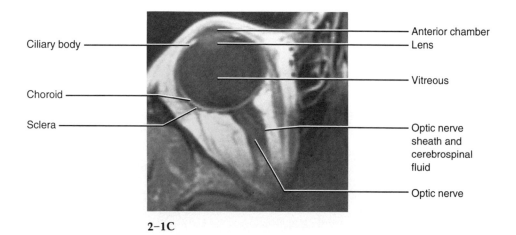

Ciliary body

Choroid

Sclera

Anterior chamber

Lens

Vitreous

Optic nerve sheath and cerebrospinal fluid

Optic nerve

2–1C

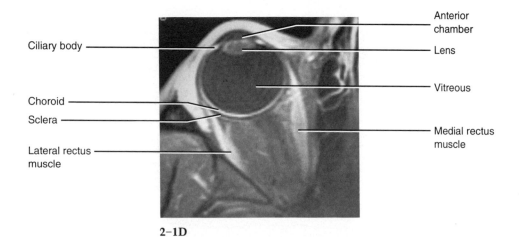

Ciliary body

Choroid

Sclera

Lateral rectus muscle

Anterior chamber

Lens

Vitreous

Medial rectus muscle

2–1D

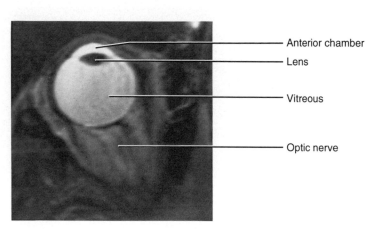

Anterior chamber

Lens

Vitreous

Optic nerve

2–1E

Chapter 2: Anatomic Considerations **21**

ANATOMY OF THE ORBIT

FIGURE 2-2 *Normal Orbit*

A through F, Serial contiguous 3-mm thick slices. Axial T1W images progress from the inferior portion (*A*) to the superior portion (*F*) of the orbit.

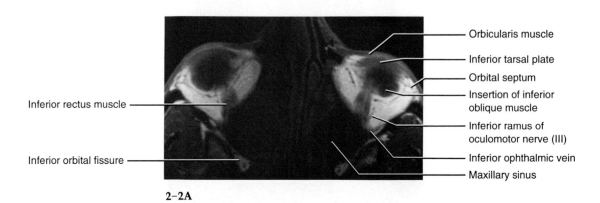

Inferior rectus muscle

Inferior orbital fissure

Orbicularis muscle

Inferior tarsal plate

Orbital septum

Insertion of inferior oblique muscle

Inferior ramus of oculomotor nerve (III)

Inferior ophthalmic vein

Maxillary sinus

2-2A

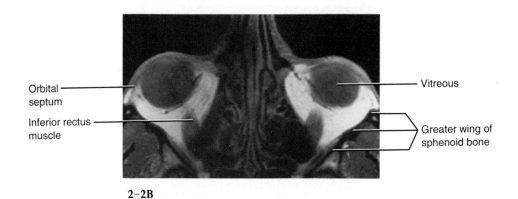

Orbital septum

Inferior rectus muscle

Vitreous

Greater wing of sphenoid bone

2-2B

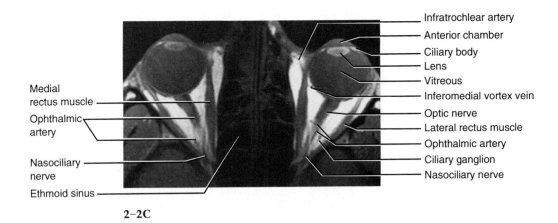

Medial rectus muscle

Ophthalmic artery

Nasociliary nerve

Ethmoid sinus

Infratrochlear artery

Anterior chamber

Ciliary body

Lens

Vitreous

Inferomedial vortex vein

Optic nerve

Lateral rectus muscle

Ophthalmic artery

Ciliary ganglion

Nasociliary nerve

2-2C

(continued)

FIGURE 2–2 *Normal Orbit* (continued)

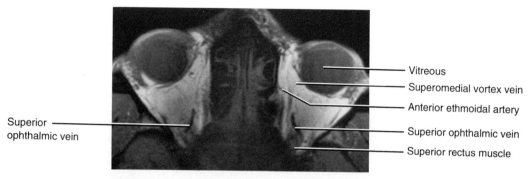

Superior ophthalmic vein

Vitreous
Superomedial vortex vein
Anterior ethmoidal artery
Superior ophthalmic vein
Superior rectus muscle

2–2D

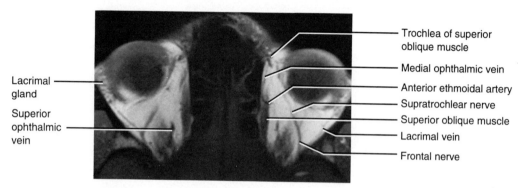

Lacrimal gland
Superior ophthalmic vein

Trochlea of superior oblique muscle
Medial ophthalmic vein
Anterior ethmoidal artery
Supratrochlear nerve
Superior oblique muscle
Lacrimal vein
Frontal nerve

2–2E

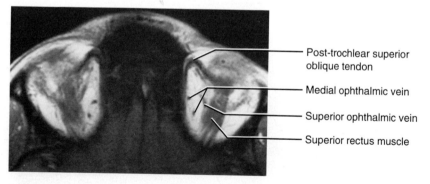

Post-trochlear superior oblique tendon
Medial ophthalmic vein
Superior ophthalmic vein
Superior rectus muscle

2–2F

FIGURE 2-3 *Normal Orbit*
A through G, Serial contiguous 3-mm thick slices. Coronal T1W images progress from the anterior portion (*A*) to the posterior portion (*G*) of the orbit.

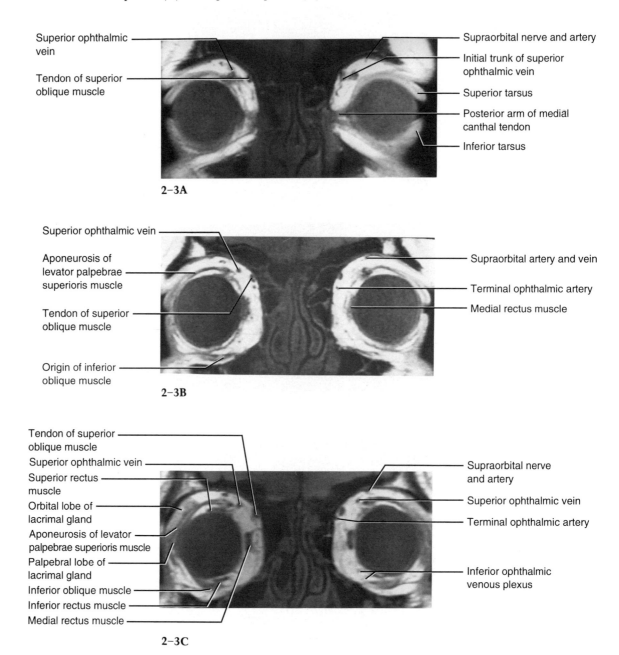

Superior ophthalmic vein

Tendon of superior oblique muscle

Supraorbital nerve and artery

Initial trunk of superior ophthalmic vein

Superior tarsus

Posterior arm of medial canthal tendon

Inferior tarsus

2-3A

Superior ophthalmic vein

Aponeurosis of levator palpebrae superioris muscle

Tendon of superior oblique muscle

Origin of inferior oblique muscle

Supraorbital artery and vein

Terminal ophthalmic artery

Medial rectus muscle

2-3B

Tendon of superior oblique muscle

Superior ophthalmic vein

Superior rectus muscle

Orbital lobe of lacrimal gland

Aponeurosis of levator palpebrae superioris muscle

Palpebral lobe of lacrimal gland

Inferior oblique muscle

Inferior rectus muscle

Medial rectus muscle

Supraorbital nerve and artery

Superior ophthalmic vein

Terminal ophthalmic artery

Inferior ophthalmic venous plexus

2-3C

(continued)

FIGURE 2-3 *Normal Orbit* (continued)

Superior ophthalmic vein

Levator palpebrae superioris muscle

Superior rectus muscle

Superior oblique muscle

Lateral rectus muscle

Medial rectus muscle

Inferior oblique

Inferior rectus muscle

Inferior division of oculomotor nerve (III)

Supraorbital nerve and artery

Terminal ophthalmic artery

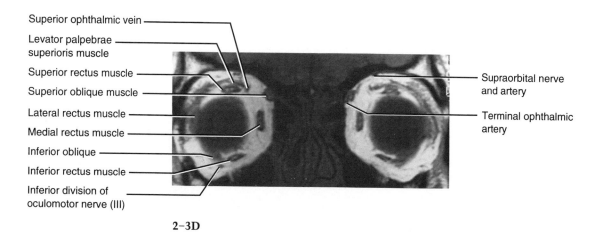

2-3D

Superior ophthalmic vein

Supraorbital artery and nerve

Levator palpebrae superioris muscle

Superior rectus muscle

Superior oblique muscle

Lateral rectus muscle

Inferior rectus muscle

Inferior division of oculomotor nerve (III)

Supraorbital nerve and artery

Lacrimal nerve, artery, and vein

Intermuscular membrane

2-3E

Levator palpebrae superioris muscle

Superior rectus muscle

Superior ophthalmic vein

Superior oblique muscle

Medial rectus muscle

Lateral rectus muscle

Inferior rectus muscle

Frontal nerve and artery

Lacrimal artery, vein, and nerve

Nasociliary nerve

Ophthalmic artery

Maxillary sinus

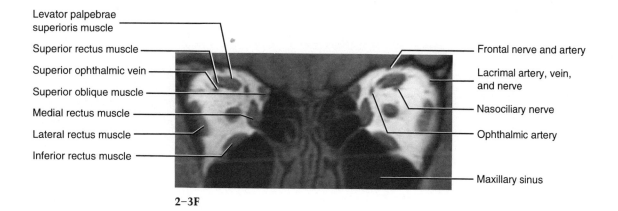

2-3F

(continued)

FIGURE 2–3 *Normal Orbit* (continued)

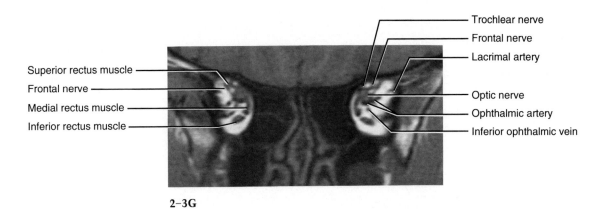

Superior rectus muscle

Frontal nerve

Medial rectus muscle

Inferior rectus muscle

Trochlear nerve

Frontal nerve

Lacrimal artery

Optic nerve

Ophthalmic artery

Inferior ophthalmic vein

2–3G

FIGURE 2-4 *Normal Orbit*
A through C, Serial 3-mm thick slices. Sagittal (*A*) and parasagittal (*B* and *C*) T1W images.

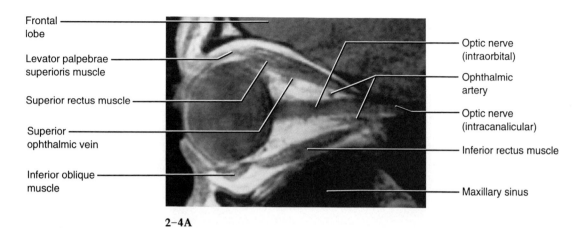

Frontal lobe

Levator palpebrae superioris muscle

Superior rectus muscle

Superior ophthalmic vein

Inferior oblique muscle

Optic nerve (intraorbital)

Ophthalmic artery

Optic nerve (intracanalicular)

Inferior rectus muscle

Maxillary sinus

2-4A

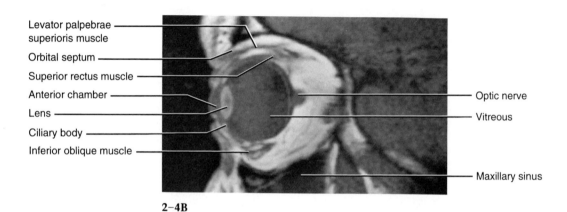

Levator palpebrae superioris muscle

Orbital septum

Superior rectus muscle

Anterior chamber

Lens

Ciliary body

Inferior oblique muscle

Optic nerve

Vitreous

Maxillary sinus

2-4B

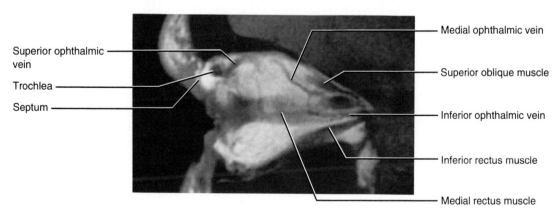

Superior ophthalmic vein

Trochlea

Septum

Medial ophthalmic vein

Superior oblique muscle

Inferior ophthalmic vein

Inferior rectus muscle

Medial rectus muscle

2-4C

FIGURE 2–5 *Normal Orbit*
Axial T2W image.

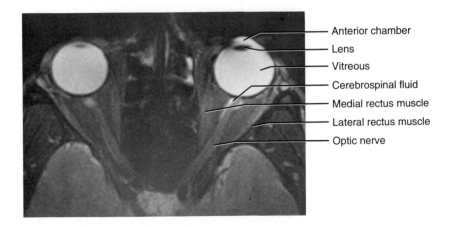

Anterior chamber
Lens
Vitreous
Cerebrospinal fluid
Medial rectus muscle
Lateral rectus muscle
Optic nerve

Part Two | Disorders of the Globe

MRI of the Eye and Orbit,
by Patrick De Potter, Jerry A. Shields, and Carol L. Shields.
J. B. Lippincott Company, Philadelphia © 1995.

3
Congenital Anomalies

PATRICK DE POTTER

JERRY A. SHIELDS

CAROL L. SHIELDS

PERSISTENT HYPERPLASTIC PRIMARY VITREOUS

Clinical and Pathological Features

Persistent hyperplastic primary vitreous (PHPV) is a congenital anomaly that is usually unilateral and that can be present at birth. PHPV is one of the most common lesions that simulate retinoblastoma. However, PHPV usually can be differentiated from retinoblastoma on the basis of history, ocular examination, and ancillary studies. Leukokoria is noted in the affected microphthalmic eye during the first days or weeks after birth. Examination of the anterior segment reveals that the ciliary processes are drawn into a contracting, retrolental, loose, fibrovascular mass attached to a cataractous lens. B-scan ultrasonography and computed tomography (CT) usually demonstrate a retrolental mass associated with remnants of the persistent hyaloid and absence of calcification in a microphthalmic eye. However, differentiation of retinoblastoma from PHPV is not always possible on CT examination.

MR Features

PHPV has MR features that differ from those of retinoblastoma (see Tables 7–1 and 7–3). Thus, differentiation of retinoblastoma from PHPV is possible with contrast-enhanced magnetic resonance imaging (MRI).

The varied manifestations of PHPV are well identified on MRI. The fibrovascular retrolental mass appears hypointense on T1-weighted (T1W) and T2-weighted (T2W) images. The vitreous has been noted to be hyperintense on T1W and T2W images in the absence of retinal detachment. Tractional retinal detachment can occur. The detached retina may have a tubular image arising from the optic disk and reaching the retrolental mass, or it may form a falciform fold from a point eccentric to the optic nerve. The gliotic retinal tissue is hypointense on T1W and T2W images. The subretinal fluid is usually hyperintense on both spin echo images. A gravitational fluid–fluid level may be seen, which probably corresponds to the presence of hemorrhage in the subretinal space. After administration of gadolinium ethylenetriamine penta-acetic acid (Gd-DTPA), the retrolental mass may demonstrate enhancement (Fig. 3–1).

BIBLIOGRAPHY

De Potter P, Shields JA, Shields CL. Computed tomography and magnetic resonance imaging of intraocular lesions. *Ophthalmol Clin North Am.* 1994; 7:333–346.

De Potter P, Flanders AE, Shields JA, Shields CL. Magnetic resonance imaging of intraocular tumors. *Int Ophthalmol Clin.* 1993; 33:37–45.

De Potter P, Flanders AE, Shields JA, Shields CL, Gonzales CF, Rao VM. The role of fat suppression technique and gadopentetate dimeglumine in magnetic resonance imaging evaluation of intraocular tumors and simulating lesions. *Arch Ophthalmol.* 1994; 112: 340–348.

Mafee MF. Magnetic resonance imaging: Ocular pathology. In: Newton TH, Bilaniuk LT, eds. *Radiology of the Eye and Orbit.* New York: Raven Press; 1990, Chap. 3.

Mafee MF, Goldberg MF. Persistent hyperplastic primary vitreous: Role of computed tomography and magnetic resonance. *Radiol Clin North Am.* 1987; 25:683–692.

Mafee MF, Goldberg MF, Greenwald MF, Schulman J, Malmed A, Flanders AE. Retinoblastoma and simulating lesions: Role of CT and MR imagining. *Radiol Clin North Am.* 1987; 25:667–682.

Manschot WA. Persistent hyperplastic primary vitreous. *Arch Ophthalmol.* 1958; 59:188–203.

Reese AB. Persistence and hyperplasia of the primary vitreous: The Jackson Memorial Lecture. *Am J Ophthalmol.* 1955; 40:317–331.

Schulman JA, Peyman GA, Mafee MF, Lawrence L, Bauman AE, Goldman A, Kurwa B. The use of magnetic resonance imaging in the evaluation of retinoblastoma. *J Pediatr Ophthalmol Strabismus.* 1986; 23:144–147.

Shields JA, Shields CL. *Intraocular Tumors. A Textbook and Atlas.* Philadelphia: WB Saunders; 1992.

FIGURE 3-1 *Bilateral Persistent Hyperplastic Primary Vitreous*

A 2-month-old girl presented with bilateral leukokoria 1 week after birth.

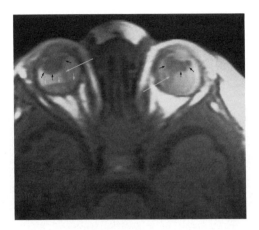

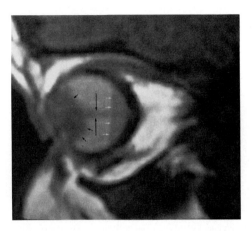

3-1A Axial T1W image. Both eyes developed total retinal detachment. The subretinal fluid appears hyperintense, and a hypointense retrolental mass (*short black arrows*) is noted bilaterally. A fluid–fluid level is seen in the right eye, probably corresponding to gravitational layering of serosanguineous fluid in the subretinal space (*short white arrows*). The retina, which is drawn by traction, shows a tubular hypointense signal (*long arrows*) in the subretinal space.

3-1B Sagittal T1W image of the right orbit. Note the retrolental mass (*short black arrows*) that is contiguous with the tubular image (*long arrows*) of the detached retina. The gravitational fluid–fluid level (*white arrows*) assumes a vertical position in the sagittal plane (with the patient in a supine position).

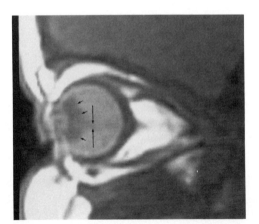

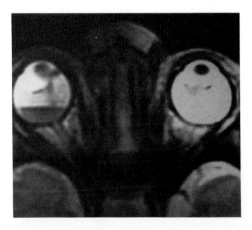

3-1C Sagittal T1W image of the left eye. Note the retrolental mass (*short arrows*) and the detached retina (*long arrows*).

3-1D Axial T2W image. The subretinal fluid appears hyperintense. The retrolental mass and the detached retina remain hypointense. The decreased signal intensity of the serosanguineous fluid on T1W and T2W suggests acute subretinal hemorrhage.

(continued)

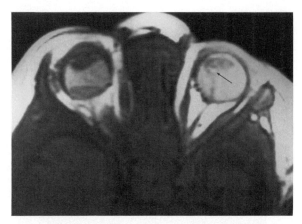 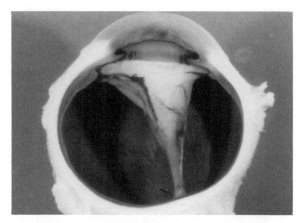

3–1E Axial Gd-DTPA–enhanced T1W image. Note the minimal enhancement (*arrow*) of the retrolental mass in the left eye. No enhancement is detected in the right eye. Only 1 cc of gadopentetate dimeglumine was administered.

3–1F Photograph of a grossly sectioned globe with PHPV. Note the stalk of totally detached retina reaching the retrolental mass.

MRI of the Eye and Orbit,
by Patrick De Potter, Jerry A. Shields, and Carol L. Shields.
J. B. Lippincott Company, Philadelphia © 1995.

4

Retinal Detachment

PATRICK DE POTTER

CAROL L. SHIELDS

JERRY A. SHIELDS

RHEGMATOGENOUS RETINAL DETACHMENT

Clinical and Pathological Features

The term retinal detachment is used to define a separation of the neurosensory retina from the retinal pigment epithelium. Accumulation of subretinal fluid is a feature of all retinal detachments. There are four major types of retinal detachment: rhegmatogenous, tractional, combined tractional and rhegmatogenous, and serous/hemorrhagic retinal detachment. The most common form is rhegmatogenous detachment, which results from a full-thickness retinal hole or tear. Retinal detachment can also be produced by mechanical traction forces that pull the retina away from the underlying retinal pigment epithelium. Some retinal detachments combine a rhegmatogenous and tractional component. Retinal detachments can occur in the absence of a retinal tear and vitreoretinal traction. Separation of the sensory retina from the retinal pigment epithelium results in an increase in the protein concentration and number of large molecules in the subretinal space. The protein concentration of the subretinal space increases with time.

MR Features

The appearance of rhegmatogenous retinal detachment on magnetic resonance imaging (MRI)
depends on the amount of proteinaceous material in the subretinal space. The detached retina may appear as a V-shaped, nonshifting structure with its apex at the optic disk and its extremities extending toward the ciliary body. With respect to the vitreous, the subretinal space is seen as an area of isointense to hyperintense signal on T1-weighted (T1W) images and isointense signal on T2-weighted (T2W) images (Fig. 4–1, *A* and *B*). There is no enhancement of the subretinal space or enhancing choroidal or retinal lesions after Gd-DTPA administration. These MR features are different from those of uveal melanoma (see Tables 6–1 and 6–3) or retinoblastoma (see Tables 7–1 and 7–3).

EXUDATIVE NONRHEGMATOGENOUS RETINAL DETACHMENT

Clinical and Pathological Features

Secondary exudative nonrhegmatogenous retinal detachments are the result of an accumulation of subretinal proteinaceous or lipoproteinaceous fluid. This fluid accumulation is caused by a choroidal or retinal inflammatory process, neoplasm, or vascular or fibroproliferative lesion.

MR Features

The MRI appearance of exudative nonrhegmatogenous retinal detachment varies with the amount of exudation in the subretinal space and with the degree of organization of the subretinal material. The localized exudative retinal detachment secondary to choroidal or retinal neoplasm appears as a semilunar high signal intensity on T1W and T2W images (Figs. 4–2, A and B). When the retinal detachment is total, it appears with a characteristic V-shaped high signal intensity on T1W and T2W images. Because of the low signal intensity of the vitreous on T1W images, the exudative nonrhegmatogenous retinal detachment, with its high signal intensity, may be easily identified. However, on T2W images, the hyperintensity of the subretinal fluid and the vitreous often makes their differentiation impossible. The signal intensity of the exudative retinal detachment is usually higher than that of the rhegmatogenous retinal detachment owing to the increased proteinaceous content of the former.

After Gd-DTPA administration, the exudative non-rhegmatogenous retinal detachment does not enhance. This lack of enhancement allows differentiation between choroidal or retinal neoplasms and secondary retinal detachment (Fig. 4–2C). Gd-DTPA–enhanced MRI is most helpful in differentiating subretinal fluid from the causative lesion (see Tables 6–1, 6–3, 7–1, and 7–3).

HEMORRHAGIC RETINAL DETACHMENT

Clinical and Pathological Features

Hemorrhagic retinal detachment may occur secondary to trauma, to a choroidal or retinal neoplasm, or to other diseases of the fundus that predispose the individual to vascular proliferation and hemorrhage (macular degeneration, diabetic retinopathy, peripheral exudate hemorrhagic chorioretinopathy). A growing choroidal melanoma may break through Bruch's membrane and produce retinal and vitreous hemorrhage. Among the other causes producing hemorrhagic retinal detachment, proliferative age-related macular degeneration (central or peripheral) may simulate choroidal melanoma (see Chapter 7). Rupture of intraretinal arterial macroaneurysm can also produce secondary hemorrhagic detachment. Use of aspirin or anticoagulants may predispose these patients to a massive hemorrhage. When the media are clear, fluorescein angiography is a very helpful ancillary study for differentiating hemorrhagic detachment from a choroidal melanoma.

MR Features

Gd-DTPA–enhanced MRI is helpful when opaque media preclude a view of the posterior pole. The MRI appearance of hemorrhagic retinal detachment varies with the chronicity of the hemorrhage. Acute hemorrhagic retinal detachment appears isointense on T1W images and markedly hypointense on T2W images with respect to the vitreous. Subacute retinal hemorrhage appears with a high signal intensity on T1W images and low to high signal intensity on T2W images owing to the presence of methemoglobin (Figs. 4–3, A and B; 4–4, A through C; and 4–5) These precontrast MR features are identical to those of uveal melanoma in the adult population (see Tables 6–1 and 6–2) and of retinoblastoma in children (see Tables 7–1 and 7–2). In its chronic stage, hemorrhagic retinal detachment is seen as an area of hyperintensity decreasing to marked hypointensity on both T1W and T2W images as a result of the accumulation of ferritin and hemosiderin.

On Gd-DTPA–enhanced T1W images, the hemorrhagic retinal detachment does not enhance, unlike an underlying choroidal or retinal tumor, which will enhance (Fig. 4–4D) (see Tables 6–1 and 7–1). Therefore, contrast-enhanced MRI is very helpful in differentiating subacute hemorrhagic retinal detachment from uveal melanoma in adults and from retinoblastoma in children.

BIBLIOGRAPHY

Chignell AH, Carruthers M, Rahi AHS. Clinical, biochemical, and immunoelectrophoretic study of subretinal fluid. Br J Ophthalmol. 1971; 55:525–532.

De Potter P, Flanders AE, Shields JA, Shields CL. Magnetic resonance imaging of intraocular tumors. Int Ophthalmol Clin. 1993; 33:37–45.

De Potter P, Flanders AE, Shields JA, Shields CL, Gonzales CF, Rao VM. The role of fat suppression technique and gadopentetate dimeglumine in magnetic resonance imaging evaluation of intraocular tumors and simulating lesions. Arch Ophthalmol. 1994; 112:340–348.

De Potter P, Shields JA, Shields CL. Computed tomography and magnetic resonance imaging of intraocular lesions. Ophthalmol Clin North Am. 1994; 7: 333–346.

Landers MB, Hjelmeland LM. Types of pathogenetic mechanisms of retinal detachment. In: Ryan SJ,

Glaser BM, Michels RG, eds. *Retina, Surgical Retina.* 1989:105–109.

Mafee MF. Magnetic resonance imaging: Ocular pathology. In: Newton TH, Bilaniuk LT, eds. *Radiology of the Eye and Orbit.* New York. Raven Press; 1990, Chap. 3.

Mafee MF, Peyman GA. Retinal and choroidal detachments: Role of magnetic resonance imaging and computed tomography. *Radiol Clin North Am.* 1987; 25:487–507.

Shields JA, Augsburger JJ, Brown GC, Stephens RF. The differential diagnosis of posterior uveal melanoma. *Ophthalmology.* 1980; 87:518–522.

Shields JA, Shields CL. Differential diagnosis of posterior uveal melanoma. In: Shields JA, Shields CL, eds. *Intraocular Tumors. A Textbook and Atlas.* Philadelphia: WB Saunders; 1992: 137–153.

Straatsma BR, Foos RY, Kreiger AE. Rhegmatogenous retinal detachment. In: Tasman W, Jaeger EA, eds. *Duane's Clinical Ophthalmology.* Vol. 3. 1989, Chap. 27.

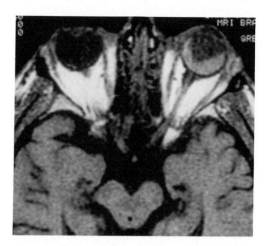

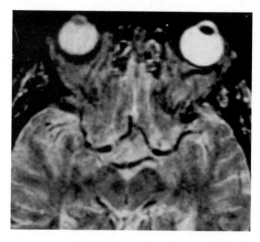

4-1A Axial T1W image. A V-shaped fluid collection shows an increased signal intensity with respect to the vitreous. The V-shaped configuration is produced by the total retinal detachment. The high signal intensity of the subretinal fluid is caused by its high proteinaceous content.

4-1B Axial T2W image. The subretinal space becomes hyperintense and isointense with respect to the vitreous.

FIGURE 4-2 *Exudative Nonrhegmatogenous Retinal Detachment*
Choroidal melanoma produced secondary exudative nonrhegmatogenous retinal detachment in the left eye.

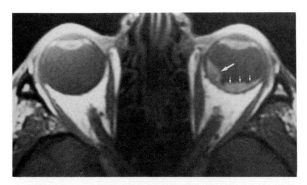

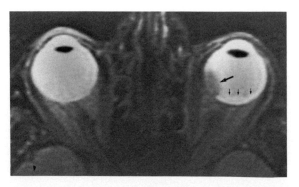

4-2A Axial T1W image. The choroidal melanoma (*long arrow*), located nasally to the optic disk, and the associated exudative retinal detachment (*short arrows*), located temporally to the optic disk, are both hyperintense with respect to the vitreous.

4-2B Axial T2W image. The signal intensity of the choroidal melanoma is hypointense (*long arrow*), but the subretinal fluid (*short arrows*) remains hyperintense.

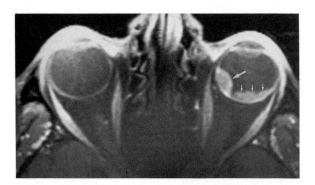

4-2C Fat-suppressed axial Gd-DTPA–enhanced T1W image. The tumor (*long arrow*) demonstrates moderate heterogeneous enhancement, but the exudative subretinal fluid (*short arrows*) does not enhance.

A 46-year-old woman presented with sudden decreased vision in the left eye 8 days before undergoing MRI studies.

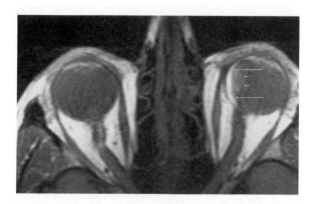 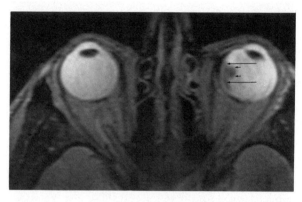

4–3A Axial T1W image. A lenticular collection of blood beneath the retinal pigment epithelium (*long arrows*) shows high signal intensity compared to the less hypointense dome-shaped collection beneath the sensory retina (*short arrows*).

4–3B Axial T2W image. Both subretinal pigment epithelium and subretinal blood appear hypointense with respect to the vitreous. The MR features of the subacute hemorrhagic retinal pigment epithelial detachment (*long arrows*) are related to the presence of intracellular methemoglobin. The subretinal hemorrhage (*short arrows*) is more acute.

FIGURE 4-4 *Hemorrhagic Retinal Detachment*
A 46-year-old patient presented with hemorrhagic retinal detachment and vitreous hemorrhage secondary to traumatic injury occurring 14 days before the ocular findings, which simulated choroidal melanoma in the right eye.

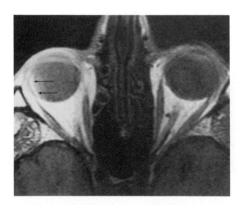

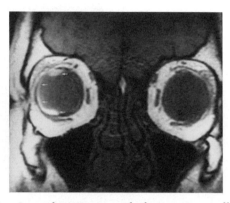

4-4A Axial T1W image. A subretinal crescent-shaped fluid collection is noted in the temporal region. The collection is markedly hyperintense (*arrows*) with respect to the vitreous. The vitreous shows a higher signal intensity than that of the left eye because of the vitreous hemorrhage.

4-4B Coronal T1W image. The hyperintense collection extends from the superior to the inferior portion of the right eye (*arrows*).

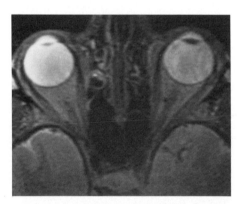

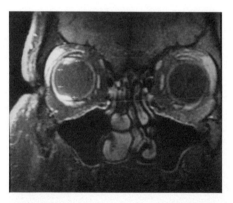

4-4C Axial T2W image. The fluid collection remains hyperintense in signal intensity, and therefore is no longer able to be differentiated from the high signal intensity of the vitreous. This is consistent with subacute hemorrhage and extracellular methemoglobin. Note the increased signal intensity of the vitreous in the right eye owing to the vitreous hemorrhage.

4-4D Fat-suppressed coronal Gd-DTPA–enhanced T1W image. The crescent-shaped fluid collection (*arrows*) does not show enhancement.

(continued)

FIGURE 4-4 *Hemorrhagic Retinal Detachment* (continued)

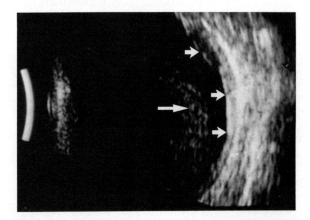

4-4E B-scan ultrasonography. The shallow hemorrhagic retinal detachment (*short arrows*) appears more echogenic in its inferior portion than in its superior portion. Note the vitreous echoes from the vitreous hemorrhage (*long arrow*).

FIGURE 4-5 *Hemorrhagic Retinal Detachment*

A 45-year-old patient with advanced proliferative diabetic retinopathy in the left eye presented with a 15-day history of hemorrhagic tractional retinal detachment and hemorrhage between the back of the vitreous body and the front of the retina (retrohyaloid space).

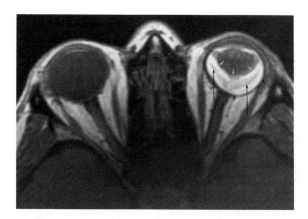 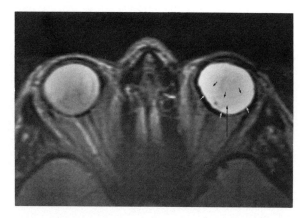

4-5A Axial T1W image. The V-shaped subretinal fluid collection (*short black arrows*), which is suggestive of total retinal detachment appears with a high signal intensity. It is separated from the hyperintense retrohyaloid hemorrhage (*short white arrows*) by a V-shaped line corresponding to the detached thickened retina (*long black arrows*). Note the apex of the V arising from the optic disk. (From Orbit. In: Rao VM, Flanders AE, Tom BM, eds. *MRI and CT Atlas of Correlative Imaging in Otolaryngology*. London: Martin Dunitz; 1992:329.)

4-5B Axial T2W image. Both the subretinal (*short white arrows*) and preretinal (*short black arrows*) hemorrhage remain hyperintense in signal intensity, which is suggestive of subacute hemorrhage and extracellular methemoglobin. The V-shaped detached retina (*long black arrow*), with its low signal intensity, separates them. The core of the vitreous cavity has a slightly lower signal intensity than the preretinal hemorrhage.

MRI of the Eye and Orbit,
by Patrick De Potter, Jerry A. Shields, and Carol L. Shields.
J. B. Lippincott Company, Philadelphia © 1995.

5

Inflammatory Disorders

PATRICK DE POTTER

CAROL L. SHIELDS

JERRY A. SHIELDS

POSTERIOR SCLERITIS

Clinical and Pathological Features

Scleritis is an uncommon inflammatory disorder of the sclera that may lead to the loss of the eye as a result of deteriorating vision, severe pain, or even perforation of the globe. Scleritis can be classified as anterior or posterior. Posterior scleritis is the rarest form of scleritis, primarily affecting women. Most commonly, there is a gradual onset of blurred vision with hyperopic changes in the affected eye associated with severe pain. External examination may reveal limitation of extraocular movements and proptosis. On ophthalmoscopic examination, optic disk edema and exudative retinal detachment can be seen. Posterior scleritis is classified into two forms: acute and chronic. Both types are characterized by thickened sclera and choroid with choroidal folds. Nodular posterior scleritis appears as an elevated mass simulating amelanotic choroidal melanoma.

Histopathologic examination reveals two predominant, grossly different types. The nodular type is a classic example of focal or zonal necrotizing granulomatous inflammation surrounding a discrete sequestrum of scleral collagen. In the diffuse type (brawny scleritis), which is sometimes seen in patients with rheumatoid arthritis, large areas of scleral collagen are surrounded by granulomatous inflammation, causing diffuse thickening of the sclera. Ultrasonography reveals a thickened choroidal-scleral complex with high internal reflectivity and retrobulbar edema. Orbital computed tomography (CT) shows a thickened sclera that may enhance with administration of a contrast agent.

MR Features

Based on our magnetic resonance imaging (MRI) experience, nodular scleritis appears as an elevated mass with low signal intensity and isointense signal with respect to the vitreous on T1-weighted (T1W) images (see Figs. 5–1A, 5–2A). On T2-weighted (T2W) images, the tumor shows a hypointense signal with respect to the vitreous (Figs. 5–1B and 5–2B). After Gd-DTPA administration, nodular posterior scleritis demonstrates no or minimal enhancement (Figs. 5–1, C and D; and 5–2, C and D). These MR features are different from those of choroidal melanoma (see Tables 6–1 and 6–3).

Diffuse posterior scleritis appears as a diffuse thickening of the sclera, mainly located at the posterior pole, with an isointense to slightly hyperintense signal with respect to vitreous on T1W images (Figs. 5–3, A and B). On T2W images, the lesion becomes hypointense with respect to vitreous (Fig. 5–3C). On Gd-DTPA–enhanced T1W images, the mass shows moderate to marked enhancement relating to the degree of inflammation (Fig. 5–3, D and E). Associated intraocular and orbital features, such as exudative retinal detachment, optic disk edema, and orbital inflammation, can be evaluated with MRI.

VOGT-KOYANAGI-HARADA SYNDROME

Clinical and Pathological Features

Vogt-Koyanagi-Harada (VKH) syndrome is a unilateral or bilateral uveitis with exudative retinal detachment associated with systemic manifestations (alopecia, poliosis, vitiligo, dysacusis) and other central nervous system signs and symptoms (cerebrospinal fluid pleocytosis, meningeal signs). It appears to have a predilection for oriental or black patients. Diffuse choroiditis with serous retinal detachment is well documented by fluorescein angiography.

Histopathologically, VKH syndrome resembles sympathetic ophthalmia, with granulomatous inflammation within the uveal tract and formation of multiple focal granulomas called Dalen-Fuchs nodules.

MR Features

On precontrast MR studies, VKH syndrome presents as unilateral or bilateral diffuse thickening of the posterior uveal tract with exudative retinal detachment. The thickened, inflamed, posterior choroid shows a uniform hyperintense signal with respect to the vitreous and the overlying exudative retinal detachment on T1W images (Fig. 5–4A). On T2W images, the high signal intensity of the thickened choroid is hypointense with respect to the high signal intensity of the vitreous and secondary retinal detachment (Fig. 5–4B). The high signal intensity of the subretinal fluid depends on its proteinaceous content. Gd-DTPA–enhanced T1W images demonstrate moderate enhancement of the thickened posterior uvea with no enhancement of the subretinal fluid (Fig. 5–4, C and D).

BIBLIOGRAPHY

Benson WE, Shields JA, Tasman WS, Crandall AS. Posterior scleritis. *Arch Ophthalmol.* 1979; 97:1482–1486.

Berger B, Reeser F. Retinal pigment epithelial detachments in posterior scleritis. *Am J Ophthalmol.* 1980; 90:604–606.

Chan CC, Palestine AG, Nussenblatt RB. Sympathetic ophthalmia and Vogt-Koyanagi-Harada syndrome. In: Tasman W, Jaeger EA, eds. *Duane's Clinical* Ophthalmology. Vol. 4. 1989, Chap. 51.

De Potter P, Flanders AE, Shields JA, Shields CL. Magnetic resonance imaging of intraocular tumors. *Int Ophthalmol Clin.* 1993; 33:37–45.

De Potter P, Flanders AE, Shields JA, Shields CL, Gonzales CF, Rao VM. The role of fat suppression technique and gadopentetate dimeglumine in magnetic resonance imaging evaluation of intraocular tumors and simulating lesions. *Arch Ophthalmol.* 1994; 112: 340–348.

Forster RK. Endophthalmitis. In: Tasman W, Jaeger EA, eds. *Duane's Clinical Ophthalmology.* Vol. 4, 1989, Chap. 24.

Lubin JR, Ni C, Albert DM. A clinicopathological study of the Vogt-Koyanagi-Harada syndrome. *Int Ophthalmol Clin.* 1982; 22:141–156.

Mafee MF, Peyman GA. Retinal and choroidal detachments: Role of magnetic resonance imaging and computed tomography. *Radiol Clin North Am.* 1987; 25:487–507.

Portnoy SL, Franklin R. Scleritis. In: Ryan SJ, Schachat AP, Murphy RB, Patz A, eds. *Retina.* St. Louis. CV Mosby; 1989:663–670.

Singh G, Guthoff R, Foster CS. Observations on long-term follow-up of posterior scleritis. *Am J Ophthalmol.* 1986; 101:570–575.

Smith RE, Nozik RA. Endophthalmitis. In: Smith RE, Nozik RA, eds. *Uveitis.* Baltimore. Williams & Wilkins; 1987:101–105.

Smith RE, Nozik RA. Vogt-Koyanagi-Harada syndrome. In: Smith RE, Nozik RA, eds. *Uveitis.* Baltimore. Williams & Wilkins; 1987:162–165.

Snyder DA, Tessler HH. Vogt-Koyanagi-Harada syndrome. *Am J Ophthalmol.* 1980; 90:69–75.

Spencer WH. Sclera. In: Spencer WH, Font RL, Green WR, Howes EL, Jakobiec FA, Zimmerman LE, eds. *Ophthalmic Pathology. An Atlas and Textbook.* Philadelphia. WB Saunders; 1986:406–407.

Watson P. Diseases of the sclera and episclera. In: Tasman W, Jaeger EA, eds. *Duane's Clinical Ophthalmology.* Vol. 4. 1984, Chap. 23.

FIGURE 5-1 *Nodular Anterior Scleritis*

A 46-year-old man presented with redness and thickening of the sclera nasally and temporally in the left eye. No etiology was found after a complete systemic work-up. Biopsy of the lesion revealed nongranulomatous inflammatory elements.

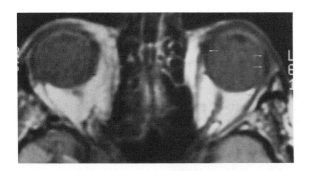

5-1A Axial proton density-weighted image. The scleral inflammation has a 360-degree equatorial location (*arrows*) and has a low signal intensity with respect to the vitreous.

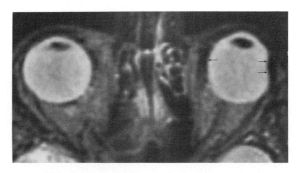

5-1B Axial T2W image. The thickened sclera (*arrows*) remains markedly hypointense, as in the T1W image as well (not shown). The inflammatory process appears to involve the medial and lateral muscles at their scleral insertion.

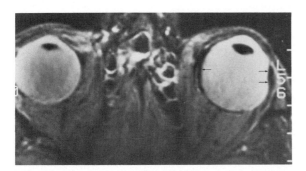

5-1C Axial Gd-DTPA–enhanced T2W image. The scleral thickening (*arrows*) remains hypointense with no enhancement.

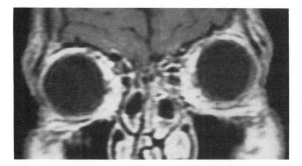

5-1D Coronal Gd-DTPA–enhanced T1W image. No enhancement of the lesion is demonstrated. The low signal intensity of the scleral inflammatory infiltrate is not distinguishable from the low signal intensity of the vitreous.

(continued)

FIGURE 5-1 *Nodular Anterior Scleritis* (continued)

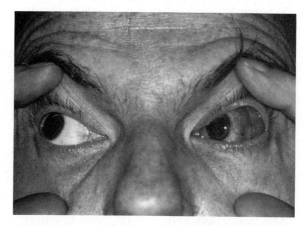

5-1E A photograph shows the redness and infiltration of the sclera temporally in the left eye.

FIGURE 5–2 *Nodular Posterior Scleritis*

A 34-year-old woman presented with idiopathic nodular posterior scleritis in the left eye simulating a choroidal melanoma. Ophthalmoscopically, the lesion was amelanotic with no associated subretinal fluid.

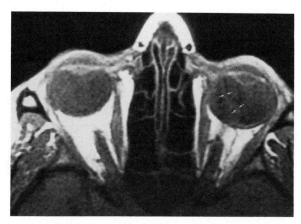

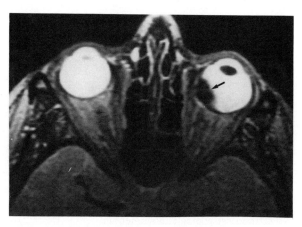

5–2A Axial T1W image. The mass shows an isointense signal with respect to the vitreous. The overlying thickened choroid (*arrows*) appears as a curvilinear area with minimal hyperintense signal.

5–2B Axial T2W image. The lesion (*arrow*) becomes hypointense with respect to the vitreous.

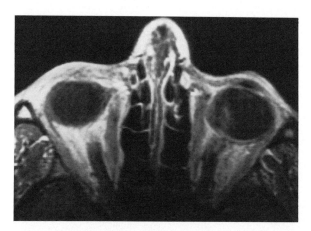

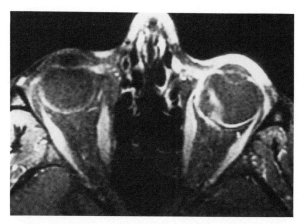

5–2C Axial Gd-DTPA–enhanced T1W image. The lesion demonstrates minimal enhancement. Enhancement is also documented along the internal margin of the lesion, an area corresponding to the thickened, inflamed choroid.

5–2D Fat-suppressed axial Gd-DTPA–enhanced T1W image. The enhancement of the irregular thickened choroid is more pronounced.

(continued)

FIGURE 5–2 *Nodular Posterior Scleritis* (continued)

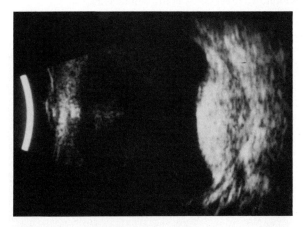

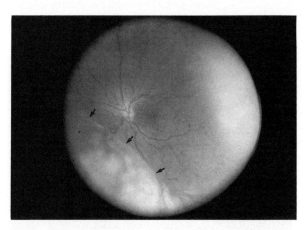

5–2E B-scan ultrasonography reveals a dome-shaped, acoustically solid, subretinal lesion that is 7.0 mm thick. No retrobulbar edema is documented.

5–2F A wide-angle photograph shows the elevated amelanotic mass (*arrows*) in the inferonasal quadrant.

FIGURE 5–3 *Diffuse Posterior Scleritis*

A 44-year-old patient presented with bilateral diffuse posterior scleritis and orbital inflammation.

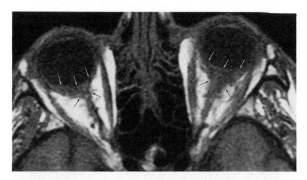

5–3A Axial T1W image. Bilateral thickening of the posterior wall with secondary subretinal fluid (*white arrows*) is characterized by a mild hyperintense signal with respect to the vitreous. Inflammation of the intraconal fat producing a hypointense signal surrounds bilaterally the distal portion of the optic nerve (*black arrows*).

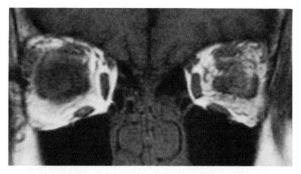

5–3B Coronal T1W image. The intraconal orbital fat inflammatory infiltrate encircles both optic nerve sheath complexes. Note the reticular pattern of the orbital fat.

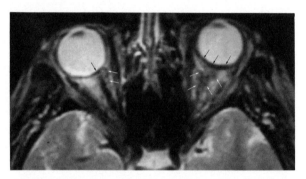

5–3C Axial T2W image. The thickened posterior sclera becomes hypointense (*black arrows*) with respect to the overlying subretinal fluid and vitreous, which both appear hyperintense. The scleral thickening is more prominent in the left eye. The retro-ocular inflammation in the left and right intraconal spaces remains hypointense (*white arrows*).

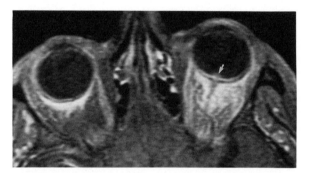

5–3D Fat-suppressed axial Gd-DTPA–enhanced T1W image. The inflamed scleral tissue and adjacent retro-ocular orbital fat show enhancement bilaterally. The intraconal enhancement extends along the left optic nerve. Note the optic disk swelling in the left eye (*arrow*).

(continued)

FIGURE 5–3 *Diffuse Posterior Scleritis* (continued)

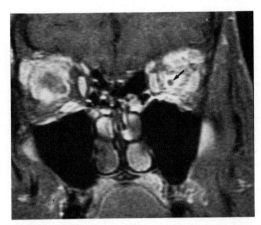

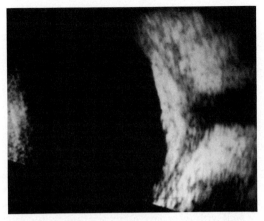

5–3E Fat-suppressed coronal Gd-DTPA–enhanced T1W image. Note the bilateral marked enhancement of the perioptic nerve inflammatory infiltrate. The left optic nerve does not enhance (*arrow*).

5–3F B-scan ultrasonography. The left eye shows the pathognomonic T sign (*on end*) associated with retroscleral edema.

FIGURE 5-4 *Bilateral Vogt-Koyanagi-Harada Syndrome*
A 26-year-old Asian patient presented with bilateral Vogt-Koyanagi-Harada syndrome.
(Courtesy of Oscar Kallay, M.D., Brussels, Belgium.)

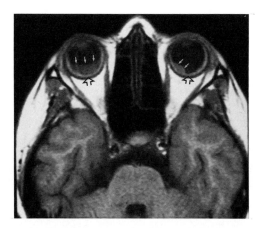

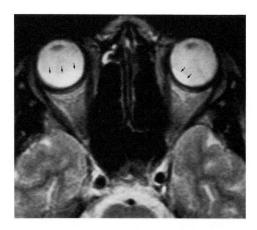

5-4A Axial T1W image. The bilateral thickened choroid has a regular curvilinear hyperintense signal (*open arrows*) with respect to the vitreous. The associated exudative bilateral retinal detachment (*short arrows*) shows a hyperintense signal with respect to the vitreous, but the signal is hypointense with respect to the inflammatory thickening of the choroid.

5-4B Axial T2W image. The choroid becomes hyperintense, as does the subretinal fluid. However, the high proteinaceous content of the exudative retinal detachment shows a higher signal intensity (*arrows*).

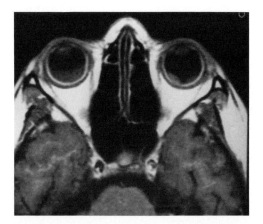

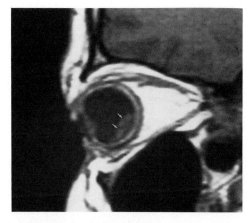

5-4C Axial Gd-DTPA–enhanced T1W image. The thickened choroid demonstrates moderate enhancement bilaterally. The associated subretinal fluid does not enhance.

5-4D Sagittal Gd-DTPA–enhanced T1W image. The nonenhancement of the secondary retinal detachment of the left eye is well visualized (*arrows*).

MRI of the Eye and Orbit,
by Patrick De Potter, Jerry A. Shields, and Carol L. Shields.
J. B. Lippincott Company, Philadelphia © 1995.

6

Tumors of the Uvea

PATRICK DE POTTER

JERRY A. SHIELDS

CAROL L. SHIELDS

UVEAL MELANOCYTIC TUMORS

CHOROIDAL NEVUS

Clinical and Pathological Features

A choroidal nevus is a benign melanocytic tumor of the choroid. It appears as a flat or minimally elevated lesion. Nevi can vary in diameter, but in our experience, they are usually less than 2.0 mm thick. Although most choroidal nevi are clinically pigmented, they can be amelanotic. The presence of orange pigment on the tumor surface and subretinal fluid may suggest activity of the lesion and constitutes risk factors for transformation into malignant melanoma.

Choroidal nevus can contain four types of cells: polyhedral nevus cells, slender spindle nevus cells, plump fusiform and dendritic cells, and balloon cells. No cellular atypia is found in choroidal nevus. Ultrasonography demonstrates an acoustically hollow or solid sessile mass with low-to-medium internal reflectivity.

A choroidal nevus should be managed by observation and serial fundus photography. Most nevi require no treatment. However, evidence of documented growth should be considered a clinical sign of early malignant transformation, in which case treatment should be instituted.

MR Features

Because of the minimal elevation of choroidal nevi, it is very difficult to detect these tumors using magnetic resonance imaging (MRI). However, the melanin content of a choroidal nevus makes its detection easier. Tumors with high melanin content demonstrate decreased T1 and T2 values compared with those of amelanotic tumors. Therefore, pigmented choroidal nevi present with a hyperintense signal on T1-weighted (T1W) images and a hypointense signal on T2-weighted (T2W) images with respect to the vitreous (Fig. 6–1, *A* and *B*). Amelanotic choroidal nevi are usually undetected due to their isointense signal to the vitreous on T1W and T2W images. After Gd-DTPA administration and with fat-suppression technique, a choroidal nevus shows minimal to moderate enhancement on T1W images (Fig. 6–1*C*). These MR features are also found in choroidal melanoma (Tables 6–1 and 6–2). Fat-suppression techniques and Gd-DTPA enhancement appear to be most helpful in detecting a choroidal nevus. However, based on our experience, melanocytic lesions with thicknesses of less than 1.8 mm cannot be detected by contrast-enhanced MRI with fat-suppression technique.

Our experience indicates that indirect ophthalmoscopy, ultrasonography (Fig. 6–1*D*), and fluorescein angiography are the most important diagnostic

TABLE 6-1 *MR Features of Choroidal Lesions with Thicknesses Greater than 1.8 mm on Spin Echo Sequences*

	Signal Intensity of Lesion with Respect to the Vitreous		Degree of Lesion Enhancement after Gd-DTPA
	T1WI	T2WI	
Choroidal nevus	Iso/Hyper	Iso/Hypo	+/++
Choroidal melanoma	Hyper	Iso/Hypo	+/+++
Choroidal metastasis	Hyper	Iso/Hypo	+
Choroidal hemangioma	Iso/Hyper	Iso	++++
Choroidal leiomyoma	Hyper	Iso/Hypo	+++/++++
Choroidal osteoma	Hyper	Hypo	−/+++
Choroidal hemangiopericytoma	Hyper	Hypo	+++
Acute choroidal hemorrhage	Iso	Hypo	−
Subacute choroidal hemorrhage	Hyper	Hypo/Iso	−
Chronic choroidal hemorrhage	Iso	Hypo	−

T1WI, T1-weighted image; *T2WI*, T2-weighted image; *Gd-DTPA*, gadolinium diethylenetriamine penta-acetic acid; *iso*, isointense; *hyper*, hyperintense; *hypo*, hypointense.

modalities for detecting and evaluating choroidal nevi. Contrast-enhanced MRI studies do not allow a differential diagnosis between choroidal nevus and small choroidal melanoma. Therefore, routine MRI studies are not recommended for evaluating choroidal nevus.

CHOROIDAL MELANOMA

Clinical and Pathological Features

Malignant melanoma of the ciliary body and choroid (posterior uvea) is the most common primary intraocular malignant disease. The incidence of malignant melanoma of the choroid has been

TABLE 6-2 *Intraocular Lesions (with Thicknesses > 1.8 mm) in Adults That Can Have MR Features Identical to Those of Choroidal Melanoma on Nonenhanced MRI*

Choroidal nevus
Choroidal metastasis
Choroidal hemangiopericytoma
Choroidal osteoma
Uveal leiomyoma
Uveal melanocytoma
Subacute choroidal hemorrhage
Subacute hemorrhagic retinal detachment (age-related macular degeneration)
Retinal capillary hemangioma
Retinal gliosis
Adenoma of the nonpigmented ciliary body epithelium

estimated to be 5.2 to 7.5 cases per million per year. Malignant melanomas of the uvea are particularly rare in blacks and Asians. Most posterior uveal melanomas are diagnosed in middle-aged or elderly patients (at a mean age of 53 years), and they generally have no hereditary pattern.

Clinically, posterior uveal melanoma may exhibit different degrees of pigmentation and growth patterns. Although most uveal malignant melanomas are pigmented, the degree of pigmentation can vary considerably. Some tumors may be partially pigmented and partially nonpigmented. Ciliary body and choroidal melanoma may grow in either a nodular or a diffuse pattern. A nodular uveal melanoma may exhibit a well-circumscribed ovoid or dome-shaped appearance. As the tumor grows, Bruch's membrane can be ruptured, and the tumor may assume a mushroom or collar-button shape. The mushroom-shaped configuration is very suggestive of choroidal melanoma and is clearly evident on ophthalmoscopic and ultrasonographic examination. The diffuse choroidal melanoma may be more difficult to recognize on ophthalmoscopic examination because of the poorly circumscribed, diffuse thickening of the uvea and the lack of distinct nodular elevation. In the ciliary body, diffuse malignant melanoma may extend for 360 degrees and exhibit a ring pattern. Diffuse uveal melanomas are usually associated with extensive secondary retinal detachment and a high incidence of extraocular extension.

Uveal melanomas are usually divided into three groups: spindle cell melanoma, epithelioid cell melanoma, and mixed cell melanoma. It is impossible to recognize the tumor cell type clinically. Tumor necrosis is often seen in larger melanomas that have broken Bruch's membrane. The presence of orange pigment on the tumor surface is highly suggestive of malignant transformation and is related to the accumulation of clumps of macrophages containing lipofuscin and melanin granules at the level of the retinal pigment epithelium. Posterior uveal melanoma often invades the sclera and can extend through the sclera to produce extrascleral extension. Posterior extraocular extension can be very difficult to detect and can remain unrecognized until the patient develops proptosis or signs of panophthalmitis. The factors associated with a poor systemic prognosis include: (1) older age of the patient, (2) large tumor basal diameter (>15 mm), (3) anterior location of the tumor in the ciliary body, (4) presence of epithelioid cells, and (5) extraocular extension.

The diagnosis of posterior uveal melanoma can be challenging for the ophthalmologist. Among the imaging studies, fluorescein angiography and A- and B-scan ultrasonography are commonly used and are most helpful in differentiating melanoma from simulating lesions. Fluorescein angiographic features of uveal melanoma are not pathognomonic and vary depending on the size, pigmentation, and growth pattern of the tumor. With A-scan ultrasonography, posterior uveal melanoma shows low to medium internal reflectivity with decreasing amplitude (angle Kappa). B-scan studies demonstrate a dome- or mushroom-shaped choroidal mass, usually with acoustic hollowness and choroidal excavation. Ultrasonography can be very helpful in detecting small degrees of extraocular extension. Computed tomography (CT) is less commonly used, but may be helpful in differentiating simulating lesions by detecting calcification within the tumor. Radioactive phosphorus uptake test and fine-needle aspiration biopsy are very valuable surgical diagnostic adjuncts when other noninvasive methods are inconclusive.

MR Features

Uveal melanoma is particularly amenable to MR evaluation because of the paramagnetic properties of melanin. Because melanin-free radicals produce paramagnetic proton relaxation enhancement, both T1 and T2 relaxation times of choroidal melanoma are shorter in the presence of melanin than in its absence. Therefore, uveal melanoma characteristically demonstrates a hyperintense signal with respect to the vitreous on T1W weighted images and a hypointense signal on T2W images (Figs. 6–2, A and B; 6–3, A and B; 6–5A; 6–6, A and B; 6–7, A through C; 6–8, A through C; 6–9A). If melanin content was the only histologic factor responsible for these MR features, the signal intensity of melanotic uveal melanoma would be correlated to the degree of pigmentation of these tumors. Indeed, several studies have documented these MR characteristic features of uveal melanoma. This "hyperintense signal on T1W images and hypointense signal on T2W images" pattern of uveal melanoma detected on MRI (at 1.5 T) has been reported to be between 72% and 100%. A study of 15 uveal melanomas using a 0.5-T unit reported diverse appearances of uveal melanomas, with a combination of T1 hyperintensity and T2 hyperintensity and isointensity of the tumor with respect to the vitreous. The use of a 0.5-T scanner may explain this spectrum of MR appearances. Tumor necrosis, blood, or altered blood products might also explain the heterogeneity of tumor signal observed with MRI.

The authors' experience with 43 uveal melanomas has shown that 95% of them demonstrate the characteristic MR features of T1 hyperintensity and T2 hypointensity. However, in 5%, choroidal melanoma may show hyperintensity on T1W images and isointensity on T2W images with respect to the vitreous at 1.5 T (see Fig. 6–4, A and B). We have also found that the degree of pigmentation of uveal melanoma is not significantly associated with the brightness of the tumor on unenhanced T1W images, suggesting that the amount of melanin is not the only histologic factor related to the signal features of uveal melanomas. Clinically, amelanotic choroidal melanoma can show minimal to moderate hyperintensity on T1W images and hypointensity on T2W weighted images (see Fig. 6–6, A and B).

Fat-suppression technique improves contrast difference in signal intensity of choroidal melanoma and associated retinal detachment by expanding the dynamic range of the image (see Figs. 6–7B and 6–8B).

Gadolinium–diethylenetriamine penta-acetic acid (Gd-DTPA)–enhanced T1W images, with or without fat suppression, are superior in detecting and delineating uveal melanomas, as they show increased contrast-to-noise ratios compared to noncontrast T1W and T2W images. Based on the authors' experience, choroidal melanoma demonstrates minimal to moderate enhancement after Gd-DTPA administration (see Figs. 6–7, D and E; 6–8, D and E; and 6–9B). Large uveal melanomas, and particularly ciliochoroidal melanomas, show greater enhancement than do smaller uveal melanomas.

On noncontrast T1W images, the choroidal melanoma and the secondary retinal detachment appear hyperintense with respect to the vitreous (Figs. 6–8, *A* and *B;* and 6–9*A*). On Gd-DTPA–enhanced T1W images, with or without fat-suppression technique, the contrast enhancement of the tumor increases its signal intensity above that of the subretinal fluid, which is not enhanced (see Figs. 6–8, *D* and *E* and 6–9*B*). Based on the authors' series, the tumor intensity enhancement occurring after Gd-DTPA administration was not statistically associated with the degree of tumor pigmentation.

The authors' experience suggests that postcontrast T1W images with fat-suppression technique are most helpful in detecting and delineating small uveal melanomas. In the authors' series of 43 uveal melanomas, all tumors, including those with a thickness exceeding 1.8 mm, were detected on Gd-DTPA–enhanced T1W images with fat suppression.

In the adult population, other benign and malignant choroidal neoplasms, as well as retinal lesions, may show the same MR features as choroidal melanoma on noncontrast MRI (see Tables 6–1 and 6–2). Based on the authors' experience, it is very difficult to differentiate choroidal metastasis from choroidal melanoma using noncontrast MRI. However, nonenhanced MR features of choroidal hemangioma and acute and chronic hemorrhage are different from those of choroidal melanoma (see Tables 6–1 and 6–3). On postcontrast MRI, the intensity of tumor enhancement varies among these lesions and helps to differentiate choroidal melanoma from choroidal metastasis or choroidal leiomyoma (see Table 6–1). Based on the authors' limited experience, choroidal leiomyoma demonstrates marked enhancement, choroidal melanoma shows moderate enhancement, choroidal metastasis exhibits minimal enhancement, and retinal

TABLE 6–3 *Intraocular Lesions (with Thickness > 1.8 mm) in Adults with MR Features That Differ from Those of Choroidal Melanoma on Nonenhanced MRI*

Circumscribed choroidal hemangioma
Posterior nodular scleritis
Exudative nonrhegmatogenous retinal detachment
Rhegmatogenous retinal detachment
Acute choroidal hemorrhage
Chronic choroidal hemorrhage
Acute hemorrhagic retinal detachment
Chronic hemorrhagic retinal detachment

and choroidal detachment do not enhance after Gd-DTPA administration (see Table 6–1).

MRI also proved to be useful in detecting extraocular extension of uveal melanoma and massive optic nerve invasion. Extraocular extension of uveal melanoma usually appears as a well-circumscribed area with low signal intensity on T1W images and isointensity to low signal intensity on T2W images with respect to orbital fat (Fig. 6–10, *A* through *C*). After Gd-DTPA administration, the extraocular extension exhibits minimal to moderate enhancement (Fig. 6–10, *D* and *E*). In the authors' experience, ultrasonography appears to be as accurate as MRI in detecting extraocular extension (Fig. 6–10*F*). However, MRI provides more information for defining the preferred treatment approach to large extraocular extension (surgical orbital exenteration versus modified enucleation). Contrast-enhanced MRI may help differentiate extraocular extension from nonenhancing fibrotic scar tissue adjacent to the sclera after plaque radiotherapy (Fig. 6–11, *A* through *D*).

MELANOCYTOMA

Clinical and Pathological Features

Melanocytoma, or magnocellular nevus, is a deeply pigmented benign tumor that can occur in the uvea and in the substance of the optic nerve. Because melanocytomas are sometimes clinically misdiagnosed as malignant melanoma, it is important to consider the racial predisposition of these two tumors. Approximately 50% of melanocytomas occur in blacks, whereas the incidence of uveal malignant melanoma in blacks is less than 1%. For this reason, a pigmented elevated lesion found in a black patient on fundus examination is more suggestive of melanocytoma than of malignant melanoma.

Uveal melanocytoma is quite similar to uveal nevus and melanoma, and it may be impossible to differentiate them clinically. Melanocytoma of the optic disk appears as a black elevated mass with fibrillated margins and is located eccentrically on the optic nerve head. An adjacent choroidal component of the melanocytoma is present in 50% of cases. Although melanocytoma of the optic disk shows little tendency to grow, slow enlargement of the tumor has been documented in 15% of patients. Malignant transformation is extremely rare.

Uveal melanocytoma and melanocytoma of the optic disk are composed of deeply pigmented, benign, oval or round cells with abundant cytoplasm and a high content of melanin.

MR Features

Because of their melanin content, uveal melanocytoma and melanocytoma of the optic disk show a hyperintense signal on T1W images and a hypointense signal on T2W images with respect to vitreous (Fig. 6–12, A and B). Based on our experience, minimal enhancement is seen after Gd-DTPA administration (Fig. 6–12C). These MR features are identical to those of choroidal melanoma (see Tables 6–1 and 6–2). Therefore, MRI is not very helpful in differentiating choroidal melanoma from melanocytoma.

UVEAL METASTASIS

Clinical and Pathological Features

It is currently believed that cancer metastatic to the uvea is the most common intraocular malignant disease. However, many cases are never diagnosed because ocular examination is not routinely performed on patients with systemic metastatic disease. Uveal metastasis most commonly originates from primary breast and lung carcinomas in women and from lung and gastrointestinal tract carcinomas in men. In 18% to 25% of patients, the location of the primary tumor is never found.

The choroid is the most common site of carcinoma metastatic to the eye. About 40% of metastatic lesions to the choroid are partially located between the temporal retinal vascular arcades. Choroidal metastasis typically appears as a yellow-creamy, placoid, or dome-shaped lesion, associated in 75% of cases with secondary shifting retinal detachment. With the exception of choroidal metastasis from skin melanoma, choroidal metastases are amelanotic or minimally pigmented. Metastatic tumors to the uvea have a tendency to occur bilaterally and to be multifocal. This clinical presentation helps the ophthalmologist to differentiate metastatic lesion from primary amelanotic uveal melanoma. Metastatic carcinoma to the optic disk is rare, and usually represents extension of the juxtapapillary choroidal metastasis into the optic nerve head.

The histopathologic appearance of a metastatic carcinoma to the uvea depends partly on the features of the primary tumor. Usually, the tumor has a placoid or diffuse configuration with either glandular acini or cords of tumor cells retained from the primary tumor. Immunohistochemistry or electron microscopy may be necessary to determine the primary origin of the tumor.

Fluorescein angiography has some limited value in differentiating choroidal metastasis from other amelanotic choroidal lesions. A-scan ultrasonography will reveal a lesion with irregular medium internal reflectivity. On B-scan ultrasonography, choroidal metastasis usually exhibits an ovoid or dome-shaped choroidal mass with medium-to-high acoustic solidity and no appreciable choroidal excavation. A shifting retinal detachment may be demonstrated. Based on our experience, orbital CT is of little help in evaluating patients with choroidal metastasis. In the instances in which noninvasive methods of diagnosis are not helpful, fine-needle aspiration biopsy is indicated to guide therapeutic decisions.

MR Features

Metastatic lesions to the uvea demonstrate varying signal intensities on MRI. Reports of small series of metastatic carcinoma involving the uvea have shown a combination of T1 hyperintensity/isointensity and T2 hypointensity/isointensity with respect to the vitreous. The authors have found that metastatic choroidal tumors involving the uvea are relatively hyperintense with respect to vitreous on T1W images and relatively hypointense on T2W images (Figs. 6–13, A and B; 6–14, A and B; 6–15, A and C; and 6–16, A and B). Therefore, uveal metastatic tumors may share the same MR features as other pigmented or amelanotic intraocular lesions (see Tables 6–1 and 6–2).

Gd-DTPA–enhanced T1W images help to differentiate tumor from secondary retinal detachment. Moreover, our experience suggests that the enhancement of metastatic choroidal tumor is not as marked as that seen with choroidal melanoma, choroidal hemangioma, or choroidal leiomyoma (Figs. 6–15, B and C; 6–16C, and 6–17). This minimal enhancement after Gd-DTPA administration may be helpful in differentiating choroidal metastasis from choroidal melanoma or uveal leiomyoma, which present similar MRI characteristics on nonenhanced T1W and T2W images (see Table 6–1). Gd-DTPA–enhanced T1W images with fat-suppression technique are most helpful in detecting small metastatic choroidal lesions (thickness > 1.8 mm) by expanding the dynamic range of the image (see Fig. 6–17). Gd-DTPA–enhanced MRI evaluation of an eye suspected to contain uveal metastasis is particularly indicated in order to image the brain and detect intracranial metastasis (see Fig. 6–17).

UVEAL VASCULAR TUMORS

CIRCUMSCRIBED CHOROIDAL HEMANGIOMA

Clinical and Pathological Features

The circumscribed choroidal hemangioma is a benign vascular tumor of the choroid that is not associated with the facial nevus flammeus or other variants of the Sturge-Weber syndrome. On ophthalmoscopic examination, the tumor appears as a fairly well-defined, amelanotic, red-orange mass, mainly located posterior to the equator. The lesion can be almost indistinguishable from the normal choroid. Fibrous metaplasia of the overlying retinal pigment epithelium forms white deposits on the tumor surface. The retina over a circumscribed choroidal hemangioma often develops cystoid degeneration. However, localized or total secondary retinal detachment can occur.

Histopathologically, the circumscribed choroidal hemangioma may be classified as predominantly capillary, predominantly cavernous, or a mixed type. Overlying cystic changes of the retina, as well as fibrous or osseous metaplasia of the retinal pigment epithelium, may occur.

On fluorescein angiography, the rapid linear hyperfluorescence of the tumor during the prearterial or the early arterial phases is rather characteristic of choroidal hemangioma. On late frames, there is intraretinal hyperfluorescence secondary to leakage of the dye into the cystoid spaces within the retina. A-scan ultrasonography demonstrates high internal reflectivity with no choroidal excavation. On B-scan ultrasonography, the lesion appears as a dome-shaped choroidal mass with internal acoustic solidity.

MR Features

Although circumscribed choroidal hemangioma can demonstrate a signal of variable intensity on nonenhanced T1W images, it characteristically appears with a low signal intensity, and is isointense to slightly hyperintense with respect to the vitreous on nonenhanced T1W images (Figs. 6-18, A and D; 6-19, A and B; and 6-20A). On T2W images, choroidal hemangioma shows an increased signal, which is isointense to the hyperintense vitreous (Figs. 6-18B; 6-19C; and 6-20B). These MR features are helpful in differentiating choroidal hemangioma from choroidal melanoma or metastasis (see Tables 6-1 and 6-3).

On Gd-DTPA–enhanced T1W images, with or without fat suppression, circumscribed choroidal hemangioma shows marked enhancement (Figs. 6-18, C and D; 6-19, D and E; and 6-20C). This contrast enhancement improves detection of tumors that cannot be seen on nonenhanced T1W and T2W images because of their isointense signal relative to the vitreous. Gd-DTPA enhancement of the tumor increases the tumor's signal intensity above that of the associated secondary exudative retinal detachment, which does not enhance (Fig. 6-20C).

CHOROIDAL HEMANGIOPERICYTOMA

Clinical and Pathological Features

Intraocular hemangiopericytomas are very rare tumors. These tumors arise from the pericytes and are usually found in the peritoneum and lower extremities. In the eye, they appear as an amelanotic choroidal or ciliary body mass with overlying cystic retinal spaces. The malignant potential of hemangiopericytomas is variable and unpredictable. Histopathologic examination reveals a tumor composed of sinusoidal vascular channels separated by spindle-shaped cells. Immunochemical studies test positive for vimentin.

MR Features

Supraciliary hemangiopericytoma has been described as being markedly hyperintense compared to the vitreous on T1W images and hypointense on T2W images (Fig. 6-21, A and B). Although the MR signal characteristics of the tumor, when compared to those of the vitreous, can be suggestive of uveal melanoma (see Tables 6-1 and 6-2), the tumor appears slightly hyperintense with respect to white matter on T1W images and markedly hyperintense on T2W images. This MR pattern relative to the white matter is different from that described for uveal melanoma.

MISCELLANEOUS UVEAL TUMORS

CHOROIDAL OSTEOMA

Clinical and Pathological Features

Choroidal osteoma is a benign, ossifying tumor of the choroid that is typically found unilaterally (75%) in young, healthy females in the second or third decade of life. The tumor usually appears as a yellow-white-orange, oval or round, juxtapapillary lesion with characteristically well-defined scalloped or geographic margins.

Histopathologic examination reveals that choroidal osteoma is formed by mature bone with intertrabecular marrow spaces containing loose fibrovascular elements, mast cells, and foamy, vacuolated, mesenchymal cells with absence of hematopoietic tissues. Fluorescein angiography confirms the histopathologically documented vascularity of the choroidal osteoma. Ultrasonography and CT are most helpful in detecting a calcified, highly reflective plaque of bone density.

MR Features

Characteristically, cortical bone shows low signal intensity on T1W and T2W images. One would expect, then, that the bony plaque in the choroid would have a low signal intensity. However, the authors reported one case of choroidal osteoma that had a high signal intensity on T1W images and a low signal intensity on T2W images, simulating choroidal melanoma (see Tables 6–1 and 6–2, and Fig. 6–22, A through C). On Gd-DTPA–enhanced T1W images, the choroidal osteoma enhances markedly (Fig. 6–22D). The histopathologic features of choroidal osteoma with the presence of fatty marrow in the intertrabecular spaces explain these MR findings. Based on the authors' experience, contrast-enhanced MRI does not help in differentiating choroidal osteoma (with thicknesses > 1.8 mm) from choroidal melanoma. Three other cases of choroidal osteoma were imaged without detecting increased signal intensity at the level of the choroid suggestive of fatty marrow. These three lesions were less than 1.8 mm in thickness.

UVEAL LEIOMYOMA

Clinical and Pathological Features

Uveal leiomyoma is a rare benign tumor of smooth muscle origin which can arise in the iris, ciliary body, or choroid. In the ciliary body, the tumor has a predilection for a supraciliary location. The tumor may simulate amelanotic choroidal melanoma on the basis of clinical appearance and ancillary studies. Light and electron microscopy and immunohistochemistry usually confirm the diagnosis of leiomyoma when the tumor is obtained after either enucleation or tumor resection.

MR Features

Although one case report has described a choroidal leiomyoma with hyperintense signal on T1W and T2W images, the authors' experience with two histologically proven mesectodermal leiomyoma of the ciliary body did not confirm these findings. In these two cases, the ciliary body leiomyoma appeared hyperintense with respect to the vitreous on

nonenhanced T1W images and hypointense on T2W images (Figs. 6–23, A through C, and 6–24, A and B). On Gd-DTPA–enhanced T1W images with or without fat suppression technique, the tumor showed marked enhancement (Fig. 6–24, C and D). Based on the authors' experience, nonenhanced MRI does not help in differentiating uveal leiomyoma from uveal melanoma (see Tables 6–1 and 6–2).

BIBLIOGRAPHY

Bloom PA, Ferris JD, Laidlaw DAH, Goddard PR. Magnetic resonance imaging. Diverse appearances of uveal malignant melanomas. *Arch Ophthalmol.* 1992; 110:1105–1111.

Bond JB, Haik BG, Mihara F, Gupta KL. Magnetic resonance imaging of choroidal melanoma with and without gadolinium contrast enhancement. *Ophthalmology.* 1991; 98:459–466.

Brown HH, Brodsky MC, Hembree K, Mrak RE. Supraciliary hemangiopericytoma. *Ophthalmology.* 1991; 98: 378–382.

Chambers RB, Davidorf FH, McAdoo JF, Chakeres DW. Magnetic resonance imaging of uveal melanomas. *Arch Ophthalmol.* 1987; 105:917–921.

De Potter P, Flanders AE, Shields JA, Shields CL. Magnetic resonance imaging of intraocular tumors. *Int Ophthalmol Clin.* 1993; 33:37–45.

De Potter P, Flanders AE, Shields JA, Shields CL, Gonzales CF, Rao VM. The role of fat suppression technique and gadopentetate dimeglumine in magnetic resonance imaging evaluation of intraocular tumors and simulating lesions. *Arch Ophthalmol.* 1994; 112:340–348.

De Potter P, Gonzalez CF, Flanders AE, Shields JA, Shields CL. Imaging studies of intraocular tumors. In: Alberti WE, Sagerman RH, eds. *Radiotherapy of Intraocular and Orbital Tumors.* Berlin: Springer Verlag; 1993;295–309.

De Potter P, Shields JA, Shields CL. Computed tomography and magnetic resonance imaging of intraocular lesions. *Ophthalmol Clin North Am.* 1994; 7: 333–346.

De Potter P, Shields JA, Shields CL, Ras VM. Magnetic resonance imaging in choroidal osteoma. *Retina.* 1991; 11:221–223.

De Potter P, Shields JA, Shields CL, Santos R. Modified enucleation via lateral orbitotomy for choroidal melanoma with orbital extension: A report of two cases. *Ophthalmic Plast Reconstr Surg.* 1992; 8:109–113.

De Potter P, Shields JA, Shields CL, Yannuzzi LA, Fisher YE, Rao VM. Unusual MRI findings in metastatic carcinoma to the choroid and optic nerve: A case report. *Int Ophthalmol.* 1992; 16:39–44.

Gass JD, Guerry RK, Jack RL, Harris G. Choroidal osteoma. *Arch Ophthalmol.* 1978; 96:428–443.

Gomori JM, Grossman RI, Shields JA, Augsburger JJ, Joseph PM, DeSimeone D. Choroidal melanomas: Correlation of NMR spectroscopy and MR imaging. *Radiology.* 1986; 158:443–445.

Haik BG, Saint Louis L, Smith ME, Ellsworth RM, Deck M, Friedlander M. Magnetic resonance imaging in choroidal tumors. *Ann Ophthalmol.* 1987; 19:218–238.

Mafee MF. Magnetic resonance imaging: Ocular pathology. In: Newton TH, Bilaniuk LT, ed. *Radiology of the Eye and Orbit.* New York: Raven Press; 1990, Chap. 3.

Mafee MF, Peyman GA. Retinal and choroidal detachments: Role of magnetic resonance imaging and computed tomography. *Radiol Clin North Am.* 1987; 25:487–507.

Maffe MF, Peyman GA, Peace JH, Cohen SB, Mitchell MW. Magnetic resonance imaging in the evaluation and differentiation of uveal melanoma. *Ophthalmology.* 1987; 94:341–348.

Mihara F, Gupta KL, Murayama S, Lee N, Bond JB, Haik. MR imaging of uveal melanoma: Role of pulse sequence and contrast agent. *AJNR.* 1991; 12:991–996.

Peyman GA, Mafee MF. Uveal melanoma and simulating lesions: The role of magnetic resonance imaging and computed tomography. *Radiol Clin North Am.* 1987; 25:471–486.

Peyster RG, Augsburger JJ, Shields JA, Hershey BL, Eagle RC Jr, Haskin ME. Intraocular tumors: Evaluation with MR imaging. *Radiology.* 1988; 168:773–779.

Seddon JM, Albert DM, Lavin PT, Robinson N. A prognostic factor study of disease-free interval and survival following enucleation for uveal melanoma. *Arch Ophthalmol.* 1983; 101:1894–1899.

Shields CL, Shields JA, Augsburger JJ. Choroidal osteoma. *Surv Ophthalmol.* 1988; 33:17–27.

Shields CL, Shields JA, Varenhorst M. Transscleral leiomyoma. *Ophthalmology.* 1991; 98:84–87.

Shields JA. Melanocytoma of the optic nerve head. A review. *Int Ophthalmol.* 1978; 1:31–37.

Shields JA, Shakin EP, Shields CL. Metastatic malignant tumors. In: Gold DH, Weingiest TA. *The Eye in Systemic Diseases.* Philadelphia: JB Lippincott; 1990: 299–303.

Shields JA, Shields CL. Diagnostic approaches to posterior uveal melanoma. In: Shields JA, Shields CL, eds. *Intraocular Tumors. A Textbook and Atlas.* Philadelphia: WB Saunders; 1992:155–169.

Shields JA, Shields CL, Donoso LA. Management of posterior uveal melanoma. *Surv Ophthalmol.* 1991; 36: 161–195.

Shields JA, Shields CL, Eagle RC. Mesectodermal leiomyoma of the ciliary body managed by partial lamellar iridocyclochoroidectomy. *Ophthalmology.* 1989; 96:1369–1376.

Zimmerman LE. Malignant melanoma of the uveal tract. In: Spencer WH, Font RL, Green WR, Howes EL, Jacobiec FA, Zimmerman LE, eds. *Ophthalmic Pathology. An Atlas and Textbook.* Vol. 3. 3rd ed. Philadelphia: WB Saunders; 1986:2072–2139.

FIGURE 6-1 *Choroidal Nevus*
A choroidal nevus with a thickness of 1.8 mm is located at the posterior pole of the left eye.

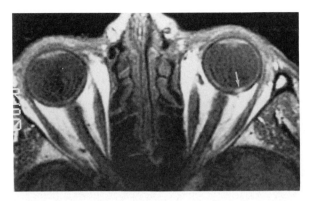

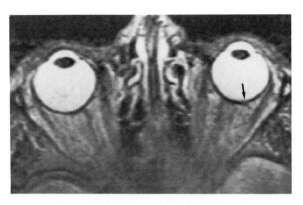

6-1A Axial T1W image. The choroidal nevus (*arrow*) shows a hyperintense signal with respect to the vitreous. No subretinal fluid is seen.

6-1B Axial T2W image. The choroidal nevus (*arrow*) appears hypointense with respect to the vitreous.

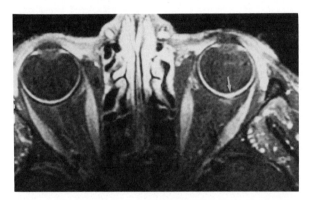

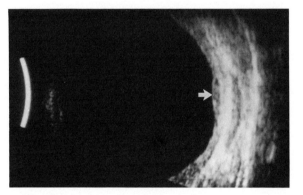

6-1C Fat-suppressed axial Gd-DTPA–enhanced T1W image. The lesion (*arrow*), as well as the uvea is seen to enhance.

6-1D B-scan ultrasonography. The lesion shows medium internal reflectivity (*arrow*). Subretinal fluid is not documented.

FIGURE 6–2 *Pigmented Choroidal Melanoma*
A dome-shaped choroidal melanoma with a thickness of 4.0 mm lies adjacent to the optic disk in the right eye.

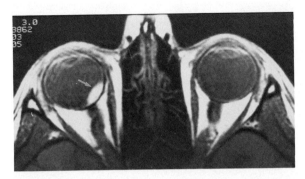 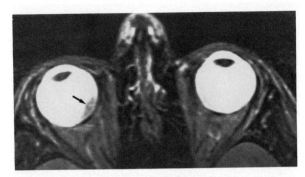

6–2A Axial T1W image. The choroidal melanoma shows a homogeneous hyperintense signal with respect to the vitreous (*arrow*).

6–2B Axial T2W image. The tumor shows a homogeneous hypointense signal with respect to the vitreous (*arrow*).

FIGURE 6-3 *Pigmented Choroidal Melanoma*
A mushroom-shaped choroidal melanoma with a thickness of 6.1 mm is located at the posterior pole of the right eye.

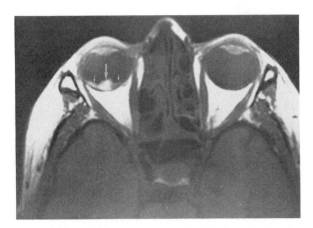

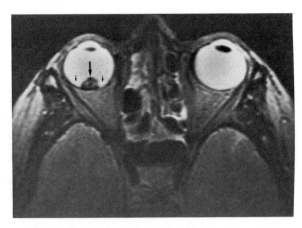

6-3A Axial T1W image. The choroidal melanoma demonstrates a heterogeneous hyperintense signal with respect to the vitreous (*long arrow*). A surrounding serous retinal detachment appears less hyperintense than the tumor (*short arrows*).

6-3B Axial T2W image. The tumor shows a heterogeneous hypointense signal (*long arrow*) compared with the high signal intensity of the vitreous and the surrounding subretinal fluid (*short arrows*). The heterogeneous signal within the tumor may be related to tumor necrosis.

FIGURE 6–4 *Pigmented Ciliochoroidal Melanoma*
A dome-shaped ciliochoroidal melanoma of the left eye measuring 7.1 mm in thickness.

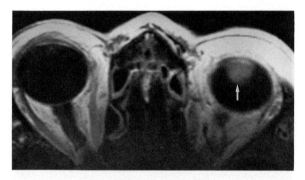

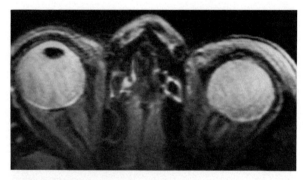

6–4A Axial T1W image. Despite its high melanin content, the tumor shows a minimally hyperintense signal with respect to the vitreous (*arrow*).

6–4B Axial T2W image. The tumor appears isointense with respect to the vitreous.

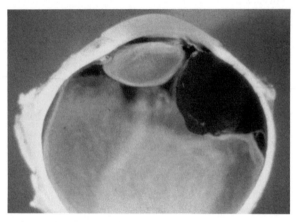

6–4C Photograph of the sectioned eye showing the pigmented ciliochoroidal melanoma.

FIGURE 6-5 *Partially Pigmented Ciliochoroidal Melanoma*
A mushroom-shaped ciliochoroidal melanoma of the left eye measuring 11.5 mm in thickness.

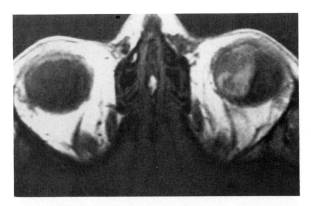

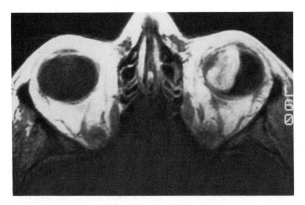

6–5A Axial T1W image. The large, mushroom-shaped ciliochoroidal tumor demonstrates a heterogeneous high signal intensity. The amelanotic base of the tumor is less hyperintense than the pigmented elevated portion (compare the histopathologic appearance of the lesion in Figure 6–5C).

6–5B Axial Gd-DTPA–enhanced T1W image. The tumor shows heterogeneous enhancement.

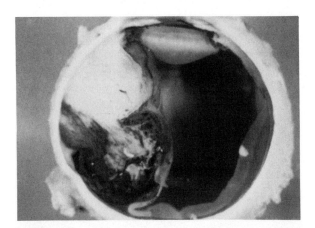

6–5C Photograph of the sectioned eye showing the intrinsic pigmentation of the tumor and the break through Bruch's membrane that produces the mushroom-shaped configuration.

FIGURE 6-6 *Amelanotic Choroidal Melanoma*

An amelanotic, dome-shaped, choroidal melanoma, measuring 7.1 mm in thickness and associated with a secondary retinal detachment, is located at the posterior pole of the right eye.

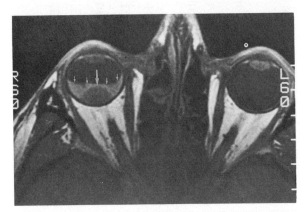

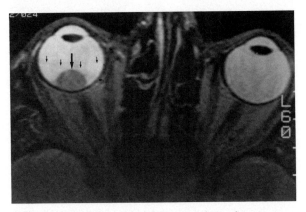

6-6A Axial T1W image. Despite its amelanotic appearance, the tumor shows a hyperintense signal (*long arrow*) with respect to the vitreous but a hypointense signal with respect to the surrounding subretinal fluid (*short arrows*). (From Orbit. In: Rao VM, Flanders AE, Tom BM, eds. *MRI and CT Atlas of Correlative Imaging in Otolaryngology.* London: Martin Dunitz; 1992: 357.)

6-6B Axial T2W image. The tumor has a hypointense signal (*long arrow*) with respect to the high signal intensity of the vitreous and the secondary retinal detachment (*short arrows*). (From Orbit. In: Rao VM, Flanders AE, Tom BM, eds. *MRI and CT Atlas of Correlative Imaging in Otolaryngology.* London: Martin Dunitz; 1992: 357.)

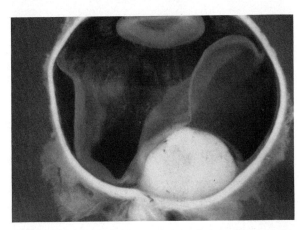

6-6C Photograph of the sectioned eye showing the amelanotic choroidal melanoma with the surrounding detached retina.

FIGURE 6-7 *Pigmented Ciliochoroidal Melanoma*
A pigmented dome-shaped ciliochoroidal melanoma of the right eye measuring 4.5 mm in thickness.

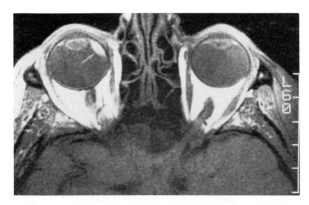

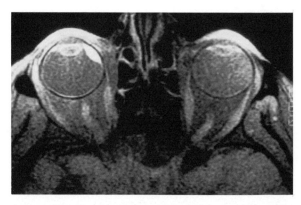

6-7A Axial T1W image. The tumor has a hyperintense signal with respect to the vitreous (*arrow*). No serous retinal detachment is detected. (From De Potter P, Flanders AE, Shields JA, Shields CL, Gonzalez CF, Rao VM. The role of fat suppression technique and gadolinium-DTPA in the evaluation of intraocular tumors and simulating lesions. *Arch Ophthalmol.* 1994; 112: 340–348. Copyright 1994, American Medical Association.)

6-7B Fat-suppressed axial T1W image. The signal intensity of the tumor appears more pronounced than that obtained without fat suppression. (From De Potter P, Flanders AE, Shields JA, Shields CL, Gonzalez CF, Rao VM. The role of fat suppression technique and gadolinium-DTPA in the evaluation of intraocular tumors and simulating lesions. *Arch Ophthalmol.* 1994; 112: 340–348. Copyright 1994, American Medical Association.)

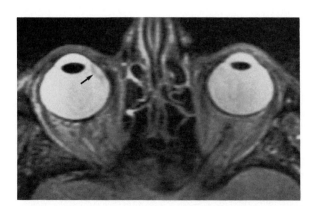

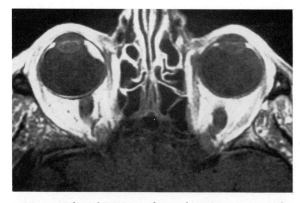

6-7C Axial T2W image. The tumor is hypointense with respect to the vitreous (*arrow*).

6-7D Axial Gd-DTPA–enhanced T1W image. The tumor demonstrates moderate enhancement. (From De Potter P, Flanders AE, Shields JA, Shields CL, Gonzalez CF, Rao VM. The role of fat suppression technique and gadolinium-DTPA in the evaluation of intraocular tumors and simulating lesions. *Arch Ophthalmol.* 1994; 112: 340–348. Copyright 1994, American Medical Association.)

(continued)

FIGURE 6–7 *Pigmented Ciliochoroidal Melanoma* (continued)

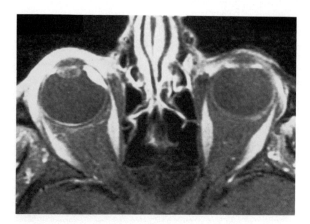

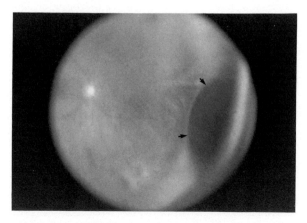

6–7E Fat-suppressed axial Gd-DTPA–enhanced T1W image. The signal intensity of the tumor enhancement is more marked than that obtained without fat suppression. (From De Potter P, Flanders AE, Shields JA, Shields CL, Gonzalez CF, Rao VM. The role of fat suppression technique and gadolinium-DTPA in the evaluation of intraocular tumors and simulating lesions. *Arch Ophthalmol.* 1994; 112:340–348. Copyright 1994, American Medical Association.)

6–7F Wide-angle fundus photograph showing the pigmented ciliochoroidal melanoma (*arrows*).

FIGURE 6-8 *Pigmented Choroidal Melanoma*
A pigmented, mushroom-shaped, juxtapapillary choroidal melanoma measuring 8.3 mm in thickness. (All figures from De Potter P, Gonzalez CF, Flanders AE, Shields JA, Shields CL. Imaging studies of intraocular tumors. In: Alberti WE, Sagerman RH, eds. *Radiotherapy of Intraocular and Orbital Tumors*. Berlin: Springer-Verlag; 1993: Chap. 38, 295–309.)

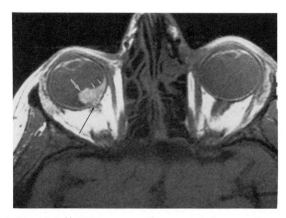

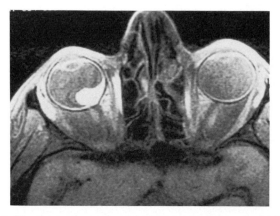

6-8A Axial T1W image. The tumor shows a hyperintense signal with respect to the vitreous (*long white arrow*). The associated surrounding retinal detachment (*short arrows*) presents with a slightly lower signal intensity than that of the tumor. Note that the tumor overhangs the optic disk with prelaminar invasion of the optic nerve (*long black arrow*).

6-8B Fat-suppressed axial T1W image. Note the high signal intensity of the tumor and the subretinal fluid, which is more pronounced than that obtained without fat suppression.

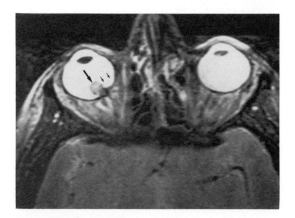

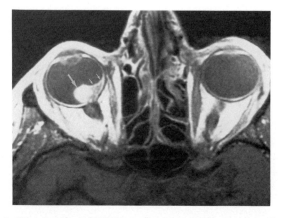

6-8C Axial T2W image. The tumor is hypointense (*long arrow*) with respect to the vitreous and the serous retinal detachment (*short arrows*).

6-8D Axial Gd-DTPA–enhanced T1W image. The tumor demonstrates moderate enhancement (*long arrow*). The secondary retinal detachment does not show enhancement (*short arrows*).

(continued)

FIGURE 6-8 *Pigmented Choroidal Melanoma* (continued)

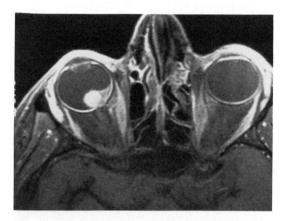

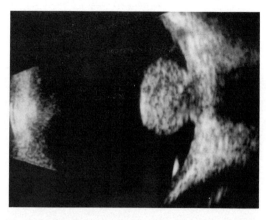

6-8E Fat-suppressed axial Gd-DTPA–enhanced T1W image. Note the improved contrast between the tumor and the subretinal fluid.

6-8F B-mode ultrasonography. The tumor overhanging the optic disk demonstrates a mushroom shape and medium internal reflectivity.

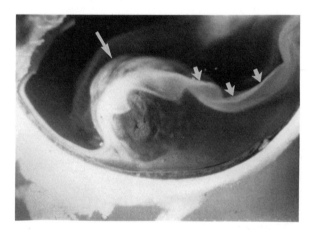

6-8G Photograph of the sectioned eye showing the mushroom-shaped, pigmented tumor (*long arrow*) and the secondary retinal detachment (*short arrows*), located nasally to the tumor.

FIGURE 6–9 *Pigmented Choroidal Melanoma*

Pigmented, dome-shaped, juxtapapillary choroidal melanoma in the left eye measuring 12 mm in thickness and associated with a secondary retinal detachment.

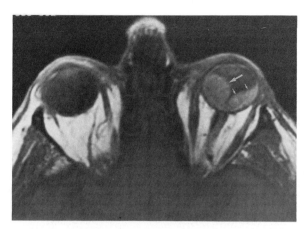 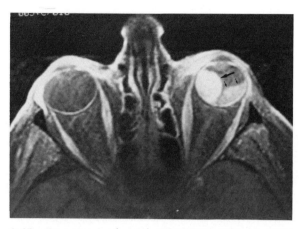

6–9A Axial T1W image. The dome-shaped tumor in the nasal portion of the eye has a hyperintense signal (*long arrow*) with respect to the vitreous but is isointense with respect to the temporal secondary retinal detachment (*short arrows*).

6–9B Fat-suppressed axial Gd-DTPA–enhanced T1W image. The tumor demonstrates moderate enhancement (*long arrow*). The secondary retinal detachment does not show enhancement (*short arrows*).

FIGURE 6–10 *Choroidal Melanoma with Extraocular Extension*

Ciliochoroidal melanoma of the left eye that was previously treated with plaque radiotherapy. There is minimally elevated tumor recurrence (1.5 mm in thickness) at the posterior margins and massive extraocular extension.

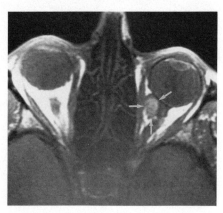

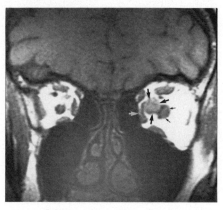

6–10A Axial T1W image. The intraocular tumor recurrence that is documented on ultrasonography is not demonstrated. The MR scans allow delineation of the hyperintense signal of the extraocular extension (*arrows*) with respect to that of the vitreous and optic nerve. The orbital mass displaces the optic nerve temporally without invading it.

6–10B Coronal T1W image. The orbital extension (*large black arrows*) has an intraconal location but does not invade the medial rectus muscle (*white arrow*) or optic nerve (*small black arrows*).

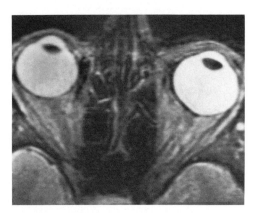

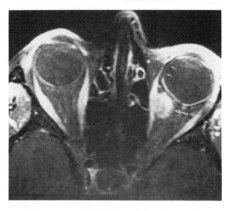

6–10C Axial T2–W image. The orbital extension has a decreased signal intensity, which is isointense with respect to orbital fat, owing to its melanin content (see Fig. 6–10G); it is, therefore, no longer seen in this plane.

6–10D Fat-suppressed axial Gd-DTPA–enhanced T1W image. The orbital extension demonstrates marked enhancement (*long arrow*). Note the lack of enhancement of the ciliochoroidal layer nasally (*short arrows*), which is attributable to ischemia from the previous plaque radiotherapy. The intraocular tumor recurrence is not demonstrated.

(continued)

FIGURE 6-10 *Choroidal Melanoma with Extraocular Extension* (continued)

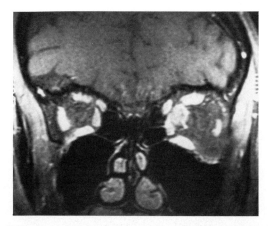

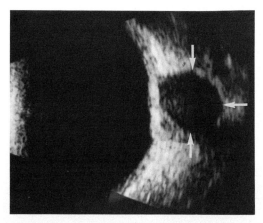

6-10E Fat-suppressed coronal Gd-DTPA-enhanced T1W image. The enhancement of the orbital tumor is heterogeneous.

6-10F B-scan ultrasonography. The intraocular tumor recurrence appears as a solid thickening of the choroid. The well-circumscribed, echolucent, orbital extension (*arrows*) is adjacent to the sclera and the optic nerve.

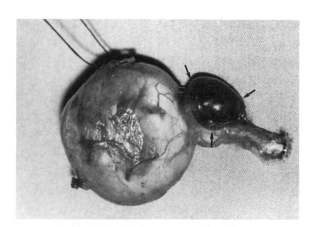

6-10G Photograph of the enucleated eye showing the deeply pigmented, well-encapsulated nodule of extraocular extension (*arrows*) adjacent to the optic nerve.

FIGURE 6–11 *Choroidal Melanoma after Plaque Radiotherapy*
An irradiated choroidal melanoma with suspected intraocular recurrence and extraocular extension in the right eye. Orbital exploration and biopsy demonstrate fibrous scar tissue.

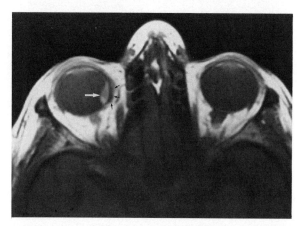

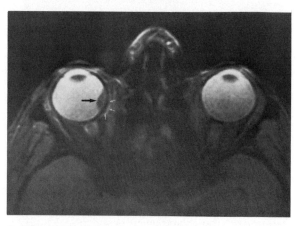

6–11A Axial T1W image. The irradiated choroidal melanoma (*long arrow*) is hyperintense with respect to the vitreous. An area of low signal intensity (*short arrows*), which suggests extraocular extension is adjacent to the sclera.

6–11B Axial gradient echo image. Both intraocular and extraocular lesions appear to have a low signal isointensity with respect to the orbital fat.

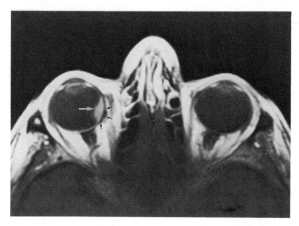

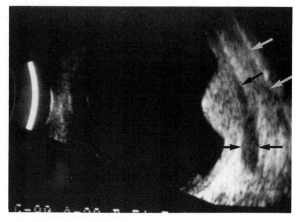

6–11C Axial Gd-DTPA–enhanced T1W image. The irradiated tumor (*long arrow*) demonstrates minimal enhancement. The orbital lesion does not enhance, which suggests fibrous scar tissue (*short arrows*). A biopsy of the orbital lesion confirmed the MR findings.

6–11D B-scan ultrasonography. The irradiated choroidal tumor shows acoustic solidity. The crescent-shaped orbital lesion demonstrates acoustic hollowness (*black arrows*) simulating extraocular extension and is located between the sclera and the medial rectus muscle (*white arrows*).

FIGURE 6-12 *Melanocytoma of the Optic Disk*

A melanocytoma with a thickness of 3.0 mm completely overhangs the optic disk.

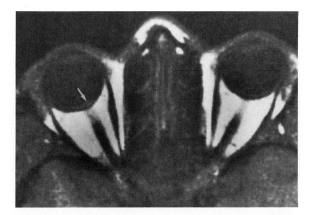

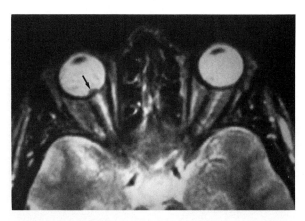

6-12A Axial T1W image. The tumor is hyperintense (*arrow*) with respect to the vitreous.

6-12B Axial T2W image. The tumor becomes hypointense (*arrow*) with respect to the vitreous.

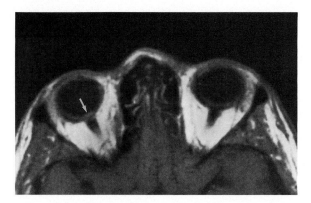

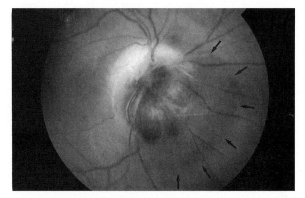

6-12C Axial Gd-DTPA–enhanced T1W image. The tumor (*arrow*) demonstrates minimal enhancement.

6-12D Fundus photograph showing the pigmented melanocytoma overhanging the optic disk and surrounded by a flat, nevoid, choroidal base (*arrows*).

FIGURE 6–13 *Choroidal Metastasis from Breast Carcinoma*
Metastatic breast carcinoma involving the choroid and located temporal to the fovea in the left eye. The lesion has a thickness of 2.5 mm.

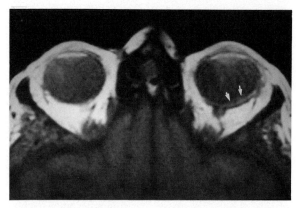

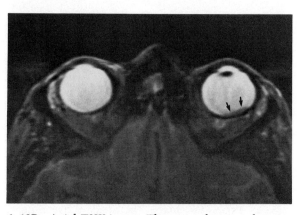

6–13A Axial T1W image. The metastatic lesion appears to be slightly hyperintense (*arrows*) with respect to the vitreous.

6–13B Axial T2W image. The tumor becomes hypointense (*arrows*) with respect to the vitreous.

FIGURE 6-14 *Choroidal and Optic Nerve Metastasis from Lung Carcinoma*
Diffuse metastatic infiltration of the choroid and optic nerve in the left eye occurred in a patient with no history of primary tumor. A systemic work-up revealed a right pleural effusion that suggested a pulmonary primary site.

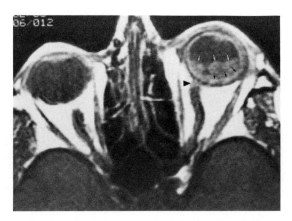

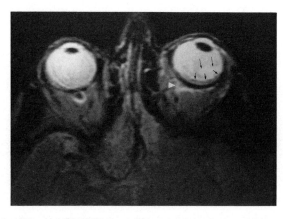

6-14A   Axial T1W image. The diffusely infiltrated choroid is hyperintense (*black arrows*) with respect to the vitreous. The secondary exudative total retinal detachment (*white arrows*) appears less hyperintense than the tumor. The retrolaminar portion of the optic nerve shows a hyperintense signal (*arrowhead*), which is suggestive of tumor infiltration of the optic nerve. (From De Potter P, Shields JA, Shields CL, Yannuzzi LA, Fisher YE, Rao VM. Unusual MRI findings in metastatic carcinoma to the choroid and optic nerve: A case report. *Int Ophthalmol.* 1992; 16:39–44. © 1992 by Kluwer Academic Publishers.)

6-14B   Axial T2W image. The metastatic lesion is hypointense (*short black arrows*) with respect to the vitreous and the subretinal fluid (*long black arrows*), which appears more hyperintense than does the vitreous. Optic nerve invasion is also evident (*arrowhead*).

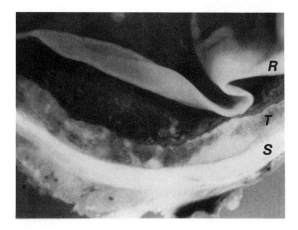

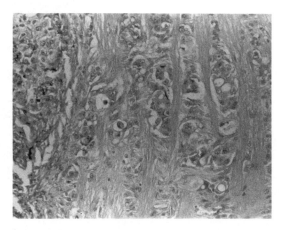

6-14C   Photograph of the sectioned eye showing the diffuse thickening of the choroid by a variably pigmented tumor. The sensory retina is detached. (*R*, retina; *S*, sclera; *T*, tumor)

6-14D   Photomicrograph showing infiltration of the lamina cribrosa by mucin-secreting adenocarcinoma cells. (Hematoxylin-eosin, ×225). (From De Potter P, Shields JA, Shields CL, Yannuzzi LA, Fisher YE, Rao VM. Unusual MRI findings in metastatic carcinoma to the choroid and optic nerve: A case report. *Int Ophthalmol.* 1992; 16:39–44. © 1992 by Kluwer Academic Publishers.)

FIGURE 6-15 *Choroidal Metastasis from Breast Carcinoma*
Metastatic breast carcinoma, located nasally to the optic disk, involving the right eye and associated with secondary retinal detachment.

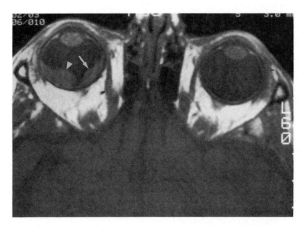

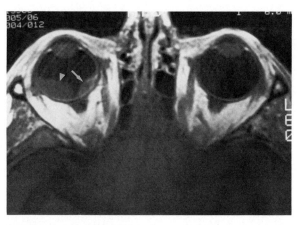

6-15A Axial T1W image. The tumor (*arrow*) is slightly hyperintense with respect to the vitreous. The associated retinal detachment (*arrowhead*) is isointense with respect to the tumor.

6-15B Axial Gd-DTPA–enhanced T1W image. The choroidal metastasis (*arrow*) demonstrates minimal enhancement. The secondary retinal detachment does not enhance (*arrowhead*).

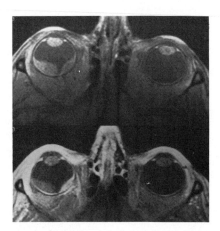

6-15C Fat-suppressed axial T1W image before [*top*] and after [*bottom*] Gd-DTPA administration. There is improved contrast between the tumor and the vitreous.

FIGURE 6–16 *Carcinoid Metastasis to the Choroid*
Bronchial carcinoid metastasis to the right eye without secondary serous subretinal fluid.

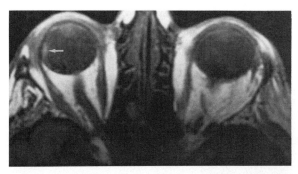

6–16A Axial T1W image. The tumor shows increased signal intensity (*arrow*) with respect to the vitreous.

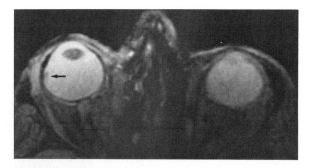

6–16B Axial gradient echo image. The tumor becomes hypointense (*arrow*).

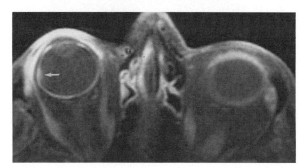

6–16C Fat-suppressed axial Gd-DTPA–enhanced T1W image. The tumor demonstrates minimal enhancement (*arrow*).

FIGURE 6–17 *Bilateral Choroidal Metastasis and Multiple Brain Metastases from Breast Carcinoma*

Fat-suppressed axial Gd-DTPA–enhanced T1W image. The infiltration of the optic disk and the nasal choroid in the right eye (*arrows*) are easily identified and show enhancement. In the left eye, the enhancing metastatic infiltrate is seen, along with the non-enhancing secondary subretinal fluid at the posterior pole (*arrowhead*). Note the multiple brain metastases that are enhanced and become visible after Gd-DTpA administration of a contrast agent.

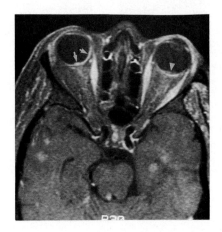

FIGURE 6–18 *Circumscribed Choroidal Hemangioma*
Circumscribed choroidal hemangioma at the posterior pole of the right eye measuring 3.0 mm in thickness.

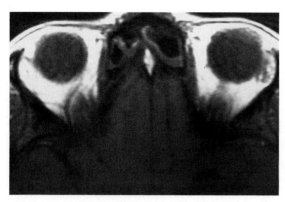

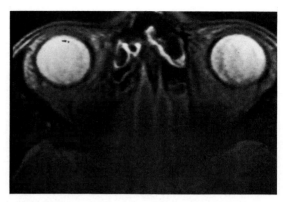

6–18A Axial T1W image. The tumor, isotense to the vitreous, is not visible.

6–18B Axial gradient echo image. The tumor is iso-intense with respect to the high signal intensity of the vitreous, and is not distinguishable.

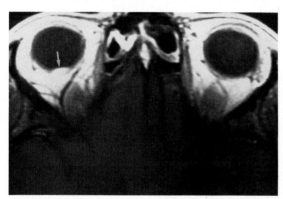

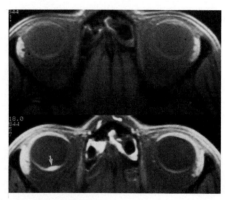

6–18C Axial Gd-DTPA–enhanced T1W image. The tumor demonstrates marked homogeneous enhancement (*arrow*).

6–18D Fat-suppressed axial T1W image before [*top*] and after [*bottom*] Gd-DTPA administration. The tumor is barely perceptible on the precontrast image. Administration of Gd-DTPA is necessary for visualization of the tumor (*arrow*).

FIGURE 6-19 *Circumscribed Choroidal Hemangioma*
Juxtapapillary, circumscribed, choroidal hemangioma of the right eye measuring 4.1 mm in thickness.

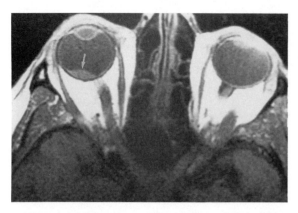

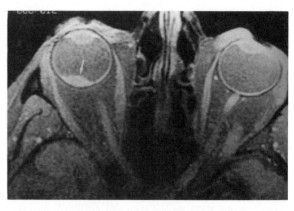

6-19A Axial T1W image. The tumor is slightly hyperintense (*arrow*) with respect to the vitreous. Note the artifact produced in the left eye by the cosmetics on the eyelid.

6-19B Fat-suppressed axial T1W image. The tumor (*arrow*) appears slightly more hyperintense than in Figure 6-19A. From Orbit. In: Rao VM, Flanders AE, Tom BM, eds. *MRI and CT Atlas of Correlative Imaging in Otolaryngology.* London: Martin Dunitz; 1992: 355.)

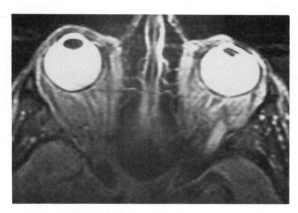

6-19C Axial T2W image. The hyperintense tumor is undiscernible from the hyperintense vitreous. From Orbit. In: Rao VM, Flanders AE, Tom BM, eds. *MRI and CT Atlas of Correlative Imaging in Otolaryngology.* London: Martin Dunitz; 1992: 355.)

(continued)

FIGURE 6-19 *Circumscribed Choroidal Hemangioma* (continued)

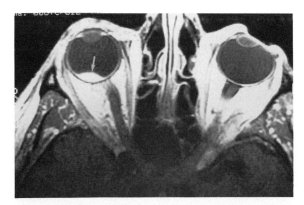

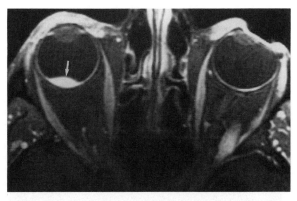

6-19D Axial Gd-DTPA–enhanced T1W image. The tumor demonstrates marked homogeneous enhancement (*arrow*). From Orbit. In: Rao VM, Flanders AE, Tom BM, eds. *MRI and CT Atlas of Correlative Imaging in Otolaryngology*. London: Martin Dunitz; 1992: 355.)

6-19E Fat-suppressed axial Gd-DTPA–enhanced T1W image. There is improved contrast between the tumor and the vitreous. From Orbit. In: Rao VM, Flanders AE, Tom BM, eds. *MRI and CT Atlas of Correlative Imaging in Otolaryngology*. London: Martin Dunitz; 1992: 355.)

FIGURE 6-20 *Circumscribed Choroidal Hemangioma*
A circumscribed choroidal hemangioma, located temporal to the fovea in the left eye, has a thickness of 4.5 mm. The tumor produced an exudative retinal detachment reaching the macula area, which explained the visual symptoms of the patient. (All figures from De Potter P, Flanders AE, Shields JA, Shields CL. Magnetic resonance imaging of intraocular tumors. *Int Ophthalmol Clin.* 1993; 33:37–45. © 1993, Little, Brown and Company.)

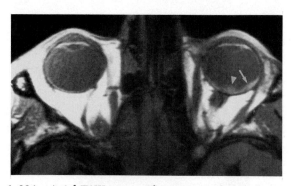 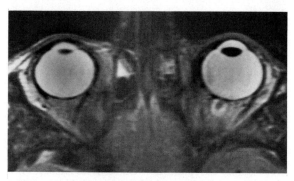

6-20A Axial T1W image. The tumor is slightly hyperintense with respect to the vitreous (*arrow*). The associated exudative retinal detachment (*arrowhead*) appears isointense to the tumor.

6-20B Axial T2-weighted image. The tumor and subretinal fluid are isointense to the vitreous.

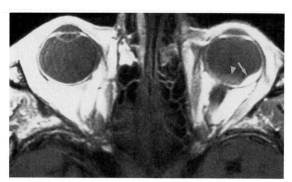

6-20C Axial Gd-DTPA enhanced T1W image. The tumor demonstrates marked homogeneous enhancement (*arrow*). The subretinal fluid does not enhance (*arrowhead*).

FIGURE 6-21 *Supraciliary Hemangiopericytoma*

A 10-year-old girl presented with a large, dome-shaped, ciliary mass measuring 9 mm in thickness and displacing the contiguous ciliary body and choroid internally. Histopathologic examination revealed a well-vascularized spindle cell proliferation with a sinusoidal pattern characteristic of hemangiopericytoma. (From Brown HH, Brodsky MC, Hembree K, Mrak RE. Supraciliary hemangiopericytoma. *Ophthalmology.* 1991; 98:379. © 1991 by the American Academy of Ophthalmology.)

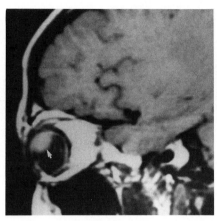

6-21A Parasagittal T1W image. The dome-shaped ciliary tumor (*arrow*) is hyperintense with respect to the vitreous.

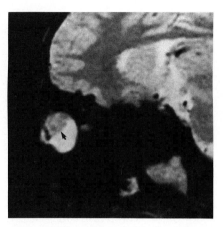

6-21B Parasagittal T2W image. The tumor (*arrow*) shows decreased signal intensity relative to the vitreous. These MR features with respect to the vitreous are identical to those of uveal melanoma.

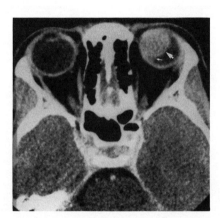

6-21C Axial contrast-enhanced CT image. The tumor (*large arrow*) appears to be homogeneously dense, whereas the associated retinal detachment, which is seen in the nasal area (*small arrow*), is less dense.

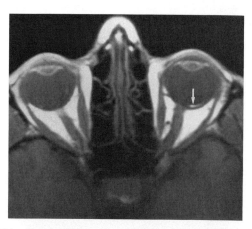

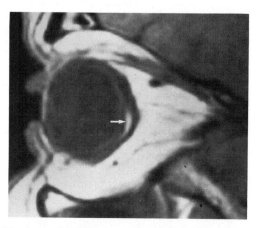

6-22A Axial T1W image. In the left eye, the high signal intensity at the level of the choroid temporal to the optic disk corresponds to the presence of fatty marrow in the intertrabecular spaces of the bony lesion (*arrow*). The tumor in the right eye is too thin to be detected. (From De Potter P, et al. Magnetic resonance imaging in choroidal osteoma. *Retina.* 1991; 11: 222. © 1991 by JB Lippincott Company.)

6-22B Sagittal T1W image. The high signal intensity of the choroidal osteoma (*arrow*) in the left eye is well visualized at the level of the choroid.

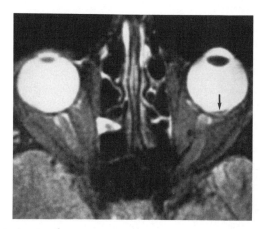

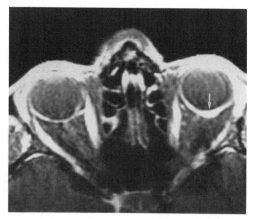

6-22C Axial T2W image. The tumor becomes hypointense (*arrow*) with respect to the vitreous because of the presence of fatty marrow. (From De Potter P, et al. Magnetic resonance imaging in choroidal osteoma. *Retina.* 1991; 11: 222. © 1991 by JB Lippincott Company.)

6-22D Fat-suppressed axial Gd-DTPA–enhanced T1W image. The tumor enhances markedly and homogeneously (*arrow*). (From De Potter P, et al. Magnetic resonance imaging in choroidal osteoma. *Retina.* 1991; 11: 222. © 1991 by JB Lippincott Company.)

(continued)

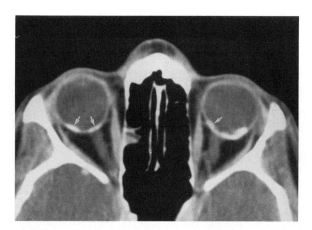

6–22E   Axial contrast-enhanced CT image. Bilateral choroidal osteomas are detected, but the lesion in the right eye, as well as the nasal portion of the lesion in the left eye (*arrows*) is too thin to be detected by MR studies.

FIGURE 6–23 *Leiomyoma of the Ciliary Body*

Ciliochoroidal tumor measuring 9.7 mm thick in the left eye of an 11-year-old girl. The tumor, which was removed by partial lamellar iridocyclochoroidectomy, proved to be a mesectodermal leiomyoma of the ciliary body. (From Shields JA, Shields CL, Eagle RC. Mesectodermal leiomyoma of the ciliary body managed by partial lamellar iridocyclochoroidectomy. *Ophthalmology.* 1989; 96: 1370–1372. © 1989 by the American Academy of Ophthalmology.)

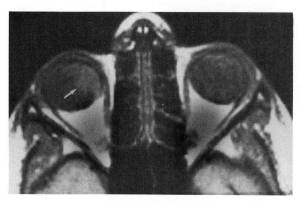

6–23A Axial T1W image. The tumor involving the ciliary body (*arrow*) is hyperintense with respect to the vitreous.

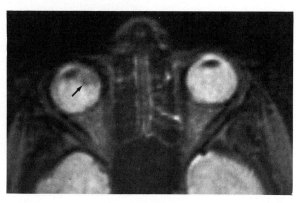

6–23B Axial T2W image. The tumor becomes hypointense (*arrow*) in relation to the high signal intensity of the vitreous.

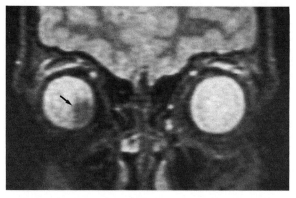

6–23C Coronal T2W image. In this plane, the inferonasal location of the tumor (*arrow*) is well appreciated.

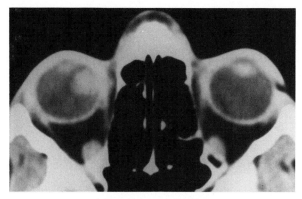

6–23D Axial contrast-enhanced CT image. The tumor involving the ciliary body appears to be hyperdense.

FIGURE 6–23 *Leiomyoma of the Ciliary Body* (continued)

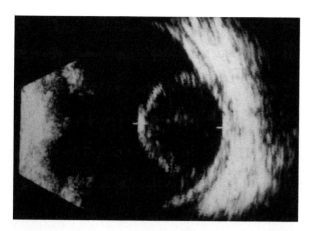

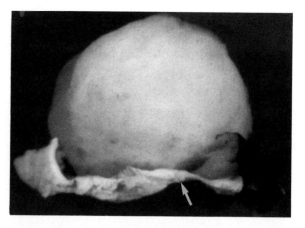

6–23E B-scan ultrasonography. The tumor has a dome-shaped and acoustically hollow configuration, simulating uveal melanoma.

6–23F Photograph of gross specimen showing the dome-shaped, amelanotic mass. Note the scleral tissue (*arrow*).

FIGURE 6-24 *Leiomyoma of the Ciliary Body and Choroid*
Ciliochoroidal leiomyoma measuring 9.3 mm thick in the left eye of a 24-year-old man.

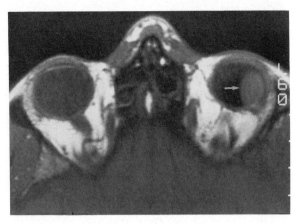

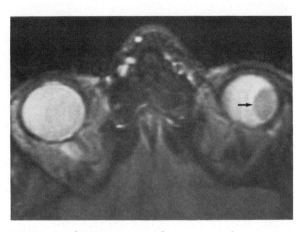

6-24A Axial T1W image. The tumor is hyperintense (*arrow*) with respect to the vitreous.

6-24B Axial T2W image. The tumor is hypointense (*arrow*) with respect to the vitreous.

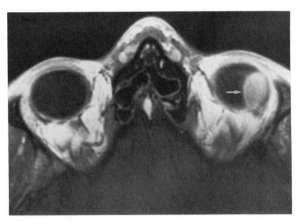

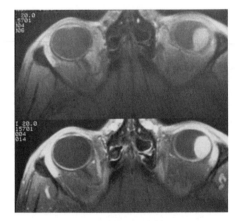

6-24C Axial Gd-DTPA–enhanced T1W image. The tumor demonstrates moderate to marked and non-homogeneous enhancement (*arrow*).

6-24D Fat-suppressed axial T1W image before [*top*] and after [*bottom*] Gd-DTPA administration. The signal intensity of the tumor is somewhat higher than that observed without fat suppression, and the enhancement of the tumor is more homogeneous and more pronounced.

MRI of the Eye and Orbit,
by Patrick De Potter, Jerry A. Shields, and Carol L. Shields.
J. B. Lippincott Company, Philadelphia © 1995.

7

Tumors and Pseudotumors of the Retina

PATRICK DE POTTER

JERRY A. SHIELDS

CAROL L. SHIELDS

RETINOBLASTOMA

Clinical and Pathological Features

Retinoblastoma is the most common intraocular malignant disease in children. The incidence of retinoblastoma is estimated to range from 1 in 15,000 to 1 in 20,000 live births. The tumor occurs bilaterally in 25% to 35% of cases. Approximately 6% of newly diagnosed cases of retinoblastoma are familial and 94% are sporadic.

The most common clinical manifestations of retinoblastoma include leukokoria and strabismus. In some cases, the initial presentation is spontaneous hyphema, pseudohypopyon, or preseptal cellulitis. On ophthalmoscopic examination, retinoblastoma can appear as a white retinal lesion in the early stage with foci of chalklike calcification. In more advanced stages, the tumor may assume either an endophytic or an exophytic pattern. In the endophytic pattern, retinoblastoma grows from the retina into the vitreous cavity with vitreous seeds and, therefore, simulates endophthalmitis. In the exophytic pattern, the tumor grows into the subretinal space, producing a secondary retinal detachment and simulating Coats' disease. The diffuse infiltrative pattern is uncommon and is characterized by a relatively flat infiltration of the retina by tumor cells, with no obvious mass.

Cytologic examination reveals that retinoblastoma can be composed of poorly differentiated to well-differentiated tumor cells. In the well-differentiated type, retinoblastoma is characterized by the presence of rosettes and fleurettes. The most important prognostic factors are optic nerve invasion, choroidal invasion, and orbital extension.

Indirect ophthalmoscopy is unquestionably the most useful tool in the diagnostic approach to retinoblastoma. On ocular A- and B-scan ultrasonography, calcification is visualized as dense echoes that remain after reducing the sensitivity. Sound attenuation is an echographic criterion that is highly suggestive of calcified retinoblastoma. Calcification has been found in more than 90% of retinoblastomas evaluated with A- and B-scan ultrasonography. If calcification is not seen on ultrasonographic examination, then computed tomography (CT) may be helpful. High-resolution, thin-section CT scanning can detect calcification within retinoblastomas with an accuracy rate of 87%. The detection of intraocular calcification in an eye with leukokoria and/or total retinal detachment in children younger than 3 years of age is virtually diagnostic of retinoblastoma until proven otherwise. CT is also a very valuable diagnostic aid to detect orbital or optic nerve invasion, as well as pinealoblastoma. However, subtle retrolaminar optic nerve invasion cannot be reliably predicted by CT.

MR Features

Magnetic resonance imaging (MRI), although less specific than CT for the detection of calcification, has proven to be useful in the differentiation of retinoblastoma from simulating lesions (Tables 7–1 and 7–3), endophytic and exophytic. Retinoblastoma demonstrates moderate hyperintensity with respect to the vitreous on T1-weighted (T1W) images and hypointensity on T2-weighted (T2W) images (Figs. 7–1, *A* through *F*; 7–2, *A* and *B*; and 7–3, *A* and *B*). Small foci of calcification visualized with ultrasonography and CT may be missed on MRI. Larger areas of tumor calcification appear markedly hypointense on both T1W and T2W images, causing heterogeneity in tumor signal (Fig. 7–1, *B* and *F*). Undifferentiated retinoblastoma may appear less hyperintense than differentiated retinoblastoma on T1W images.

After administration of gadolinium diethylene-triamine penta-acetic acid (Gd-DTPA), the tumor shows moderate to marked heterogeneous enhancement, depending on the extent of tumor necrosis (Figs. 7–1, *G* and *H*; 7–2, *C* through *E*; 7–3, *A* and *C*; and 7–4). Calcification remains markedly hypointense on Gd-DTPA–enhanced T1W images (Fig. 7–1*H*). When a secondary retinal detachment is present, the subretinal fluid remains hyperintense on T1W and T2W images and does not enhance after administration of contrast agent (see Figs. 7–1*G* and 7–2, *C* and *D*).

Because of its multiplanar capability, MRI is a sensitive study for detecting massive extension of retinoblastoma into the optic nerve substance or into the orbital tissue (Fig. 7–4). However, microscopic invasion of the optic nerve by retinoblastoma cells can be missed on MRI. MRI does not appear to be more sensitive than ultrasonography or CT in detecting minimal optic nerve invasion.

Currently, the authors recommend routine Gd-DTPA–enhanced MRI of the brain in children with bilateral and/or familial retinoblastoma in order to detect asymptomatic early pineal and parasellar tumors (trilateral retinoblastoma) (Fig. 7–5, *A* through *C*).

LESIONS SIMULATING RETINOBLASTOMA

COATS' DISEASE

Clinical and Pathological Features

Coats' disease is an idiopathic retinal vascular disorder in which telangiectasia and aneurysmal retinal vessels are associated with progressive intraretinal exudation and exudative retinal detachment. This condition is unilateral in at least 90% of cases, and it usually affects young male patients. The ophthalmoscopic appearance of the disease varies according to the stage of progression. In early stages, dilated and saccular aneurysmal changes in retinal circulation are present and are associated with exudates. In advanced stages, a total secondary exu-

TABLE 7–1 *MR Features of Retinal Lesions with Thickness Greater Than 1.8 mm on Spin Echo Sequences*

	Signal Intensity of Lesion with Respect to the Vitreous		Degree of Lesion Enhancement after Gd-DTPA
	T1WI	*T2WI*	
Retinoblastoma	Hyper	Hypo	+/+++
Coats' disease	Hyper	Iso	–
Persistent hyperplastic primary vitreous	Iso	Hypo	–/+
Retinal capillary hemangioma	Iso/Hyper	Iso/Hypo	+/++
Massive retinal gliosis (phthisis bulbi)	Iso	Hypo	–/+
Medulloepithelioma	Hyper	Iso/Hypo	+
Ocular toxocariasis	Hyper	Iso/Hypo	–/+
Adenoma of the nonpigmented cilary epithelium	Iso/Hyper	Iso/Hypo	+++
Rhegmatogenous/nonrhegmatogenous retinal detachment	Hyper	Iso	–
Hemorrhagic retinal detachment			
Acute	Iso	Hypo	–
Subacute	Hyper	Iso/Hypo	–
Chronic	Iso	Hypo	–

T1WI, T1-weighted image; *T2WI*, T2-weighted image; *Gd-DTPA*, gadolinium ethylenetriamine penta-acetic acid; Iso, isointense; Hyper, hyperintense; Hypo, hypointense.

dative retinal detachment develops, with accumulation of cholesterol particles in the subretinal space. The advanced stages of Coats' disease must be differentiated from exophytic retinoblastoma.

Fluorescein angiography reveals focal or diffuse leakage from the abnormal retinal vessels. Ultrasonography and CT studies are helpful in differentiating advanced Coats' disease from exophytic retinoblastoma by ruling out the presence of intraocular calcification and showing the V-shaped retinal detachment.

MR Features

MR studies are helpful in differentiating advanced Coats' disease from exophytic retinoblastoma (Tables 7–1 and 7–3). Because of its high proteinaceous content, the subretinal fluid appears homogeneous and is moderately to markedly hyperintense on T1W and T2W images with respect to the vitreous of the opposite eye (Figs. 7–6, *A* through *C*, and 7–7*A*). If the retina is completely detached against the lens, no residual vitreous can be seen in the affected eye. The V-shaped detached retina can be seen on both T1W and T2W images with a low signal intensity. After Gd-DPTA administration, the detached retina may show enhancement, but the subretinal fluid does not (Fig. 7–7*B*).

PERSISTENT HYPERPLASTIC PRIMARY VITREOUS

See Chapter 3 for a discussion of this disorder.

VASCULAR TUMORS OF THE RETINA

RETINAL CAPILLARY HEMANGIOMA

Clinical and Pathological Features

Capillary hemangioma of the retina can occur as an isolated tumor or as a component of the von Hippel-Lindau syndrome. In both instances, the retinal vascular tumor appears identical both clinically and pathologically. Bilaterality and multifocality imply that the lesions are part of the von Hippel-Lindau syndrome.

Retinal capillary hemangioma can have a juxtapapillary or peripheral location. The tumor appears as a reddish nodule with a dilated, tortuous, feeding artery and draining vein. In its exudative form, the retinal capillary hemangioma develops exudation surrounding the lesion or accumulating in the macula. In its vitreoretinal form, the lesion can produce vitreoretinal response with vitreous traction bands, and may be associated with tractional retinal detachment.

Fluorescein angiography is the most helpful ancillary study in confirming the diagnosis, particularly in retinal hemangioma of the optic disk that can simulate papilledema or optic neuritis.

MR Features

On MR studies, retinal capillary hemangiomas that are large enough to be successfully imaged may simulate choroidal melanoma in the adult population (Tables 6–1 and 6–2) and retinoblastoma in the pediatric population (see Tables 7–1 and 7–2). Based on the authors' experience, retinal capillary hemangioma shows a low signal intensity, which is isointense to slightly hyperintense with respect to the vitreous on T1W images (Figs. 7–8*A* and 7–9*A*). The lesion is isointense or hypointense with respect to the vitreous on T2W images (Fig. 7–8*B*). After Gd-DTPA administration, the retinal capillary hemangioma demonstrates moderate enhancement (Fig. 7–8*C* and 7–9*B*). Therefore, contrast-enhanced MRI is not very helpful in differentiating retinal capillary hemangioma from retinoblastoma or uveal melanoma.

The main role of brain MRI in a patient with retinal capillary hemangioma is to rule out the possible association with cerebellar and spinal hemangioblastoma in the von Hippel-Lindau disease. In affected asymptomatic patients, screening brain MRI studies have been recommended every 3 years up to age 50, and every 5 years thereafter.

GLIAL TUMORS OF THE RETINA

RETINAL GLIOSIS

Clinical and Pathological Features

Gliosis of the retina is both a clinical and a histopathologic finding. Massive gliosis of the retina can be seen in eyes with end-stage glaucoma, trauma, or inflammation.

TABLE 7–2 *Intraocular Lesions (with Thickness Greater Than 1.8 mm) in Children and Teenagers That Can Have MR Features Identical to Those of Retinoblastoma on Nonenhanced MRI*

Medulloepithelioma
Retinal capillary hemangioma
Uveal melanoma
Ocular toxocariasis
Subacute hemorrhagic retinal detachment

On histopathologic examination, massive gliosis of the retina is characterized by (1) segmental or total replacement of the retina by glial tissue, (2) abnormal blood vessels within the glial mass, and (3) a resultant thickening of the retina in the involved area.

Ultrasonography and CT are of limited value in demonstrating an atypical intraocular mass. Secondary calcification or localized metaplastic bone formation may be seen to simulate calcification associated with retinoblastoma.

MR Features

Based on the authors' experience, massive gliosis of the retina in a phthisical eye shows a low signal intensity on T1W and T2W images. The subretinal space shows increased signal on T1W and T2W images (Fig. 7–10, A and B). After Gd-DTPA administration, the enhancement of the retinal gliosis may vary, depending on the presence of abnormal blood vessels in the glial mass (Fig. 7–10, C and D). These MR features allow differentiation of retinoblastoma from massive gliosis in a phthisical eye in the pediatric population (see Tables 7–1 and 7–3).

MISCELLANEOUS TUMORS AND PSEUDOTUMORS OF THE RETINA

MEDULLOEPITHELIOMA

Clinical and Pathological Features

Medulloepithelioma is a congenital tumor of the nonpigmented ciliary epithelium and appears to be the second most common intraocular tumor in children after retinoblastoma. The tumor, which is usually diagnosed in children between the ages of 2 and 4 years produces a peculiar notch in the lens.

TABLE 7–3 *Intraocular Lesions (with Thickness Greater Than 1.8 mm) in Children and Teenagers with MR Features That Differ from Those of Retinoblastoma on Nonenhanced MRI*

Coats' disease
Persistent hyperplastic primary vitreous
Retinopathy of prematurity
Massive retinal gliosis (phthisis bulbi)
Rhegmatogenous/nonrhegmatogenous retinal detachment
Acute hemorrhagic retinal detachment
Chronic hemorrhagic retinal detachment

When the tumor enlarges, an observable mass can produce cataract, iris neovascularization, or glaucoma.

Medulloepithelioma may be classified as nonteratoid (diktyoma) or teratoid (teratoneuroma). Both types can present with benign and malignant features. The nonteratoid medulloepithelioma contains poorly differentiated neuroepithelial cells. The teratoid medulloepithelioma shows variable degrees of heteroplasia, along with hyaline cartilage, rhabdomyoblasts, or mesenchymal cells.

The clinical appearance of the tumor on slit lamp examination and indirect ophthalmoscopy is most helpful in establishing the diagnosis. Ultrasonography and CT show features that are similar to those of other ciliary body tumors.

MR Features

On precontrast scans, medulloepithelioma of the ciliary body shows a hyperintense signal on T1W images and an isointense or hypointense signal on T2W images with respect to the vitreous (Fig. 7–11, A and B). After Gd-DTPA administration, the tumor demonstrates moderate to marked enhancement (Fig. 7–11, C and D). Ciliary body medulloepithelioma can share the same MR features as those of uveal melanoma (see Table 6–1) and retinoblastoma in the pediatric population (see Tables 7–1 and 7–2). Therefore, contrast-enhanced MRI does not help in differentiating these lesions.

ADENOMA OF THE NONPIGMENTED CILIARY EPITHELIUM

Clinical and Pathological Features

Acquired epithelial tumors of the ciliary body can arise from the nonpigmented or the pigmented epithelium of the ciliary body. These tumors are usually benign, but can produce a subluxated lens or cataract, and may be locally invasive. These tumors do not cast a shadow when the ciliary region is transilluminated. Histologically, they are composed of proliferating cords of well-differentiated cells that resemble the nonpigmented ciliary epithelium.

MR Features

Based on the authors' experience, the adenoma of the nonpigmented ciliary body epithelium has a low signal intensity, which is isointense or slightly hyperintense with respect to the vitreous on T1W images (Figs. 7–12, A and B, and 7–13A). On T2W images, the tumor may appear isointense or slightly hypointense in relation to the vitreous (Figs. 7–12C and 7–13*B*). However, after Gd-DTPA administration, the lesion shows marked enhancement (Figs. 7–12*D* and 7–13, *C* and *D*). These MR features may be identical to those of ciliary body melanoma in the adult population (see Tables 6–2 and 7–1). Therefore, MRI studies do not help to differentiate between adenoma of the nonpigmented ciliary body epithelium and ciliary body melanoma.

AGE-RELATED MACULAR DEGENERATION

Clinical and Pathological Features

Proliferative age-related macular degeneration (disciform macular degeneration, central exudative hemorrhagic chorioretinopathy) is the most common etiology of blindness in elderly people. The serous and hemorrhagic detachment of the retina and retinal pigment epithelium is caused by choroidal neovascularization. Blood in the subretinal space can simulate choroidal melanoma, but age-related macular degeneration is characterized by subretinal exudation, blood, and breakdown products of blood, which produce a variegated gray or yellow color. In some cases, massive hemorrhage can occur, leading to confusion with large elevated choroidal melanoma. Blood can break through the internal limiting membrane of the retina, producing vitreous hemorrhage and obscuring the view of the posterior pole.

Histopathologic examination reveals hemorrhagic detachment of the retina or retinal pigment epithelium, or both, with degeneration of the outer retinal layers and degeneration and proliferation of the retinal pigment epithelium. Fluorescein angiography is most helpful for establishing the diagnosis of age-related macular degeneration. However, in cases of overlying vitreous hemorrhage, ultrasonography becomes useful. Ultrasonography shows a subretinal mass with low-to-high internal reflectivity, depending on the presence of organized blood.

MR Features

MRI can be helpful in cases in which vitreous hemorrhage obscures the view of the fundus and when ultrasonography does not differentiate subretinal blood from choroidal melanoma. Based on the authors' experience, hemorrhagic detachment of the retina and retinal pigment epithelium particularly that seen with age-related macular degeneration are not detected when the thickness of the lesion is less than 2.0 mm. MR features vary with the paramagnetic qualities of acute hemorrhage as compared with subacute and chronic hemorrhage. In the acute stage, the hemorrhagic detachment of

the retina appears to have a low signal intensity on T1W and T2W images with respect to the vitreous. In the subacute stage, because of the presence of methemoglobin, the lesion becomes hyperintense on T1W images and hypointense to hyperintense on T2W images (Fig. 7–14, *A* through *C*). These MR features may simulate uveal melanoma (see Tables 6–1 and 6–2). Chronic hemorrhagic retinal detachment appears with a low signal intensity on both T1W and T2W images owing to the presence of the less paramagnetic hemosiderin. On nonenhanced MRI, acute and chronic hemorrhagic detachment of the retina may be differentiated from choroidal melanoma.

After Gd-DTPA administration, neither hemorrhagic detachment of the retina nor of the retinal pigment epithelium usually enhances (Fig. 7–14 *D*). Although precontrast MRI studies do not help to differentiate subacute hemorrhagic retinal and/or retinal pigment epithelium detachment in age-related macular degeneration from choroidal melanoma, the lack of enhancement in age-related macular degeneration on postcontrast MR scans helps to establish the diagnostic approach.

BIBLIOGRAPHY

Benhamou E, Borges J, Tso MO. Magnetic resonance imaging in retinoblastoma and retinocytoma: A case report. *J Pediatr Ophthalmol Strabismus.* 1989; 26: 276–280.

Char DH, Hedges TR, Norman D. Retinoblastoma: CT diagnosis. *Ophthalmology.* 1984; 91:1347–350.

De Potter P, Flanders AE, Shields JA, Shields CL. Magnetic resonance imaging of intraocular tumors. *Int Ophthalmol Clin.* 1993; 33:37–45.

De Potter P, Flanders AE, Shields JA, Shields CL, Gonzales CF, Rao VM. The role of fat suppression technique and gadopentetate dimeglumine in magnetic resonance imaging evaluation of intraocular tumors and simulating lesions. *Arch Ophthalmol.* 1994; 112: 340–348.

De Potter P, Shields CL, Shields JA. Clinical variations of trilateral retinoblastoma: A report of 13 cases. *J Pediatr Ophthalmol Strabismus.* 1994; 31:26–31.

De Potter P, Shields JA, Shields CL. Computed tomography and magnetic resonance imaging of intraocular lesions. *Ophthalmol Clin North Am.* 1994; 7:333–346.

Gass JDM. Pathogenesis of disciform detachment of the neuroepithelium. Part III. Senile disciform macular degeneration. *Am J Ophthalmol.* 1967; 63:617–644.

Haik BG. Advanced Coats' disease. *Trans Am Ophthalmol Soc.* 1991; 89:371–476.

Haik BG, Saint Louis L, Smith ME, Ellsworth RM, Abramson OH, Cahill P, Deck M, Coleman J. Magnetic resonance imaging in the evaluation of leucocoria. *Ophthalmology.* 1985; 92:1143–1152.

Hennis H, Saunders R, Shields JA. Malignant teratoid medulloepithelioma of the ciliary body. *J Clin Neuro-Ophthalmol.* 1990; 10:291–292.

Koch A, Gerke E, Höpping W. Echography in retinoblastoma. *Graefes Arch Clin Exp Ophthalmol.* 1983; 221:27–30.

Lieb WE, Shields JA, Eagle RC, Kwa D, Shields CL. Cystic adenoma of the pigmented ciliary epithelium: Clinical, pathologic and immunohistopathologic findings. *Ophthalmology.* 1990; 97:1489–1493.

Mafee MF. Magnetic resonance imaging: Ocular pathology. In: Newton TH, Bilaniuk LT, eds. *Radiology of the Eye and Orbit.* New York: Raven Press; 1990, Chap. 3.

Mafee MF, Goldberg MF, Cohen SB, Golsis ED, Safran M, Chekuri L, Raofi G. Magnetic resonance imaging versus computed tomography of leukocoric eyes and use of in vitro proton magnetic resonance spectroscopy of retinoblastoma. *Ophthalmology.* 1989; 96:865–976.

Mafee MF, Goldberg MF, Greenwald MF, Schulman J, Malmed A, Flanders AE. Retinoblastoma and simulating lesions: Role of CT and MR imaging. *Radiol Clin North Am.* 1987; 25:667–682.

Mafee MF, Peyman GA. Retinal and choroidal detachments: Role of magnetic resonance imaging and computed tomography. *Radiol Clin North Am.* 1987; 25:487–507.

Maher ER, Moore AT. von Hippel-Lindau disease. *Br J Ophthalmol.* 1992; 76:743–745.

Peyster RG, Augsburger JJ, Shields JA, Hershey BL, Eagle RC, Haskin ME. Intraocular tumors: Evaluation with MR imaging. *Radiology.* 1988; 168:773–779.

Ridely ME, Shields JA, Brown GC, Tasman W. Coats' disease: Evaluation and management. *Ophthalmology.* 1982; 89:1381–1387.

Schulman JA, Peyman GA, Mafee MF, et al. The use of magnetic resonance imaging in the evaluation of retinoblastoma. *J. Pediatr Ophthalmol Strabismus.* 1986; 23:144–147.

Shields CL, Shields JA, Baez KA, Cater J, De Potter P. Choroidal invasion of retinoblastoma: Metastatic potential and clinical risk factors. *Br J Ophthalmol.* 1993; 77:544–548.

Shields CL, Shields JA, Baez KA, De Potter P, Cater J. Optic nerve invasion of retinoblastoma. *Cancer.* 1994; 73:692–698.

Shields JA, Augsburger JJ, Brown GC, Stephens RF. The differential diagnosis of posterior uveal melanoma. *Ophthalmology.* 1980; 87:543–548.

Shields JA, Decker WL, Sanborn GE, Augsburger JJ, Goldberg RE. Presumed acquired retinal hemangiomas. *Ophthalmology.* 1983; 90:1292–1300.

Shields JA, Shields CL. *Intraocular Tumors. A Textbook and Atlas.* Philadelphia: WB Saunders; 1992.

Shields JA, Shields CL. The phakomatoses. In: Nelson LB, Calhoun JC, Harley RD, eds. *Pediatric Ophthalmology.* 3rd ed. Philadelphia: WB Saunders; 1991: 427–443.

Shields JA, Stephens RF. Ultrasonography in pediatric ophthalmology. In: Harley RD, ed. *Pediatric Ophthalmology.* 2nd ed. Philadelphia: WB Saunders; 1982:145–154.

Tasman W. Late complications of retrolental fibroplasia. *Ophthalmology.* 1979; 86:1724–1740.

Till P, Ossoinig KC. Ten years study on clinical echography in intraocular disease. *Bibl Ophthalmol.* 1975; 83:49–62.

Welch RB. von Hippel-Lindau disease: The recognition and treatment of early angiomatosis retinae and the use of cryosurgery as an adjunct to therapy. *Trans Am Ophthalmol Soc.* 1970; 68:367–424.

Yanoff M, Zimmerman LE, Davis RL. Massive gliosis of the retina. *Int Ophthalmol Clin.* 1971; 11:211–229.

Zimmerman LE. The remarkable polymorphism of tumors of the ciliary epithelium. Part 1. The Norman McAlister Gregg Lecture. *Trans Aust Coll Ophthalmol.* 1970; 2:114–125.

Zimmerman LE. Retinoblastoma and retinocytoma. In: Spencer WH, Font RL, Green WR, Howes EL, Jacobiec FA, Zimmerman LE, eds. *Ophthalmic Pathology. An Atlas and Textbook.* Vol. 2. 3rd ed. Philadelphia: WB Saunders; 1985:1292–1351.

Zimmerman RA, Bilaniuk LT. Computed tomography in the evaluation of patients with bilateral retinoblastomas. *J Comput Tomogr.* 1979; 3:251–257.

FIGURE 7-1 *Bilateral Endophytic/Exophytic Retinoblastoma*

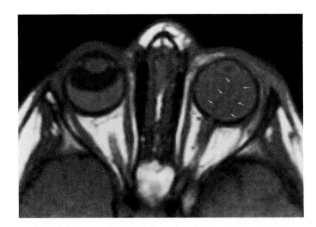

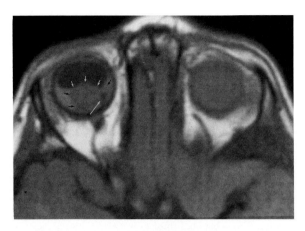

7-1A Axial T1W image. The vitreous cavity in the left eye is hyperintense. The tumor (*arrows*) shows a low signal intensity with respect to the surrounding subretinal fluid. In the right eye, the subtotal retinal detachment is hyperintense with respect to the vitreous. The left optic nerve appears to be normal.

7-1B Axial T1W image at a higher level than in *A*. In the right eye, the retinoblastoma (*short arrows*) shows a heterogeneous signal that is slightly less hyperintense than the surrounding subretinal fluid. The area of low signal intensity corresponds to calcification (*long arrow*). The right optic nerve appears to be normal.

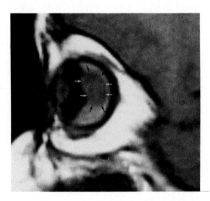

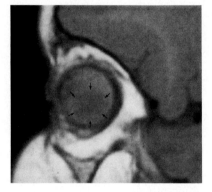

7-1C Parasagittal T1W image of the right orbit. The tumor (*arrows*) is hypointense with respect to the surrounding subretinal fluid, but hyperintense with respect to the vitreous.

7-1D Parasagittal T1W image of the left orbit. The tumor, located inferiorly (*arrows*), is hypointense with respect to the surrounding subretinal fluid.

(continued)

FIGURE 7–1 *Bilateral Endophytic/Exophytic Retinoblastoma* (continued)

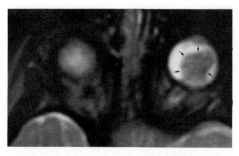

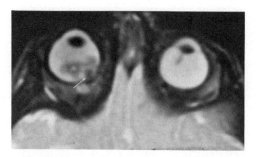

7–1E Axial T2W image at the same level as in *A*, with the head slightly tilted. The retinoblastoma in the left eye has a heterogeneous, low signal intensity (*arrows*), which is hypointense compared to the increased signal of the surrounding subretinal fluid.

7–1F Axial T2W image at a slightly lower level than in *B*, with the head slightly tilted. The tumor in the right eye is hypointense. The focus of low signal intensity within the tumor (*arrow*) corresponds to calcification.

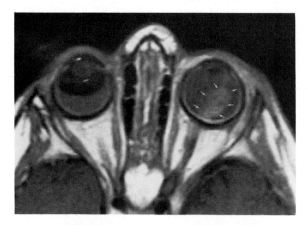

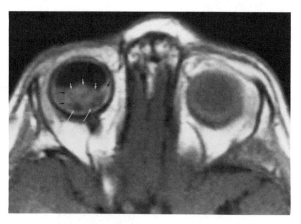

7–1G Axial Gd-DTPA–enhanced T1W image at the same level as in *A*. In the left eye, the tumor, which was barely seen on the precontrast scan, demonstrates heterogeneous enhancement (*arrows*). The subretinal fluid does not enhance.

7–1H Axial Gd-DTPA–enhanced T1W image at the same level as in *B*. The tumor in the right eye demonstrates heterogeneous enhancement (*short arrows*). The nonenhancing foci within the retinoblastoma suggest calcification (*long arrows*).

(continued)

FIGURE 7–1 *Bilateral Endophytic/Exophytic Retinoblastoma* (continued)

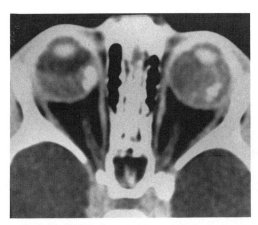

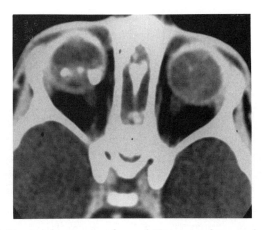

7–1I Axial contrast-enhanced CT scan at the same level as in *A*. Bilateral calcification is easily detected on CT, but is not seen on MR scans.

7–1J Axial contrast-enhanced CT scan at the same level as in *B*. The intraocular calcification in the right eye, located nasally, has a low signal intensity on MR scans (see *B*, *F*, and *H*).

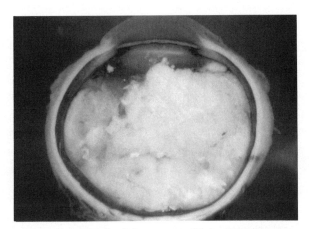

7–1K Photograph of the sectioned left eye showing the vitreous cavity filled with retinoblastoma.

FIGURE 7–2 *Unilateral Exophytic Retinoblastoma*

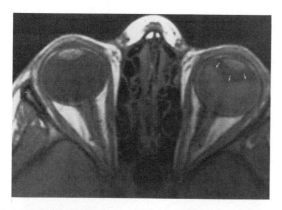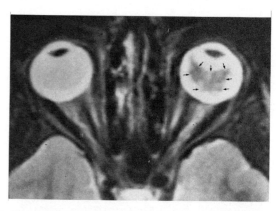

7–2A Axial T1W image. The exophytic tumor and the secondary retinal detachment in the left eye show an increased signal intensity (*arrows*) with respect to the vitreous. (From Orbit. In: Rao VM, Flanders AE, Tom BM, eds. *MRI and CT Atlas of Correlative Imaging in Otolaryngology*. London: Martin Dunitz; 1992:368.)

7–2B Axial T2W image. The tumor has a heterogeneous, hypointense signal (*arrows*) with respect to the hyperintense vitreous and the subretinal fluid. (From Orbit. In: Rao VM, Flanders AE, Tom BM, eds. *MRI and CT Atlas of Correlative Imaging in Otolaryngology*. London: Martin Dunitz; 1992: 368.)

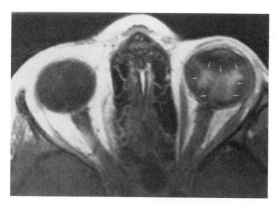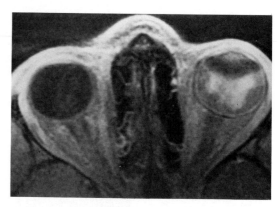

7–2C Axial Gd-DTPA–enhanced T1W image. The tumor demonstrates moderate enhancement (*arrows*). The surrounding subretinal fluid does not enhance. (From Orbit. In: Rao VM, Flanders AE, Tom BM, eds. *MRI and CT Atlas of Correlative Imaging in Otolaryngology*. London: Martin Dunitz; 1992:368.)

7–2D Fat-suppressed axial Gd-DTPA–enhanced T1W image. The degree of enhancement of the tumor and the signal of the subretinal fluid are more pronounced.

(continued)

FIGURE 7-2 *Unilateral Exophytic Retinoblastoma* (continued)

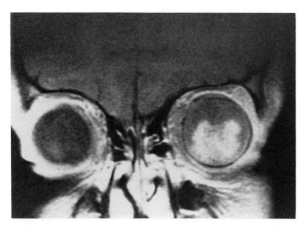

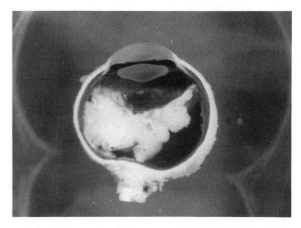

7-2E Fat-suppressed coronal Gd-DTPA–enhanced T1W image. The enhancement of the tumor is heterogeneous.

7-2F Photograph of the sectioned left eye showing the exophytic retinoblastoma with the associated retinal detachment.

FIGURE 7–3 *Unilateral Endophytic Retinoblastoma*

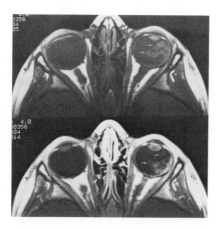

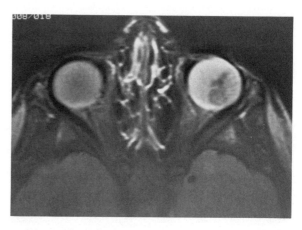

7–3A Axial precontrast [*top*] and postcontrast [*bottom*] T1W image. The retinoblastoma in the left eye appears as a heterogeneous, hyperintense mass with respect to the vitreous. Vitreous seeding (*arrows*) overlies the tumor. After Gd-DTPA administration, the tumor shows moderate heterogeneous enhancement. The retinoblastoma seeds in the vitreous do not enhance.

7–3B Axial T2W image. The tumor has a heterogeneous, hypointense signal with respect to the vitreous.

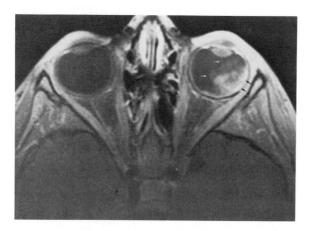

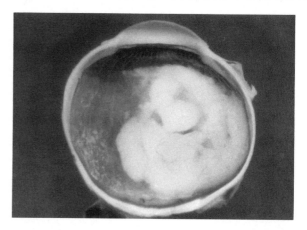

7–3C Fat-suppressed axial Gd-DTPA–enhanced T1W image. Note the marked enhancement at the base of the tumor (*black arrows*). The vitreous seeding is not enhanced (*white arrows*).

7–3D Photograph of the sectioned left eye showing the endophytic retinoblastoma with vitreous seeding.

FIGURE 7–4 *Unilateral Exophytic Retinoblastoma with Optic Nerve Invasion*
Axial Gd-DTPA–enhanced T1W image. The exophytic retinoblastoma (*arrows*) demonstrates marked enhancement. The surrounding subretinal fluid does not enhance. The enhancement seen within the retrolaminar portion of the optic nerve suggests optic nerve invasion (*arrowhead*). (Courtesy of Barrett G Haik, MD, New Orleans, LA; From Ainbinder D, et al. The role of Gd-DTPA enhanced magnetic resonance imaging in the staging of retinoblastoma. *Ophthalmology*. In press. © 1994 by the American Academy of Ophthalmology.)

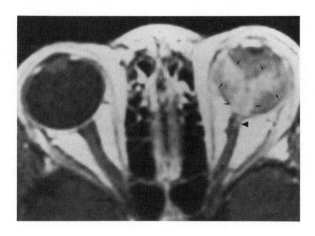

FIGURE 7–5 *Bilateral Retinoblastoma with Pinealoblastoma*
The pinealoblastoma was found on routine MR studies 8 months after the diagnosis of bilateral retinoblastoma in a 2-year-old girl. At the time of diagnosis of bilateral retinoblastoma, the right eye was treated with external beam irradiation, and the left eye was enucleated.

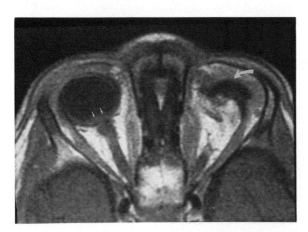

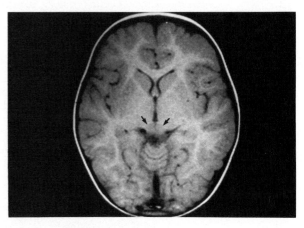

7–5A Axial Gd-DTPA–enhanced T1W image. The regressed retinoblastoma (*arrows*) in the right eye does not demonstrate enhancement after radiation treatment. Note the signal void produced by the polymethylmethacrylate sphere in the anophthalmic left socket (*curved arrow*). No sign of tumor recurrence is noted.

7–5B Axial T1W image. The pinealoblastoma (*arrows*) is slightly hypointense with respect to the cerebral white matter. There is no secondary hydrocephalus.

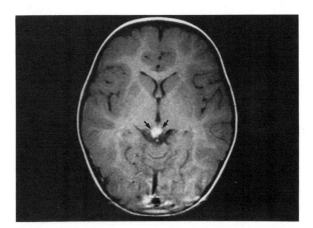

7–5C Axial Gd-DTPA–enhanced T1W image. The tumor demonstrates marked enhancement (*arrows*).

FIGURE 7–6 *Unilateral Coats' Disease*

A 2-year-old girl presented with a 3-month history of leukokoria of the left eye.

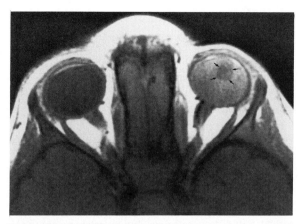

7–6A Axial T1W image. The left eye shows an increased signal intensity compared to the right eye because of the total exudative retinal detachment and its high proteinaceous content. The remaining vitreous (*arrows*) is hypointense behind the lens.

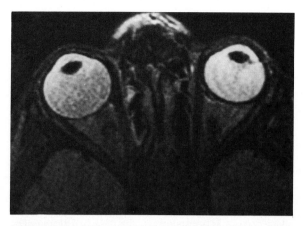

7–6B Axial T2W image. The subretinal fluid and vitreous are both hyperintense.

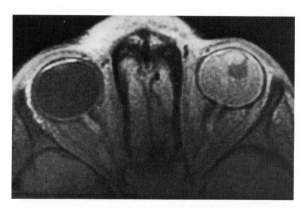

7–6C Fat-suppressed axial T1W image. The signal intensity of the subretinal fluid in the left eye is more pronounced than in the right.

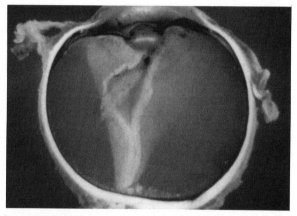

7–6D Photograph of a sectioned eye with Coats' disease showing the total retinal detachment and the proteinaceous content of the subretinal space.

FIGURE 7–7 *Unilateral Coats' Disease*
A 3-year-old boy presented with leukokoria of the right eye. (Courtesy of David H Abramson, MD, New York, NY.)

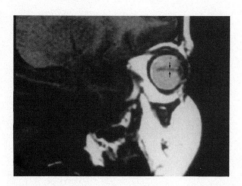

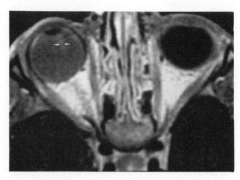

7–7A Sagittal T1W image. The hypointense tubular signal (*arrows*) corresponds to the detached retina. The proteinaceous subretinal fluid is hyperintense.

7–7B Axial Gd-DTPA–enhanced T1W image. The detached retina demonstrates minimal enhancement (*arrows*), but the subretinal fluid does not enhance. The lens is displaced anteriorly by the bullous exudative retinal detachment.

FIGURE 7–8 *Retinal Capillary Hemangioma*
A 16-year-old patient presented with bilateral multiple retinal capillary hemangiomas without cerebral involvement.

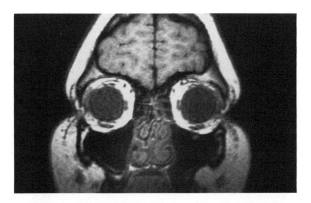

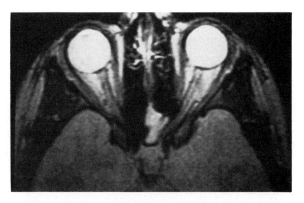

7–8A Coronal T1W image. The largest retinal capillary hemangioma (measuring 2.7 mm thick on ultrasonography) is located temporally on the horizontal meridian in the right eye and is isointense with respect to the vitreous. It is, therefore, not identified. The other retinal hemangiomas are also too small to be identified.

7–8B Axial T2W image. The same lesion in the right eye is isointense with respect to the hyperintense vitreous.

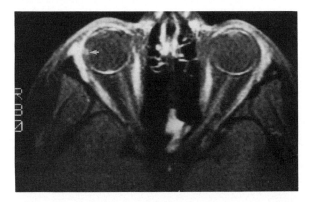

7–8C Fat-suppressed axial Gd-DTPA–enhanced T1W image. The largest retinal capillary hemangioma in the right eye demonstrates moderate enhancement (*arrow*).

FIGURE 7–9 *Retinal Capillary Hemangioma*

A 12-year-old patient presented with von Hippel-Lindau disease and bilateral retinal capillary hemangioma. The right eye was enucleated because of complications of total retinal detachment secondary to the retinal hemangioma. In the left eye, a retinal capillary hemangioma with a thickness of 2.5 mm is located superotemporally at the equator.

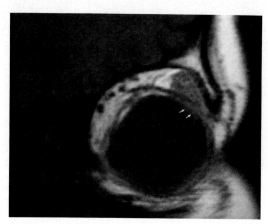

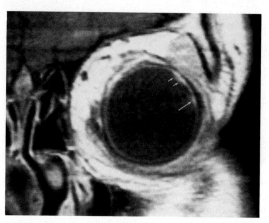

7–9A Coronal T1W image. The retinal capillary hemangioma shows a mildly hyperintense signal with respect to the vitreous. No retinal detachment is noted. The lesion is isointense relative to the vitreous on T2W images (not shown).

7–9B Coronal Gd-DTPA–enhanced T1W image. The vascular tumor demonstrates moderate enhancement (*short arrows*). A second retinal hemangioma (thickness of 1.8 mm) that was not seen on precontrast studies shows minimal enhancement (*long arrow*).

FIGURE 7–10 *Massive Gliosis*
A 13-year-old patient presented with massive retinal gliosis in the phthisical left eye.

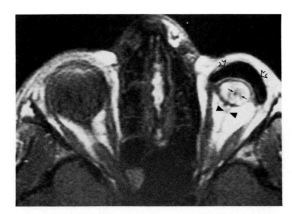

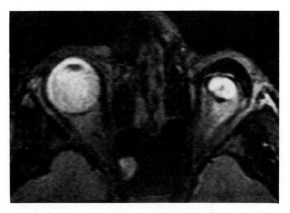

7–10A Axial T1W image. The microphthalmic left eye has a heterogeneous signal intensity. The peripheral hyperintense signal is probably produced by proteinaceous material within the subretinal space. The central hypointense signal corresponds to retinal gliosis (*black arrow*). The optic nerve sheath complex appears small in size (*arrowheads*). Note the signal void produced by the prosthetic device (*open arrows*).

7–10B Axial T2W image. The peripheral portion of the phthisical eye is hyperintense and the central core is hypointense.

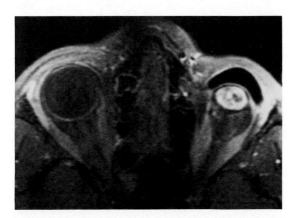

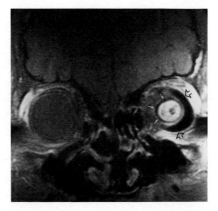

7–10C Fat-suppressed axial Gd-DTPA–enhanced T1W image. The gliotic tissue does not enhance.

7–10D Fat-suppressed coronal Gd-DTPA–enhanced T1W image. Note the chemical shift artifact (*white arrows*) and the signal void of the prosthetic device (*open arrows*).

FIGURE 7-11 *Ciliary Body Medulloepithelioma*
A 13-year-old patient presented with medulloepithelioma of the ciliary body in the right eye.

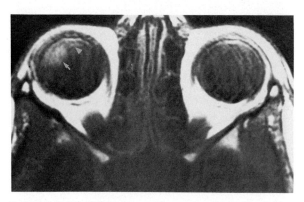

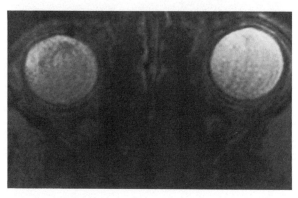

7-11A Axial T1W image. The tumor (*arrow*) appears hyperintense with respect to the vitreous. Associated subretinal fluid with hyperintense signal (*arrowhead*) is located nasally to the tumor.

7-11B Axial gradient echo image. The tumor is isointense with respect to the hyperintense vitreous.

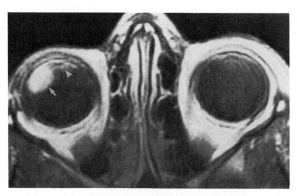

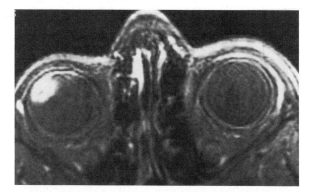

7-11C Axial Gd-DTPA–enhanced T1W image. The mass (*arrow*) shows marked enhancement. Note that the subretinal fluid does not enhance (*arrowhead*).

7-11D Fat-suppressed axial Gd-DTPA–enhanced T1W image. The enhancement of the tumor is more pronounced in this image.

FIGURE 7–12 *Adenoma of the Nonpigmented Ciliary Body Epithelium*
A 69-year-old woman was found on routine examination to have an amelanotic ciliary body tumor in the left eye. The tumor was successfully removed by partial lamellar scleroiridociliochoroidectomy.

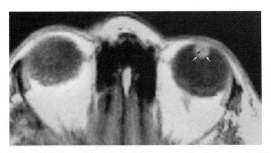

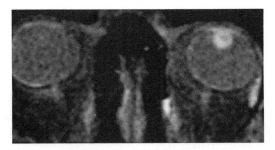

7–12A Axial T1W image. The ciliary body mass (*white arrows*) has a heterogeneous intensity pattern. The central portion of the mass (*black arrow*) has a low signal intensity, which is isointense with respect to the vitreous and which corresponds to a cystic cavity. The peripheral rim is hyperintense and is composed of tumor ciliary body cells.

7–12B Fat-suppressed T1W image. The contrast between the tumor and the vitreous is more pronounced in this image.

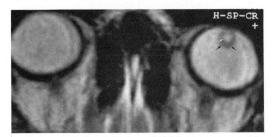

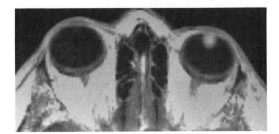

7–12C Axial T2W image. The peripheral cellular portion (*black arrows*) of the tumor becomes hypointense with respect to the vitreous. The central cystic portion (*white arrow*) is hyperintense.

7–12D Axial Gd-DTPA–enhanced T1W image. The tumor demonstrates marked enhancement with pooling of the contrast agent in the central cyst.

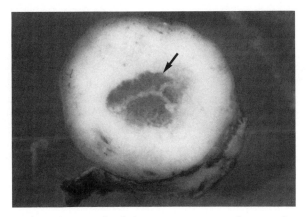

7–12E Photograph of the gross specimen showing the amelanotic ciliary body mass with the central cystic cavity (*arrow*).

FIGURE 7–13 *Adenoma of the Nonpigmented Ciliary Body Epithelium*
A 31-year-old patient presented with adenoma of the nonpigmented ciliary epithelium in the left eye, producing subluxation of the lens.

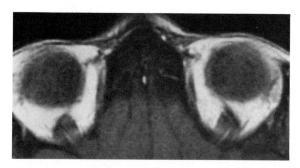

7–13A Axial T1W image. The tumor is isointense with respect to the vitreous and, therefore, is not detected. There is no associated retinal detachment.

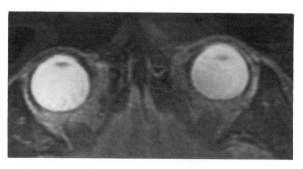

7–13B Axial T2W image. The tumor is isointense in relation to the vitreous and is, therefore, not detected.

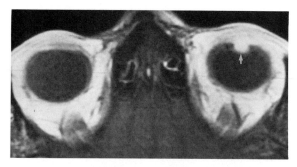

7–13C Axial Gd-DTPA–enhanced T1W image. The tumor demonstrates marked enhancement (*arrow*).

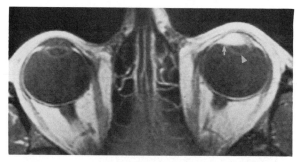

7–13D Axial Gd-DTPA–enhanced T1W image at a lower level. The enhancing tumor (*arrow*) extends into the anterior chamber and produces mild subluxation of the lens (*arrowhead*).

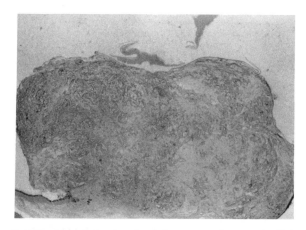

7–13E Photomicrograph of the resected tumor (colloidal iron without hyaluronidase) showing the marked staining of the mucoid material.

FIGURE 7–14 *Age-Related Macular Degeneration*
A 70-year-old patient presented with vitreous hemorrhage in the left eye obscuring the view of the posterior pole. A subretinal mass in the macular region is demonstrated by ultrasonography. A macular disciform scar is found in the right eye.

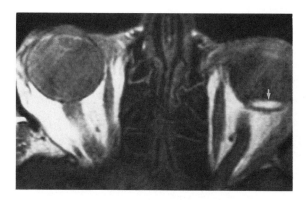

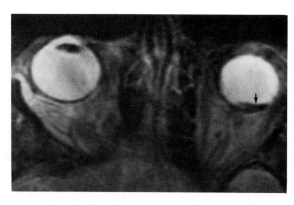

7–14A Axial T1W image. A subretinal mass (*arrow*) shows a marked hyperintense signal with respect to the vitreous. The vitreous hemorrhage is not identified.

7–14B Axial T2W image. The lesion (*arrow*) becomes hypointense with respect to the vitreous. This suggests the presence of intracellular methemoglobin.

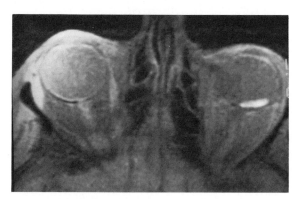

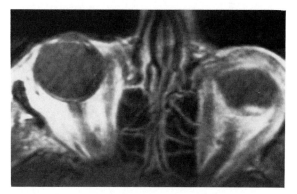

7–14C Fat-suppressed axial T1W image. The hyperintense signal of the subacute hemorrhagic retinal detachment appears more pronounced in this image.

7–14D Axial Gd-DTPA–enhanced T1W image. Contrary to choroidal melanoma, which shows the same MR features on precontrast studies as postcontrast studies, the hemorrhagic retinal detachment does not enhance.

(continued)

Chapter 7: Tumors and Pseudotumors of the Retina **115**

FIGURE 7-14 *Age-Related Macular Degeneration* (continued)

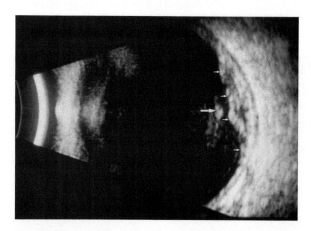

7-14E B-scan ultrasonography. A subretinal lesion with irregular surface (*short arrows*) shows a relatively high internal reflectivity. Vitreous echoes (*long arrow*) are suggestive of vitreous hemorrhage.

Part Three | Disorders of the Orbit

MRI of the Eye and Orbit,
by Patrick De Potter, Jerry A. Shields, and Carol L. Shields.
J. B. Lippincott Company, Philadelphia © 1995.

8
Congenital Anomalies

PATRICK DE POTTER

JERRY A. SHIELDS

CAROL L. SHIELDS

DEVELOPMENTAL ANOMALIES

ANOPHTHALMOS AND MICROPHTHALMOS

Clinical and Pathological Features

Congenital anophthalmos is a very rare ocular condition that is most often bilateral. Microphthalmos is usually a unilateral condition. True anophthalmos occurs when the primary optic vesicle fails to grow out from the cerebral vesicle during early embryologic development. In many cases, its etiology remains obscure, but in some cases, environmental agents, such as maternal viral infection (rubella), a deficiency or excess of vitamin A, or chemical agents (lithium, selenium, Trypan Blue), have been implicated in the pathogenesis of this abnormality. Extreme microphthalmos may be difficult to distinguish from anophthalmos. The orbits and eyelids are usually small but well formed. In addition to a complete ophthalmologic evaluation, all patients with anophthalmos or microphthalmos should have a careful history review, genetic workup, and physical examination.

In anophthalmos, histopathologic examination reveals no ocular tissue. However, the extraocular muscles may be present and well developed. In microphthalmos, the eye is present, but it is small, usually malformed, and often associated with a coloboma and orbital cyst (see the section that follows entitled Colobomatous Cyst).

MR Features

The role of magnetic resonance imaging (MRI) in congenital anophthalmos is mainly to evaluate the orbital content and the presence of extraocular muscles if surgery is contemplated. In congenital microphthalmos, it is important to evaluate the microphthalmic eye and rule out the presence of a concealed, attached, herniated, cystlike mass (microphthalmos with cyst) or retinoblastoma (Fig. 8–1, *A* and *B*).

CYSTIC LESIONS

DERMOID CYST

Clinical and Pathological Features

Dermoid cyst is the most common cystic lesion involving the orbital region. It can be located in the brow region, in which case it is usually diagnosed early in life. Deeper orbital dermoid cysts remain asymptomatic until later in life. These cysts have a propensity for the superotemporal orbital quadrant and present as slowly progressive, painless masses. Large dermoid cysts may rupture spontaneously, producing an intense inflammatory reaction. Dermoid cysts are believed to develop from embryonic entrapment of surface epidermis, particularly along the zygomaticofrontal suture.

Histopathologic examination reveals that the dermoid cyst is a rounded, cystic, epithelium-lined mass. Flakes of keratin and sebum secretion are present in the cystic lumen. The presence of adnexal elements, such as hair shafts or sebaceous or sweat glands, within the cyst wall confirms the diagnosis of a dermoid cyst.

On computed tomography (CT), a dermoid cyst appears as a well-circumscribed, round-to-oval lesion with low density and a nonenhancing lumen. It can exhibit bony expansion and fossa formation secondary to slow enlargement of the tumor.

MR Features

On MRI, dermoid cysts appear as well-defined, round to oval lesions with variable signal intensity, depending upon the composition of their content. These cysts may have an isointense to hyperintense signal intensity with respect to the vitreous or extraocular muscle and isointense to hypointense sig-nal with respect to orbital fat on T1-weighted (T1W) images (Fig. 8–2A). On T2-weighted (T2W) images, dermoid cysts are isointense or hypointense with respect to the vitreous and isointense to hyperin-tense with respect to orbital fat (Fig. 8–2B; Table 8–1). The cysts may exhibit either a homogeneous or heterogeneous signal. The intensity pattern of dermoid cysts on nonenhanced MR studies is there-fore variable and can be seen with other cystic or-bital lesions (Table 8–1). The location of the tumor and the clinical presentation will help the clinician or radiologist in the differential diagnosis. In some cases, a fat-fluid level is demonstrated. The oily portion of the cyst content, which is produced by the sebaceous glands in the cyst wall, appears in the nondependent portion of the cyst as a high signal intensity on T1W images and decreased signal in-tensity on T2W images. The keratin and water con-tent of the cyst lumen in the dependent portion of the cyst has a low signal intensity on T1W images

TABLE 8–1 *MR Features of Cystic Orbital Lesions on Spin Echo Sequences*

	Signal Intensity and Appearance of Lesion with Respect to Orbital Fat		Degree of Lesion Enhancement after Gd-DTPA
	T1WI	*T2WI*	
Dermoid cyst	Hypo/Iso Homo/Hetero	Hyper/Iso Homo/Hetero	−
Acquired inclusion cyst	Hypo Homo/Hetero	Hyper Homo/Hetero	−
Chronic hematic cyst (cholesterol granuloma)	Iso Homo/Hetero	Hyper Homo/Hetero	−
Microphthalmos with cyst	Hypo Homo	Hyper Homo	−
Mucocele	Hypo/Iso Homo/Hetero	Hyper/Iso Homo/Hetero	−
Parasitic cyst	Hypo Homo	Hyper Homo	−
Lymphangioma			−/+
Lymphatic cyst	Hypo Homo	Hyper Homo	
Hemorrhagic cyst			
Acute	Hypo Homo/Hetero	Hypo Homo/Hetero	
Subacute	Iso Homo/Hetero	Hypo/Hyper Homo/Hetero	
Chronic	Hypo Homo/Hetero	Hypo Homo/Hetero	

T1WI, T1-weighted image; *T2WI*, T2-weighted image; *Gd-DTPA*, gadolinium ethylenetriamine penta-acetic acid; Hypo, hypointense; Iso, isointense; Hyper, hyperintense; Homo, homogeneous; Hetero, heterogeneous.

and a high signal intensity on T2W images (Fig. 8–2, *A* and *B*). These MR findings are highly suggestive of dermoid cysts. After administration of gadolinium diethylenetriamine penta-acetic acid (Gd-DTPA), the lumen of the dermoid cyst does not demonstrate enhancement, but the surrounding capsule does. Fat-suppressed postcontrast T1W images are most helpful in delineating dermoid cysts (Fig. 8–2*C*).

COLOBOMATOUS CYST

Clinical and Pathological Features

Colobomatous cyst (microphthalmos with cyst) is a congenital cystic mass that protrudes through a congenital defect (coloboma) in the wall of a microphthalmic eye. The coloboma is a failure of the embryonic fissure to fuse and can present at various locations along the axis from the central nervous system (CNS) to the globe. The clinical findings in microphthalmos with cyst will depend on the location of the cyst and the size of the eye and cyst. The enlarging cyst is almost always located in the inferior portion of orbit and may sometimes protrude behind the lower eyelid. Associated systemic congenital abnormalities, such as CNS, facial, and cardiac anomalies, occur in about 10% of cases.

The cyst is in continuity with the malformed small eye adjacent to the coloboma, and is lined by undifferentiated neuroectoderm. Ultrasonography and CT studies show a rounded cystic lesion adjacent to a microphthalmic eye.

MR Features

On MRI, the cystic outpouching extending from the posterior or inferior aspect of the microphthalmic eye appears as a well-defined area with an isointense or slightly hyperintense signal relative to that of the vitreous and hypointense with respect to orbital fat on T1W images (Figs. 8–3*A* and 8–4, *A* and *B*). On T2W images, the cystic lesion presents an increased signal intensity and is isointense or slightly hypointense with respect to the vitreous and hyperintense with respect to orbital fat (Figs. 8–3, *B* and *C*; 8–4*C*; Table 8–1). The signal intensity of the orbital cyst is related to its proteinaceous content. The detached retina and proliferation of glial cells display a low signal intensity on T1W and T2W images. The disorganized glial tissue demonstrates enhancement after Gd-DTPA administration (Fig. 8–3, *D*, *E*, and *F*).

SOLID LESIONS

DERMOLIPOMA

Clinical and Pathological Features

Dermolipoma may be clinically evident in the conjunctiva, but it can extend diffusely into the orbit. Dermolipoma is usually located in the superotemporal portion of the orbit anteriorly, and bulges beneath the conjunctival epithelium. Orbital CT scanning is very helpful in delineating the posterior extent of the tumor when surgical excision is contemplated. On CT examination, the tumor appears more solid than cystic, and bony involvement is not seen.

MR Features

Orbital dermolipoma is mainly composed of mature fat. On MRI, the lesion appears as a well-defined, oblong, orbital mass with a signal that is isointense to orbital fat on T1W and T2W images. The lesion becomes totally hypointense, as does the orbital fat, on fat-suppressed images (Fig. 8–5, *A* and *B*). The cartilaginous elements and glandular acini that may be found in a dermolipoma show a hypointense signal with respect to the surrounding orbital fat. MRI can be of value in delineating the posterior extent of the lesion. After Gd-DTPA administration, orbital dermolipoma does not demonstrate enhancement (Fig. 8–5*C*).

BIBLIOGRAPHY

Axelsen I. Retinoblastoma in a microphthalmic eye. *Ophthalmologica*. 1978; 176:24–26.

Bilaniuk LT, Zimmerman RA, Newton TH. Magnetic resonance imaging: Orbital pathology. In: Newton TH, Bilaniuk LT, eds. *Radiology of the Eye and Orbit*. New York: Raven Press; 1990, Chap. 5.

Blei L, Chambers JT, Liotta LA, Di Chiro G. Orbital dermoid diagnosed by computed tomographic scanning. *Am J Ophthalmol*. 1978; 85:58–61.

Chohan BS, Parmar IPS, Bhatia JN. Anterior orbital meninoencephalocele. *Am J Ophthalmol*. 1969; 68: 144–146.

De Potter P, Flanders AE, Shields CL, Shields JA. Magnetic resonance imaging of orbital tumors. *Int Ophthalmol Clin*. 1993; 33:163–173.

Garrity JA, Trautmann JC, Bartley GB, Forbes G, Bullock JD, Jones TW, Waller RR. Optic nerve sheath meningoceles. Clinical and radiographic features in 13 cases with review of the literature. *Ophthalmology*. 1990; 97:1519–1531.

Harris GJ, Dolman PJ, Simons KB. Microphthalmos with cyst. *Ophthalm Surg.* 1992; 23:432–433.

Harris GJ, Sacks JG, Weinberg PE, O'Grady RB. Cysts of the intraorbital optic nerve sheaths. *Am J Ophthalmol.* 1976; 81:656–660.

Jakobiec FA, Font RL. Congenital tumors and malformations. In: Spencer WH, Font RL, Green WR, Howes EL, Jakobiec FA, Zimmerman LE, eds. *Ophthalmic Pathology. An Atlas and Textbook.* Philadelphia: WB Saunders; 1986:2482–2496.

Mafee MF, Putterman A, Valvassori GE, Campos M, Capek V. Orbital space-occupying lesions: Role of computed tomography and magnetic resonance imaging. *Radiol Clin North Am.* 1987; 25:529–559.

Mitchell DG, Burk DL, Vinitski S, Rifkin MD. The biophysical basis of tissue contrast in extracranial MR imaging. *AJR.* 1987; 149:831–837.

Pollock JA, Newton TH, Hoyt WF. Transsphenoidal and transethmoidal encephaloceles. A review of clinical and roentgen figures in 8 cases. *Radiology.* 1968; 90:442–453.

Rootman J, Lapointe JS. Structural lesions. In: Rootman J, ed. *Diseases of the Orbit.* Philadelphia: JB Lippincott; 1988:481–523.

Sherman RP, Rootman J, Lapointe JS. Orbital dermoids: Clinical presentation and management. *Br J Ophthalmol.* 1984; 68:642–652.

Shields JA. Cystic lesions of the orbit. In: Shields JA, ed. *Diagnosis and Management of Orbital Tumors.* Philadelphia: WB Saunders; 1989:89–122.

Shields JA. Lipomatous and myxomatous tumors. In: Shields JA, ed. *Diagnosis and Management of Orbital Tumors.* Philadelphia: WB Saunders; 1989:234–242.

Shields JA, Bakewell B, Augsburger JJ, Donoso LA, Bernardino V. Space-occupying orbital masses in children. A survey of 250 consecutive biopsies. *Ophthalmology.* 1986; 193:379–384.

Shields JA, Bakewell B, Augsburger JJ, Flanagan JC. Classification and incidence of space-occupying lesions of the orbit. A survey of 645 biopsies. *Arch Ophthalmol.* 1984; 102:1606–1611.

Sullivan JA, Harms SE. Surface coil MR imaging of orbital neoplasms. *Am J Neuroradiol.* 1986; 7:29–34.

Waring GO, Roth AM, Rodrigues MM. Clinicopathologic correlation of microphthalmos with cyst. *Am J Ophthalmol.* 1976; 82:714–721.

Weiss A, Greenwald M, Martinez C. Microphthalmos with cyst: Clinical presentations and computed tomographic findings. *J Ped Ophthalmol Strabismus.* 1985; 22:6–12.

FIGURE 8-1 *Congenital Microphthalmos 5-Month-Old Girl*
(Courtesy of James A. Katowitz, M.D., Philadelphia.)

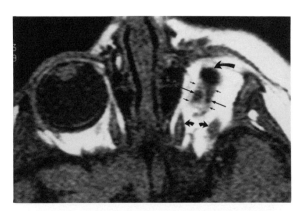

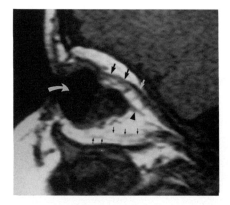

8-1A Axial T1W image. The microphthalmic eye (*short arrows*) is seen behind the prosthetic device (*long curved arrow*). The medial and lateral rectus muscles are seen in the posterior orbit (*short curved arrows*). Foci of low signal intensity (*long arrows*) correspond to fibrous or osseous metaplasia (see Fig. 8-1C).

8-1B Sagittal T1W image. The superior rectus muscle (*large arrows*) appears to be relatively normal. The inferior rectus muscle (*small arrows*) appears to be atrophic with fatty degeneration. Note the atrophic optic nerve (*arrowhead*) adjacent to the microphthalmic eye. The prosthetic device (*curved arrow*) produces a signal void.

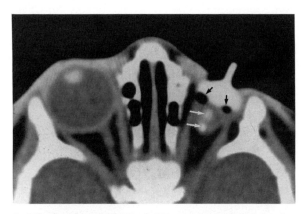

8-1C Axial nonenhanced CT scan. Note the dense foci of fibrous or osseous metaplasia (*white arrows*). Air (*black arrows*) is trapped behind the prosthetic device.

FIGURE 8–2 ***Dermoid Cyst of Conjunctival Origin***
A 37-year-old man presented with a history of painless, progressive displacement of the left eye with horizontal diplopia.

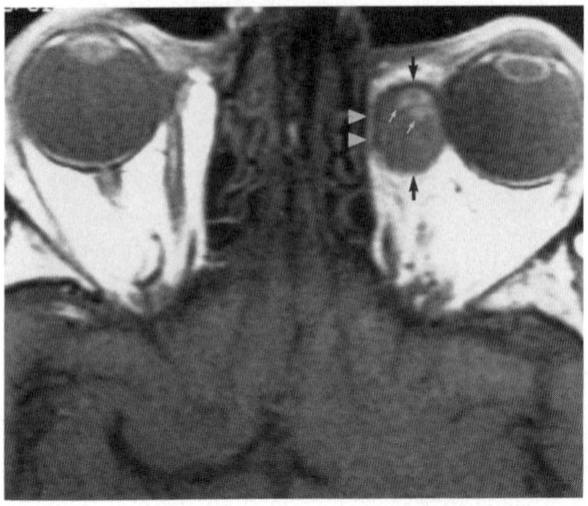

8–2A Axial T1W image. The well-defined cystic mass (*black arrows*) appears slightly hyperintense with respect to the vitreous because of its proteinaceous and water content. The oily material produced by the sebaceous glands has a comparatively higher signal intensity (*white arrows*), and is floating in the superior portion of the cyst. The ethmoid sinus is separated from the cyst by a line of orbital fat (*arrowheads*). The hypointense curvilinear line around the anterior aspect of the lesion represents chemical shift artifact. (From De Potter P, Flanders AE, Shields CL, Shields JA. Magnetic resonance imaging of orbital tumors. *Int Ophthalmol Clin*. 1993; 33:163.)

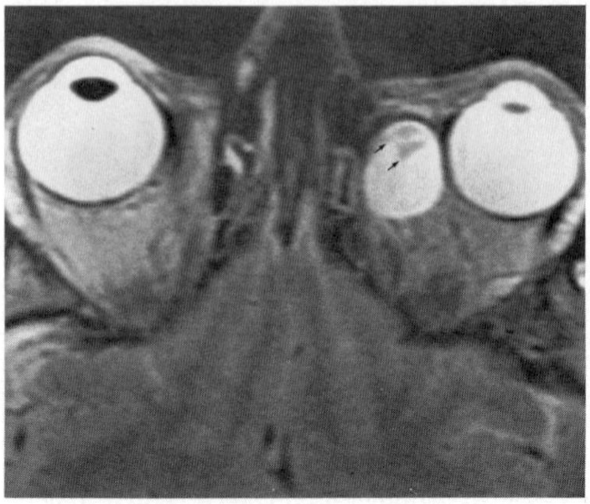

8–2B Axial T2W image. The water and proteinaceous content within the lumen of the cyst becomes hyperintense, whereas the oily sebaceous material (*arrows*) becomes hypointense. (From De Potter P, Flanders AE, Shields CL, Shields JA. Magnetic resonance imaging of orbital tumors. *Int Ophthalmol Clin*. 1993; 33:163.)

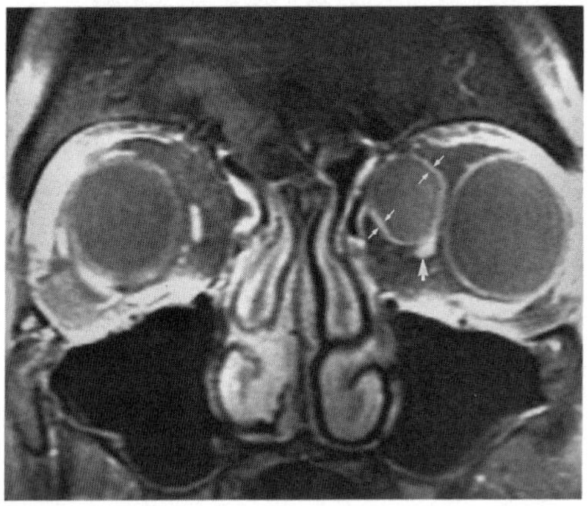

8–2C Fat-suppressed coronal Gd-DTPA–enhanced T1W image. The wall of the cyst demonstrates enhancement (*thin arrows*). The medial rectus muscle (*thick arrow*) is displaced inferiorly.

(continued)

FIGURE 8–2 *Dermoid Cyst of Conjunctival Origin* (continued)

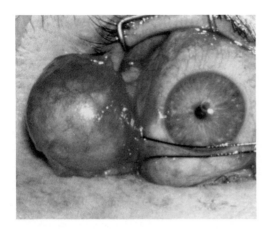

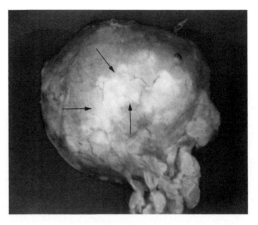

8–2D A clinical photograph shows the mass during its surgical excision via a conjunctival approach.

8–2E Gross appearance of the excised dermoid cyst showing through the thin capsule the oily sebaceous material (*arrows*) floating within proteinaceous material.

FIGURE 8-3 *Microphthalmos with Cyst*
A 3-month-old girl presented with right microphthalmos and colobomatous cyst.

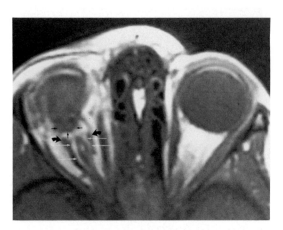

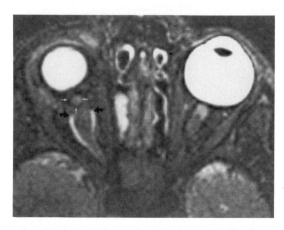

8-3A Axial T1W image. The microphthalmic right eye is contiguous with the cyst (*small black arrows*) at its posterior aspect. The optic nerve sheath complex appears to be dilated. The hyperintense linear signal (*white arrows*) within the optic nerve may represent fatty degeneration. This hyperintense signal is no longer seen on fat-suppressed images (see *B*). The hypointense linear signal (*curved arrows*) adjacent to the hyperintense linear signal likely represents cerebrospinal fluid (CSF). The microphthalmic right eye has an increased signal intensity compared to that of the opposite eye.

8-3B Axial T2W image (inversion recovery). The contents of the cyst (*arrows*) do not appear to be as hyperintense as the subretinal fluid. The hyperintense signal (*curved arrows*) adjacent to the optic nerve probably represents CSF in an arachnoid extension.

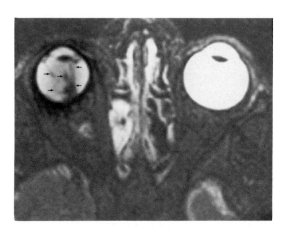

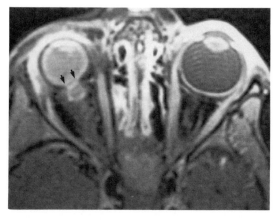

8-3C Axial T2W image (inversion recovery) at a lower level than in *B*. The detached, thickened retina and gliotic tissues produce a hypointense, V-shaped, disorganized signal (*arrows*) with respect to the increased signal of the subretinal fluid. Microphthalmos is obvious on this axial section.

8-3D Fat-suppressed axial Gd-DTPA–enhanced T1W image. The hyperintense signal of the vitreous and of the cyst lumen is more pronounced with fat suppression. Note the colobomatous defect (*arrows*) at the posterior pole.

(continued)

FIGURE 8-3 *Microphthalmos with Cyst* (continued)

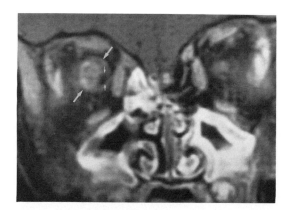

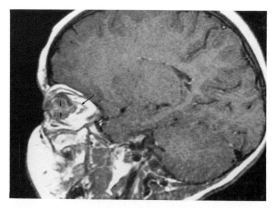

8-3E Fat-suppressed coronal Gd-DTPA–enhanced T1W image. The right optic nerve sheath complex (*long arrows*) is enlarged. The focus of low signal intensity (*short arrows*) between the optic nerve and the meninges most likely represents accumulation of CSF.

8-3F Sagittal Gd-DTPA–enhanced T1W image. The V-shaped, gliotic, detached retina (*short arrows*) demonstrates enhancement, whereas the subretinal fluid does not. The cyst is in continuity with the globe. The increased signal within the optic nerve (*long arrow*) may represent fatty degeneration.

FIGURE 8-4 *Microphthalmos with Cyst*
A 2-month-old infant presented with blue, distended, right lower eyelid. The defect, which was noted at birth, had shown progressive enlargement. (Courtesy of Gerald J. Harris, M.D., Milwaukee, WI)

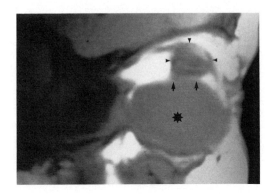

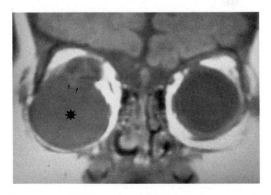

8-4A Sagittal T1W image. The microphthalmic right eye (*arrowheads*) has a heterogeneous signal intensity and is in continuity with a large orbital cyst (*) through the colobomatous defect (*arrows*). The increased signal intensity of the cyst is related to its high proteinaceous content.

8-4B Coronal T1W image. On this section, the enlargement of the right orbit is clearly evident. The dysplastic retina protrudes from the globe into the cyst cavity (*). (From Harris GJ, Dolman PJ, Simons KB. Microphthalmos with cyst. *Ophthalm Surg.* 1992; 23:432. © 1992, Slack, Inc.)

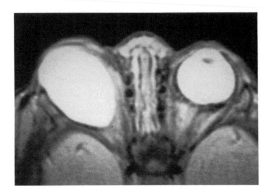

8-4C Axial T2W image at the level of the cyst. The right orbital cyst is hyperintense.

FIGURE 8-5 *Orbital Dermolipoma*

A 16-year-old girl presented with a unilateral yellow mass located superotemporally beneath the bulbar conjunctiva in the right orbit.

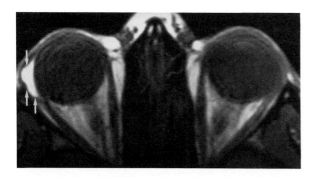

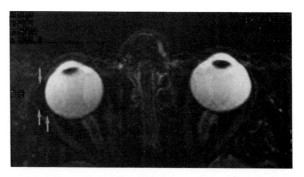

8-5A Axial T1W image. An ovoid-shaped, oblong mass (*arrows*) lies adjacent to the globe and the insertion of the lateral rectus muscle. The mass has an isointense signal relative to orbital fat. The lesion extends posteriorly to the equator of the eye.

8-5B Fast spin echo axial T2W image (FSE). The lesion becomes totally hypointense (*arrows*), as does the orbital fat.

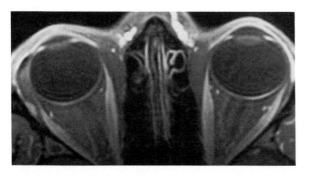

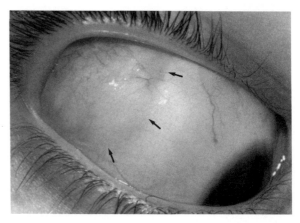

8-5C Fat-suppressed axial Gd-DTPA–enhanced T1W image. The lesion appears isointense with respect to orbital fat and does not enhance.

8-5D Clinical photograph showing the dermolipoma bulging anteriorly beneath the conjunctiva (*arrows*).

MRI of the Eye and Orbit,
by Patrick De Potter, Jerry A. Shields, and Carol L. Shields.
J. B. Lippincott Company, Philadelphia © 1995.

9

Acquired Cystic Lesions

PATRICK DE POTTER

CAROL L. SHIELDS

JERRY A. SHIELDS

IMPLANTATION EPITHELIAL CYST

Clinical and Pathological Features

Secondary or implantation cysts of the conjunctiva are similar to primary congenital cysts except that they develop after displacement of conjunctival tissue from a surgical or nonsurgical traumatic event. Conjunctival implantation cyst has been documented after enucleation, penetrating trauma to the eye, inflammation, and strabismus or retinal detachment surgery. The cyst is usually located on the bulbar or palpebral conjunctiva. In some cases, it may be located deeper in the orbit and may cause painless proptosis and diplopia.

On histopathologic examination, the secondary epithelial cyst contains nonkeratinizing conjunctival epithelium without adnexal structures. The central lumen of the cyst is filled with clear fluid, which may contain mucin if goblet cells are present.

MR Features

On magnetic resonance imaging (MRI), orbital implantation cysts of the conjunctiva appear as a well-circumscribed mass with isointense to hypointense signal with respect to the extraocular muscles and hypointense with respect to orbital fat on T1-weighted (T1W) images (Figs. 9–1, *A* and *B*; 9–2, *A* and *B*). The high cystic content of extracellular water increases the signal intensity on T2-weighted (T2W) images (Figs. 9–1*C* and 9–2*C*). The hemorrhagic contents of the epithelial cyst can be easily identified on spin echo sequences (Fig. 9–3, *A* through *C*). The content of the cyst does not enhance after administration of gadolinium diethylenetriamine penta-acetic acid (Gd-DTPA) (Figs. 9–1, *D* and *E*; 9–2, *D* and *E*; 9–3*D*) (see Table 8–1).

CHRONIC HEMATIC CYST (CHOLESTEROL GRANULOMA)

Clinical and Pathological Features

Chronic hematic cyst of the orbit is uncommon and consists of the accumulation of old blood products in a subperiosteal or intraorbital location. Contrary to chronic hematic cyst, subperiosteal hematoma refers to a recent blood collection that usually is the result of acute trauma. The clinical presentation is nonspecific, and the patient usually has a long history of painless displacement of the globe, often accompanied by diplopia. The lesion is usually caused by remote trauma. Chronic hematic cyst usually occurs in a subperiosteal location, in the temporal portion of the orbital roof.

Histopathologic examination reveals a lesion consisting of a fibrous pseudocapsule surrounding lipid-laden macrophages, chronic inflammatory

131

cells, red blood cells, hemosiderin, and cholesterol clefts. The progressive enlargement of the lesion may be attributable to recurrent hemorrhage into the cyst.

On orbital computed tomography (CT), chronic hematic cyst appears as a well-circumscribed, non-enhancing, subperiosteal lesion with associated expansion and erosion of the superotemporal aspect of the orbital roof.

MR Features

Because of the presence of blood breakdown products, the MR features of a chronic hematic cyst are usually characteristic, allowing differentiation of the lesion from soft tissue tumors of the orbit. The lesion has a high signal intensity on both T1W and T2W images. Chronic hematic cyst shows a homogeneous or heterogeneous isointense signal on T1W images and a hyperintense signal on T2W images with respect to orbital fat (Fig. 9–4, A through C). The heterogeneous appearance of the lesion may be related to the presence of secondary inflammatory granulomatous tissues. Other differential diagnoses that can conceivably have identical MR features include infected dermoids, chronic mucocles, and hemorrhagic tumors (see Table 8–1). After Gd-DTPA administration, the lesion does not enhance (Fig. 9–4D). The nonenhancement of the lesion usually rules out tumors.

MUCOCELE

Clinical and Pathological Features

A mucocele is a cystic, slowly expanding lesion that originates from the sinuses. As the lesion enlarges, it may erode through the periorbital bone into the orbit, nasopharynx, and cranial cavity. The most common sites of origin are the frontal and ethmoid sinuses. Mucocele arising in the sphenoid or maxillary sinus is rare. Characteristically, mucoceles occur in adults with a history of chronically inflamed parasinusal sinuses. Chronic headaches and visual disturbances are common complaints. Displacement of the globe, diplopia, and oculomotor dysfunction can occur. Patients with cystic fibrosis are most likely to develop ethmoidal sinus mucoceles in childhood.

Histopathologic examination reveals that mucoceles are lined by disorganized, pseudostratified, columnar epithelium with a variable degree of acute or chronic subepithelial inflammation. The lumen of the cyst contains entrapped secretory material. On CT scans the sinus is homogeneously opacified by material of soft tissue density. Dense concretions may develop centrally. The orbital extension is well defined with a smooth, bony contour and it rarely shows enhancement unless infected.

MR Features

Mucoceles may have a variable signal intensity depending on the age of the lesion (see Table 8–1). Initially, the lesion shows a low signal intensity on T1W images and a high signal intensity on T2W images owing to the high water content of the mucous secretions. In the chronic stage, the concentration of proteinaceous secretions increases as do the viscosity of the secretions and the slow resorption of water through the mucosa. The mucocele then becomes hyperintense on T1W and T2W images (Fig. 9–5, A through C) and a lesion of much longer duration (years) progressively has a low signal intensity on T1W and T2W images. If a mucopyocele is present, the infection appears to cause increased viscosity with a resulting shortening of the T1 signal. After Gd-DTPA administration, no enhancement is documented.

BIBLIOGRAPHY

Avery G, Tang RA, Close LG. Ophthalmic manifestations of mucoceles. *Ann Ophthalmol.* 1983; 15:734–737.

Bergin DJ, McCord CD, Dutton JJ, Garrett SN. Chronic hematic cyst of the orbit. *Ophthalm Plast Reconstr Surg.* 1988; 4:31–36.

Bilaniuk LT, Zimmerman RA, Newton TH. Magnetic resonance imaging: Orbital pathology. In: Newton TH, Bilaniuk LT, eds. *Radiology of the Eye and Orbit.* New York: Raven Press; 1990, Chap. 5.

De Potter P, Flanders AE, Shields CL, Shields JA. Magnetic resonance imaging of orbital tumors. *Int Ophthalmol Clin.* 1993; 33:163–173.

De Potter P, Kunin AW, Shields CL, Shields JA, Nase PK. Massive orbital cyst of the lateral rectus muscle after retinal detachment surgery. *Ophthalmol Plast Reconstr Surg.* 1993; 9:292–297.

Henderson JW, Farrow GM. *Orbital Tumors.* 2nd ed. New York; Brian C. Decker (Thieme-Stratton); 1980: Chap 4, pp 15–114.

Jakobiec FA, Font RL. Secondary tumors, mucoceles, and metastatic tumors. In: Spencer WH, Font RL, Green WR, Howes EL, Jakobiec FA, Zimmerman LE, eds. *Ophthalmic Pathology. An Atlas and Textbook.* Philadelphia: WB Saunders; 1986:2737–2765.

Johnson DW, Bartley GB, Garrity JA, Robertson DM. Massive epithelium-lined inclusion cyst after scleral buckling. *Am J Ophthalmol.* 1992; 113:439–442.

Kersten RC, Kersten JL, Bloom BR, Kulwin DR. Chronic hematic cyst of the orbit. Role of magnetic resonance imaging in diagnosis. *Ophthalmology.* 1988; 95:1549–1553.

Mafee MF, Putterman A, Valvassori GE, Campos M, Capek V. Orbital space-occupying lesions: Role of computed tomography and magnetic resonance imaging. *Radiol Clin North Am.* 1987; 25:529–559.

Milne HL, Leone CR, Kincaid MC, Brennan MW. Chronic hematic cyst of the orbit. *Ophthalmology.* 1987; 94:271–277.

Mitchell DG, Burk DL, Vinitski S, Rifkin MD. The biophysical basis of tissue contrast in extracranial MR imaging. *AJR* 1987; 149:831–837.

Morax S, Herdan ML, Chouard B. Kystes orbitaires par inclusion conjunctivale après chirurgie orbito-oculo-palpebrale. *J Fr Ophthalmol.* 1987; 10:41–49.

Rootman J. Secondary tumors of the orbit. In: Rootman J, ed. *Diseases of the Orbit.* Philadelphia: JB Lippincott; 1988:427–480.

Shields JA. Cystic lesions of the orbit. In: Shields JA, ed. *Diagnosis and Management of Orbital Tumors.* Philadelphia: WB Saunders: 1989:89–122.

Shields JA, Bakewell B, Augsburger JJ, Flanagan JC. Classification and incidence of space-occupying lesions of the orbit. A survey of 645 biopsies. *Arch Ophthalmol.* 1984; 120:1606–1611.

Som PM. Sinonasal cavity. In: Som PM, Gergeron RT, eds. *Head and Neck Imaging.* St Louis: CV Mosby; 1991: 150–159.

Sullivan JA, Harms SE. Surface coil MR imaging of orbital neoplasms. *Am J Neuroradiol.* 1986; 7:29–34.

Van Tassel P, Lee YY, Jing BS, De Pena CA. Mucoceles of the paranasal sinuses: MR imaging with CT correlation. *AJNR.* 1989: 10:607–612.

Wiot JG, Pleatman CW. Chronic hematic cysts of the orbit. *AJNR.* 1989; 10:37–39.

FIGURE 9-1 *Orbital Implantation Epithelial Cyst of the Extraocular Rectus Muscle*

A 73-year-old man presented with painless proptosis of the right eye 18 years after surgery for a retinal detachment in the same eye.

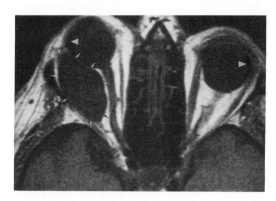

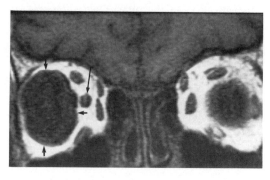

9-1A Axial T1W image. A multiloculated cystic mass (*arrows*) with an isointense signal relative to the vitreous and a slightly hypointense signal relative to the medial rectus muscle is the cause of proptosis of the right eye. The low signal intensity of the septa within the hypointense cystic mass is barely seen. The lateral rectus muscle cannot be identified. Note the signal void produced by the silicone scleral buckle (*arrow heads*) encircling both eyes.

9-1B Coronal T1W image. The cystic mass (*short arrows*) displaces the optic nerve (*long arrow*) medially. The lateral rectus muscle also cannot be identified on coronal planes. (From De Potter P, Kunin AW, Shields CL, Shields JA, Nase PK. Massive orbital cyst of the lateral rectus muscle after retinal detachment surgery. *Ophthalmol Plast Reconstr Surg.* 1993; 9:292–297. © 1993 Raven Press. Used with permission.)

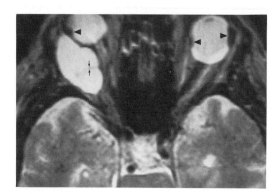

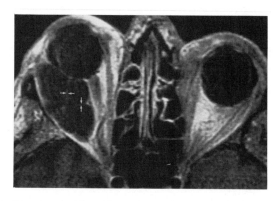

9-1C Axial T2W image. The cystic lesion becomes hyperintense with respect to the extraocular muscles and orbital fat and isointense in relation to the vitreous. The hypointense line within the lesion corresponds to a fibrous septum (*arrows*) separating cystic cavities. The signal void created by the scleral buckling (*arrowheads*) is more easily identified because of the high signal intensity of the vitreous.

9-1D Axial Gd-DTPA–enhanced T1W image. The lumen of the cyst does not enhance, but the cyst wall and internal septae demonstrate minimal enhancement (*arrows*).

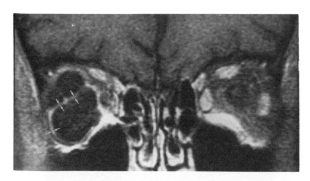

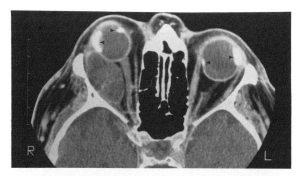

9–1E Fat-suppressed coronal Gd-DTPA–enhanced T1W image. The multicystic appearance of the lesion is well demonstrated. The enhancement of the wall and septa results in easier identification (*arrows*). (From De Potter P, Kunin AW, Shields CL, Shields JA, Nase PK. Massive orbital cyst of the lateral rectus muscle after retinal detachment surgery. *Ophthalmol Plast Reconstr Surg.* 1993; 9:292–297. © 1993 Raven Press. Used with permission.)

9–1F Axial nonenhanced CT scan. The multicystic appearance of the lesion is well visualized owing to the increased density of the fibrous septa. Note the bilateral, hyperdense, scleral buckle (*arrowheads*). (From De Potter P, Kunin AW, Shields CL, Shields JA, Nase PK. Massive orbital cyst of the lateral rectus muscle after retinal detachment surgery. *Ophthalmol Plast Reconstr Surg.* 1993; 9:292–297. © 1993 Raven Press. Used with permission.)

FIGURE 9-2 *Orbital Implantation Epithelial Cyst*

A 16-year-old boy presented with a history of progressive displacement of his right prosthesis. The right eye had been enucleated 14 years before for treatment of unilateral sporadic retinoblastoma. A polymethylmethacrylate sphere was inserted at that time.

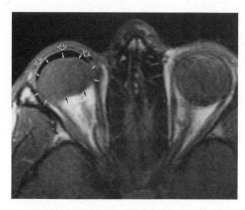

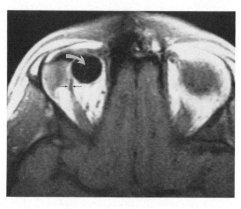

9-2A Axial T1W image. In the anophthalmic right socket, an ovoid cystic mass (*solid arrows*) shows a slightly hyperintense signal with respect to the vitreous of the opposite eye. This is probably related to the high proteinaceous content of the cyst. The lateral and medial rectus muscles reach the cyst wall. The curvilinear signal dropout (*open arrows*) corresponds to the prosthesis. On this plane, the polymethylmethacrylate sphere is not seen.

9-2B Axial T1W image at a higher level than in *A*. The signal dropout of the silastic ball implant (*curved arrow*) is displaced medially. The superior rectus muscle (*arrows*) abuts the lateral aspect of the ball.

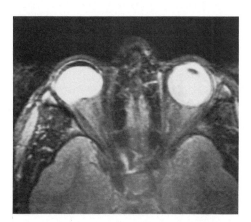

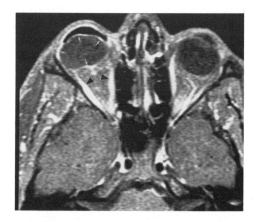

9-2C Axial T2W image. The cyst becomes markedly hyperintense, and isointense to the vitreous of the opposite eye.

9-2D Fat-suppressed axial Gd-DTPA–enhanced T1W image. The lumen of the cyst does not enhance. The thin wall of the cyst (*white arrows*), as well as the lateral and medial rectus muscles (*arrowheads*), demonstrate good enhancement.

FIGURE 9–2 *Orbital Implantation Epithelial Cyst* (continued)

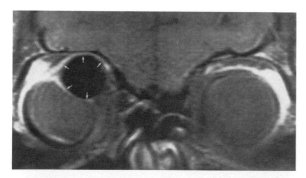

9–2E Fat-suppressed coronal Gd-DTPA–enhanced T1W image. In this plane, the anatomic relation of the cyst and the silastic ball implant is well demonstrated. The enhancing tissue surrounding the orbital implant (*arrows*) probably corresponds to secondary fibrovascular tissue wrapping around the ball.

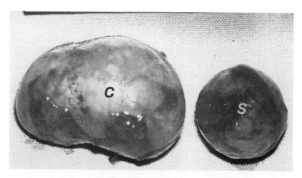

9–2F Gross appearance of the excised epithelial cyst (*C*) and the silastic ball wrapped by fibrovascular tissue (*S*).

FIGURE 9–3 *Hemorrhagic Epithelial Cyst*
A 27-year-old man presented with a 2-week history of ptosis of the left upper eyelid. There was no history of pain, prior trauma, or diplopia. There were no pilosebaceous units, other epidermal appendages, or lymphoid tissues noted on histopathologic examination.

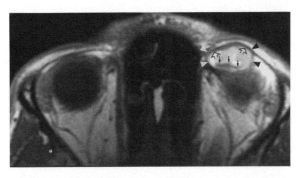

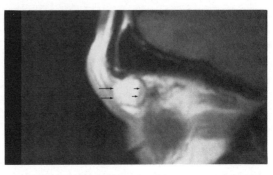

9–3A Axial T1W image. The well-circumscribed lesion (*arrowheads*) exhibits a heterogeneous signal. The predominantly heterogeneous hyperintense signal corresponds to methemoglobin suspension in subacute and chronic hemorrhage. Anteriorly, the capsule is well seen with a low signal intensity (*open arrows*). Posteriorly, the linear rim of hypointense signal (*short black arrows*) may represent chronic hemosiderin deposits.

9–3B Sagittal T1W image. A fluid-fluid level is clearly shown, with probable hemosiderin in the lower portion of the cyst (*short arrows*) and methemoglobin in the anterior portion (*long arrows*).

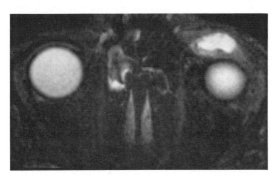

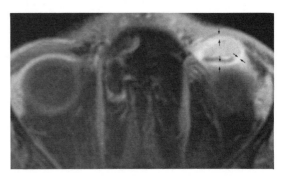

9–3C Axial T2W image (inversion recovery). The heterogeneous signal of the lesion confirms a mixture of hemorrhage in various stages.

9–3D Fat-suppressed axial Gd-DTPA–enhanced T1W image. The lumen of the cyst does not enhance but the capsule does (*arrows*).

FIGURE 9–3 *Hemorrhagic Epithelial Cyst* (continued)

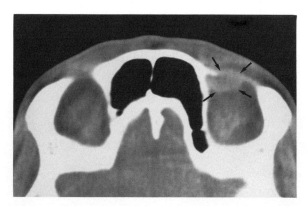

9–3E   Axial nonenhanced CT scan. The cystic lesion (*arrows*) appears to be relatively homogeneous.

FIGURE 9–4 *Chronic Hematic Cyst (Cholesterol Granuloma)*

A 25-year-old woman noted a nontender lump beneath the lateral portion of the right upper eyelid. There was no history of trauma.

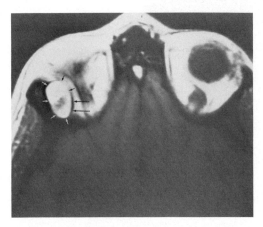

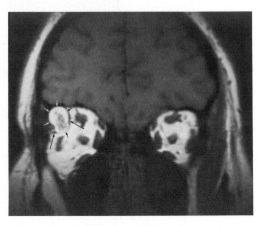

9–4A Axial T1W image. The well-circumscribed mass (*short arrows*), which has a subperiosteal location in the right lacrimal gland fossa, has a heterogeneous signal. There is evidence of bony expansion and erosion. The lesion shows a central hypointense area surrounded by a more hyperintense signal. The peripheral portion corresponds to old blood with cholesterol clefts, and the central portion probably corresponds to granulomatous, fibrous tissue, and hemosiderin. The curvilinear hypointense signal surrounding the cyst corresponds to thin, bony lamella (*long arrows*).

9–4B Coronal T1W image. The lesion (*short arrows*) does not extend intracranially. Note the signal void produced by cortical bone (*long arrows*).

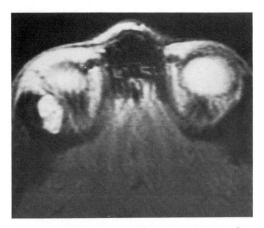

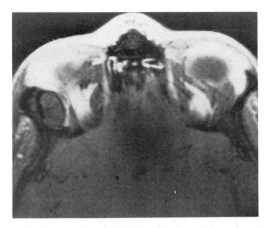

9–4C Axial T2W image. The cyst remains heterogeneously hyperintense with respect to the orbital fat. The vague central area containing granulomatous, fibrous tissue, and hemosiderin appears to be slightly hypointense compared with the peripheral portion.

9–4D Fat-suppressed (incomplete) axial Gd-DTPA–enhanced T1W image. The cyst does not demonstrate enhancement and has a low signal intensity. These MR features are probably related to the suppressed signal from the lipid-laden macrophages and cholesterol in the lesion.

(continued)

FIGURE 9–4   *Chronic Hematic Cyst (Cholesterol Granuloma)* (continued)

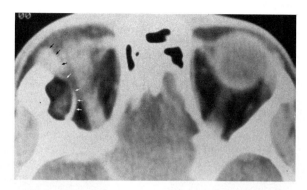

9–4E   Axial nonenhanced CT scan. The hypodense cystic lesion has resulted in expansion of the right lacrimal gland fossa and minimal erosion. The bony lamella (*white arrows*) surrounding the cyst medially is well visualized. The lacrimal gland (*black arrows*) is displaced anteriorly.

FIGURE 9–5 *Mucocele of the Frontal Sinus*
A 54-year-old man with chronic sinusitis presented with a palpable mass in the super-onasal aspect of the left orbit.

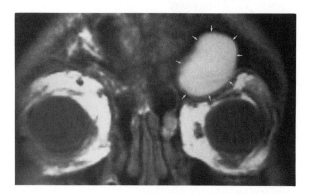

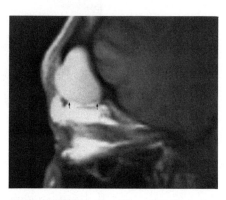

9–5A Coronal T1W image. The well-circumscribed mucocele (*arrows*), with its homogeneous hyperintense signal, has enlarged the left frontal sinus.

9–5B Sagittal T1W image. The orbital portion of the frontal sinus mucocele can be seen through the site of bony dehiscence (*arrows*).

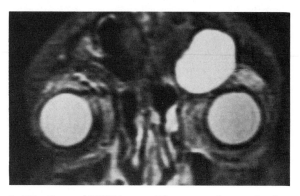

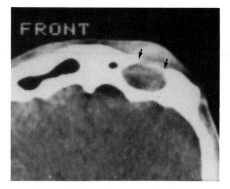

9–5C Coronal T2W image. The mucocele remains hyperintense.

9–5D Axial nonenhanced CT scan. A well-defined cystic mass is seen to fill the enlarged left frontal sinus producing bone destruction (*arrows*).

(continued)

FIGURE 9–5 *Mucocele of the Frontal Sinus* (continued)

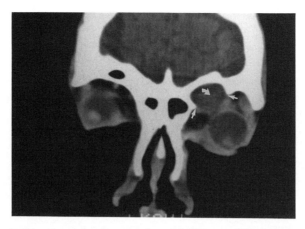

9–5E   Coronal contrast-enhanced CT scan. The homogeneous cystic mass (*curved arrow*) is eroding into the superior portion of the left orbit through a bony dehiscence (*arrows*).

MRI of the Eye and Orbit,
by Patrick De Potter, Jerry A. Shields, and Carol L. Shields.
J. B. Lippincott Company, Philadelphia © 1995.

10
Inflammatory Diseases

PATRICK DE POTTER

CAROL L. SHIELDS

JERRY A. SHIELDS

ORBITAL INFECTION

Clinical and Pathological Features

Clinically, bacterial orbital cellulitis is characterized by acute orbital pain, lid edema, chemosis, proptosis, and limited ocular movements. The patient is usually ill with fever, and often has a history of an antecedent upper respiratory tract infection, recent lid trauma, or sinus infection. Orbital cellulitis can have a preseptal, subperiosteal, intraconal, and/or extraconal location. Preseptal cellulitis is much more common than orbital cellulitis, especially in children. Clinical evaluation and computed tomography (CT) appear to be the best methods to distinguish preseptal from orbital cellulitis. CT scanning of patients with preseptal cellulitis will reveal edema of the lids and subcutaneous tissue anterior to the orbital septum. By contrast, orbital cellulitis is characterized by involvement of the tissue in the orbit itself.

In mucormycosis infections, the usual presentation is that of a rapidly progressive, orbital apex syndrome in a diabetic, immunosuppressed, or debilitated patient. The infection originates from an infection in the palate, nose, or sinuses and spreads by contiguous involvement to the orbit. In aspergillus infections, the infection usually occurs in a healthy individual, and has a much less acute course.

MR Features

Magnetic resonance imaging (MRI) in patients with mucormycosis of the orbit demonstrates inflamed orbital tissues that show decreased signal intensity on T1-weighted (T1W) images and increased signal intensity on T2-weighted (T2W) images. The inflamed sinus mucosa appears thickened, with a low signal intensity on T1W images and low to high signal intensity on T2W images. The involved sinus cavities are opacified with inflammatory exudates that are hypointense on both T1W and T2W images (Fig. 10–1, *A* through *C*). The enhancement pattern of the infectious tissue is variable (Fig. 10–1, *D* and *E*). Absence of enhancement after administration of gadolinium diethylenetriamine penta-acetic acid (Gd-DTPA) may suggest tissue infarction. Evaluation of the cavernous sinus is recommended to determine the extent of the infection.

IDIOPATHIC ORBITAL INFLAMMATION (INFLAMMATORY PSEUDOTUMOR)

Clinical and Pathological Features

The nonspecific orbital inflammatory syndromes have traditionally been termed "pseudotumors," a term used to describe a nongranulomatous idiopathic inflammatory process within the orbit. These syndromes range from a diffuse process affecting the anterior, posterior, or entire orbit to a localized process that targets a specific orbital structure, such as extraocular muscle, lacrimal gland, or sclera. In this acute form, the patient typically presents with an abrupt onset of pain, proptosis, diplopia, and sometimes, visual impairment. The chronic form may represent a sequela of acute recurrent orbital inflammation or may present insidiously as a subacute process. Acute idiopathic orbital inflammation tends to occur in younger patients with clinical and radiologic signs of sinusitis.

In nonspecific orbital inflammatory syndromes, there is a nonspecific polymorphous infiltrate of inflammatory cells—notably, neutrophils, lymphocytes, plasma cells, and macrophages—with various amounts of fibrosis depending on the chronicity. The inflammatory process may be diffuse or localized. No epithelioid cells, giant cells, or well-defined germinal centers are found. CT scanning is quite helpful in delineating the five anatomic patterns of idiopathic orbital inflammation: anterior, posterior, diffuse, lacrimal, and myositic. Although usually confined to the orbital soft tissues, idiopathic orbital inflammation can produce bone destruction or extraorbital extension.

MR Features

In the diffuse form, idiopathic orbital inflammation generally appears as an infiltrative process of the orbital fat with an intraconal and/or extraconal location and possible involvement of the lacrimal gland and extraocular muscles. It may also mold to the globe or the optic nerve sheath complex. The infiltrative process usually appears isointense or slightly hyperintense with respect to extraocular muscles and hypointense with respect to orbital fat on T1W images (Figs. 10–2A and 10–3A). On standard and fast spin echo T2W images the lesion shows variable signal intensity ranging from isointense to slightly hyperintense or markedly hyperintense (Figs. 10–2, B and C; 10–3B; and Table 10–1). Other infiltrative orbital lesions that could conceivably have MR characteristics include lymphoproliferative disorders, metastases, capillary hemangioma, and plexiform neurofibroma. However, the age of the patient, the clinical presentation and other systemic findings may help the clinician or radiologist in the diagnostic approach (Table 10–1). The acute form, which is often associated with tissue edema, shows a greater increase in signal intensity on T2W images than does the chronic sclerosing form, which usually contains more tissue fibrosis. A reticular pattern of the orbital fat is

TABLE 10–1 *MR Features of the Most Common Ill-Defined Infiltrative Orbital Lesions on Spin Echo Sequences*

	Signal Intensity and Appearance with Respect to Orbital Fat		Degree of Lesion Enhancement after Gd-DTPA
	T1WI	*T2WI*	
Acute idiopathic orbital inflammation	Hypo	Hyper	+ + +
	Homo	Homo	Homo
Chronic/sclerosing idiopathic orbital inflammation	Hypo	Iso	+
	Homo	Homo	Homo
Lymphoproliferative disorders	Hypo	Iso/Hyper	+ + +
	Homo	Homo	Homo
Metastasis	Hypo	Hyper	+/+ + +
	Homo/Hetero	Homo/Hetero	Homo/Hetero
Capillary hemangioma	Hypo	Hyper	+ + +
	Homo/Hetero	Homo/Hetero	Homo/Hetero
Plexiform neurofibroma	Hypo	Hyper	+ + +
	Homo	Homo	Homo

T1WI, T1-weighted image; *T2WI*, T2-weighted image; *Gd-DTPA*, gadolinium ethylenetriamine penta-acetic acid; Hypo, hypointense; Iso, isointense; Hyper, hyperintense; Homo, homogeneous; Hetero, heterogeneous.

highly suggestive of idiopathic orbital inflammation. The presence of bone scalloping or erosion can be detected on MR scans. In the localized form, the selected enlargement of one or more extraocular muscles (orbital myositis) may simulate dysthyroid orbitopathy (Fig. 10–4, *A* and *B*). However, in contrast to dysthyroid orbitopathy, the muscle tendons in orbital myositis are usually enlarged.

After Gd-DTPA injection, enhancement of the infiltrative process may be variable. Marked enhancement is usually seen in the acute form of the disease (Fig. 10–2, *D* and *E*). Minimal to moderate enhancement is often seen in the chronic and sclerosing type of idiopathic orbital inflammation (Fig. 10–3, *C* through *F*; Table 10–1). Delineation of the infiltrative process is best accomplished with postcontrast studies using fat suppression technique and on fast spin echo sequences. Extension to the cavernous sinus and the brain can easily be identified on postcontrast MRI studies.

DYSTHYROID ORBITOPATHY (GRAVES' DISEASE)

Clinical and Pathological Features

Dysthyroid orbitopathy (Graves' disease) is an inflammatory condition in which orbital tissues, particularly the extraocular muscles, are affected by an immune disorder with both cell-mediated and humoral components. It is the most common cause of unilateral and bilateral exophthalmos and is most prevalent in women. Dysthyroid orbitopathy may precede, follow, or coexist with hyperthyroidism or hypothyroidism. The presence of eyelid lag, upper lid retraction, and diffuse conjunctival edema and vascular injection at the insertions of the rectus muscles helps to differentiate dysthyroid orbitopathy from other conditions producing proptosis.

On histopathologic examination, the inflammation is virtually always restricted to the muscle bellies of the extraocular muscles and consists mostly of lymphocytes and plasma cells, with a scattering of mast cells in a perivascular location. Endomysial fibrosis and mucopolysaccharide deposits are evident. CT studies reveal the enlargement of one or more extraocular rectus muscles. Although the posterior and middle thirds of the muscle bellies are affected, the tendons near their insertions are usually not thickened.

MR Features

The excellent inherent soft tissue contrast of MRI provides exquisite morphologic information

regarding the involvement of the extraocular rectus muscles in dysthyroid orbitopathy. The inferior rectus muscle is the most frequently affected muscle. The medial and superior rectus-levator complex is the next most frequently involved (Figs. 10–5; 10–6, *A* through *C*; 10–7, *A* through *C*). The sparing of the tendons of the affected rectus muscles (Fig. 10–7C) helps to differentiate dysthyroid orbitopathy from idiopathic inflammatory orbital myositis or neoplastic infiltration of extraocular muscles, in which both the rectus muscles and their tendons are typically enlarged. Because of its multiplanar capability, MRI is very helpful in demonstrating the relationship of the extraocular muscles to the optic nerve at the orbital apex, particularly if surgery is contemplated (Fig. 10–7B). Muscle enhancement is best evaluated on fat suppressed Gd-DTpA enhanced T1W images.

BIBLIOGRAPHY

Armington WG, Bilaniuk LT. The radiologic evaluation of the orbit: Conal and intraconal lesions. Semin Ultrasound, CT and MR. 1988; 9:455–473.

Atlas SW, Grossman RI, Savino PJ, Sergott RC, Schatz NJ, Bosley TM, Hackney DB, Bilaniuk LT, Goldberg HI, Zimmerman RA. Surface coil MR of orbital pseudotumor. *AJNR*. 1987; 8:141–146.

Bilaniuk LT, Zimmerman RA, Newton TH. Magnetic resonance imaging: Orbital pathology. In: Newton TH, Bilaniuk LT, eds. *Radiology of the Eye and Orbit*. New York: Raven Press; 1990, Chap 5.

Centeno RS, Bentson JR, Mancuso AA. CT scanning in rhinocerebral mucormycosis and aspergillosis. *Radiology*. 1981; 140:383–389.

Frohman LP, Kupersmith MJ, Lang J, Reede D, Bergeron RT, Aleksic S, Trasi S. Intracranial extension and bone destruction in orbital pseudotumor. *Arch Ophthalmol*. 1986; 104:380–384.

Jakobiec FA, Font RL. Noninfectious orbital inflammations. In: Spencer WH, Font RL, Green WR, Howes EL, Jakobiec FA, Zimmerman LE, eds. *Ophthalmic Pathology. An Atlas and Textbook*. Philadelphia: WB Saunders; 1986:2765–2812.

Jakobiec FA, Font RL. Orbital infections. In: Spencer WH, Font RL, Green WR, Howes EL, Jakobiec FA, Zimmerman LE, eds. *Ophthalmic Pathology. An Atlas and Textbook*. Philadelphia: WB Saunders; 1986: 2812–2842.

Kennerdell JS, Dresner SC. The nonspecific orbital inflammatory syndromes. *Surv Ophthalmol*. 1984; 29: 93–103.

Mafee MF, Putterman A, Valvassori GE, Campos M, Capek V. Orbital space-occupying lesions: Role of computed tomography and magnetic resonance imaging. *Radiol Clin North Am*. 1987; 25:529–559.

Nugent RA, Rootman J, Robertson WD, Lapointe JS, Harrison PB. Acute orbital pseudotumors: Classification and CT features. *AJNR.* 1981; 2:431–436.

Rootman J, Robertson W, Lapointe JS. Inflammatory diseases. In: Rootman J, ed. *Diseases of the Orbit.* Philadelphia: JB Lippincott; 1988:143–204.

Sergott RC, Glaser JS. Graves' ophthalmopathy. A clinical and immunological review. *Surv Ophthalmol.* 1981; 26:1–21.

Shields JA. Inflammatory conditions that can simulate neoplasms. In: Shields JA, ed. *Diagnosis and Management of Orbital Tumors.* Philadelphia: WB Saunders; 1989:67–85.

Shields JA, Bakewell B, Augsburger JJ, Flanagan JC. Classification and incidence of space-occupying lesions of the orbit. A survey of 645 biopsies. *Arch Ophthalmol.* 1984; 120:1606–1611.

Stefanyszyn MA, Harley RD, Penne RB. Orbital infections. In: Nelson LB, Calhoun JH, Harley RD, eds. *Pediatric Ophthalmology.* 3rd ed. Philadelphia: WB Saunders; 1991:360–364.

Trokel SL, Jakobiec FA. Correlation of CT scanning and pathologic features of ophthalmic Graves' disease. *Ophthalmology.* 1981; 88:553–564.

Weber AL, Mikulis DK. Inflammatory disorders of the paraorbital sinuses and their complications. *Radiol Clin North Am.* 1987; 25:615–630.

FIGURE 10–1 *Mucormycosis with Orbital Involvement*
A 42-year-old diabetic woman experienced progressive right external ophthalmoplegia.
Biopsy of the right maxillary sinus confirmed mucor. (Courtesy of Mary A. Stefanyszyn,
M.D., Philadelphia.)

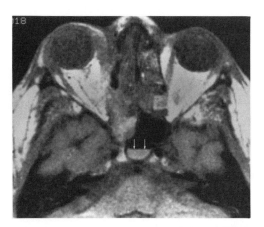

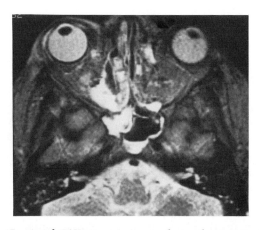

10–1A Axial T1W image. Material of heterogeneous signal intensity is seen in the ethmoid and sphenoid sinuses, as well as in the right orbit. A fluid-fluid level with high signal intensity is identified (*arrows*). The areas of increased signal intensity probably correspond to the presence of macromolecules.

10–1B Axial T2W image. A mixed signal intensity is noted secondary to the hemorrhagic and inflammatory changes. The areas of low signal intensity are due to high viscosity and lack of free water. The inflamed sphenoid mucosa is hyperintense.

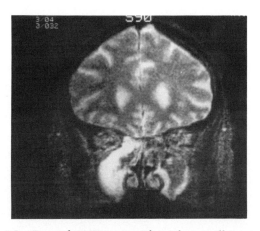

10–1C Coronal T2W image. The right maxillary sinus is filled by a hyperintense material. The inflamed mucosa of the left maxillary sinus is hyperintense.

(continued)

FIGURE 10–1 *Mucormycosis with Orbital Involvement* (continued)

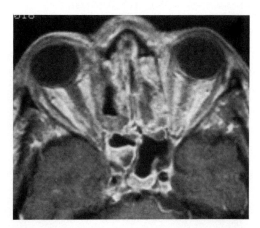 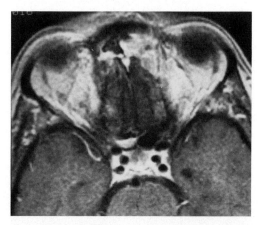

10–1D Axial Gd-DTPA–enhanced T1W image. The inflammatory tissue shows heterogeneous enhancement. Note the fluid-fluid level in the sphenoid sinus.

10–1E Axial Gd-DTPA–enhanced T1W image at the level of the cavernous sinus. The cavernous sinus appears not to be involved.

FIGURE 10-2 *Acute Idiopathic Inflammatory Orbital Pseudotumor*

A 34-year-old man presented with a history of sudden onset of painful swelling of the right upper lid associated with diplopia. His symptoms were completely alleviated with a high dose of systemic steroids.

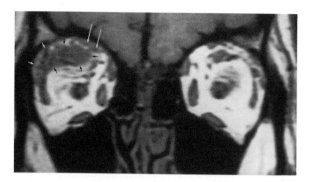

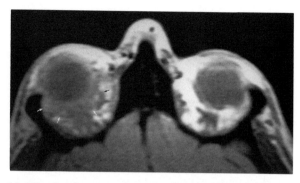

10-2A Coronal T1W image. A poorly defined infiltrative lesion (*short arrows*) with an isointense signal relative to the extraocular muscles is seen to encircle the superior rectus and levator palpebrae superioris muscles. Note the supraorbital artery and nerve (*long arrows*) and the extension to the lateral rectus muscle. The orbital roof is not involved by the process.

10-2B Axial proton density–weighted image. The orbital fat adjacent to the sclera is infiltrated by the ill-defined mass (*arrows*) that is hypointense with respect to orbital fat.

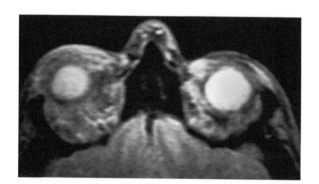

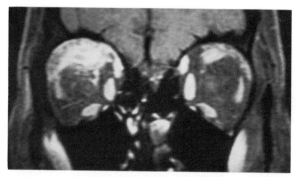

10-2C Axial T2W image. The infiltrative process remains hypointense.

10-2D Fat-suppressed coronal Gd-DTPA–enhanced T1W image. The lesion enhances markedly. The extraocular rectus muscles show normal enhancement.

(continued)

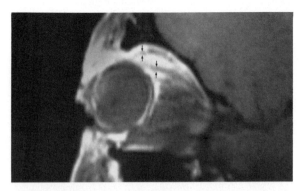

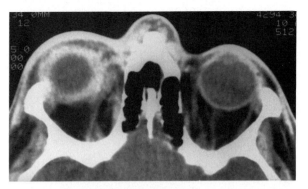

10–2E Fat-suppressed parasagittal Gd-DTPA–enhanced T1W image. The superior rectus and levator palpebrae superioris muscles (*arrows*) are slipped with the enhancing ill-defined lesion.

10–2F Axial contrast-enhanced CT scan. The sclera appears thickened by the infiltrative process.

FIGURE 10–3 *Sclerosing Idiopathic Orbital Inflammation*
A 65-year-old woman presented with a history of progressive, painless, blurred vision in the left eye with no proptosis or diplopia. Histopathologic features were consistent with sclerosing orbital inflammation. (Courtesy of Marlon Maus, M.D. and Peter J. Savino, M.D., Philadelphia.)

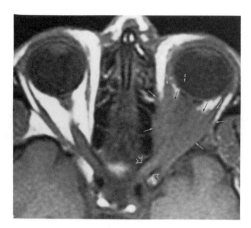

10–3A Axial T1W image. An infiltrative process with low signal intensity has an intraconal and extraconal location (*closed arrows*). The inflammatory tissue blends with the lateral and medial rectus muscles. The optic canal is not widened by the mass (*open arrows*).

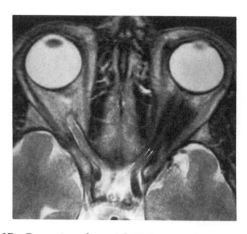

10–3B Fast spin echo axial T2W image (FSE). The ill-defined inflammatory tissue appears hypointense, and the extraocular muscles can easily be identified. The lesion extends up to the orbital entrance of the optic canal (*arrows*).

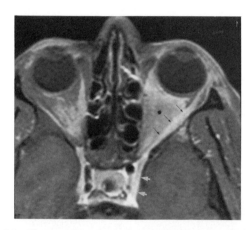

10–3C Fat-suppressed axial Gd-DTPA–enhanced T1W image at the level of the superior orbital fissure. The enhancing infiltrative process extends posteriorly to the left cavernous sinus (*white arrows*), through the superior orbital fissure. The enhancement of the inflammatory tissue (*) is less marked than that of the extraocular muscles (*black arrows*).

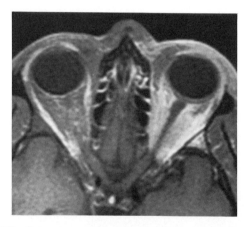

10–3D Fat-suppressed axial Gd-DTPA–enhanced T1W image at the level of the optic canal. The enhancing inflammatory tissue is well delineated at the orbital apex.

(continued)

FIGURE 10–3 *Sclerosing Idiopathic Orbital Inflammation* (continued)

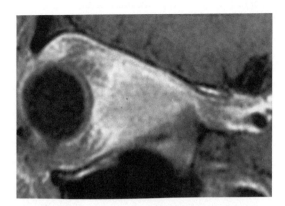

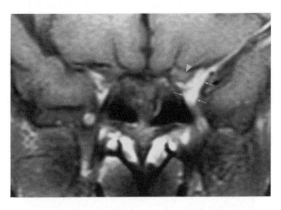

10–3E Fat-suppressed parasagittal Gd-DTPA–enhanced T1W image. The ill-defined orbital inflammatory tissue enhances homogeneously. Abnormal cavernous sinus enhancement is also seen.

10–3F Fat-suppressed coronal Gd-DTPA–enhanced T1W image. The left cavernous sinus is infiltrated by the enhancing lesion (*arrows*). The optic nerve (*arrowhead*) does not show enhancement.

FIGURE 10–4 *Idiopathic Orbital Myositis*

A 45-year-old woman presented with a history of abrupt onset of left orbital pain and vertical diplopia. Her symptoms were completely alleviated by administration of systemic steroids. (Courtesy of Antonella Boschi, M.D., Brussels, Belgium.)

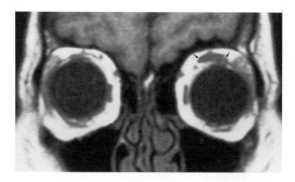 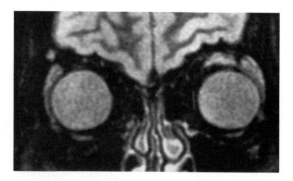

10–4A Coronal T1W image. The left superior rectus and levator palpebrae superioris muscles are slightly enlarged (*arrows*). There is no infiltration of the surrounding orbital fat. The left lacrimal gland is also slightly enlarged.

10–4B Coronal T2W image (inversion recovery). The increased signal intensity of the enlarged superior rectus and levator palpebrae superioris muscles probably reflects the presence of edema.

FIGURE 10–5 *Unilateral Dysthyroid Orbitopathy*
A 38-year-old woman presented with minimal left upper eyelid retraction. (Courtesy of Antonella Boschi, M.D., Brussels, Belgium.) A coronal T1W image demonstrates slight enlargement of the left inferior rectus muscle (*arrow*). The other extraocular rectus muscles are not involved.

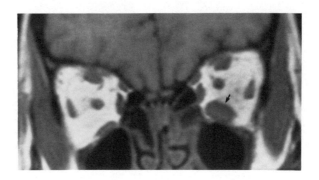

FIGURE 10-6 *Bilateral Dysthyroid Orbitopathy*
A 60-year-old woman presented with bilateral proptosis, eyelid lag, and upper eyelid retraction. (Courtesy of Antonella Boschi, M.D., Brussels, Belgium.) A coronal T1W image (A), a T2W image (inversion recovery) image (B), and a gradient echo image (C) demonstrate bilateral enlargement of the medial rectus, inferior rectus, and superior rectus-levator complex muscles. The enlarged muscles show increased signal intensity.

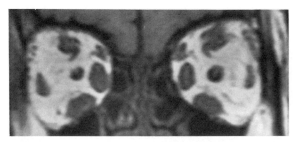

10-6A

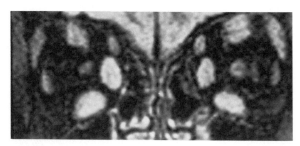

10-6B

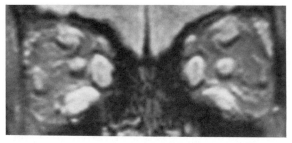

10-6C

FIGURE 10–7 *Bilateral Dysthyroid Orbitopathy*
A 70-year-old woman presented with advanced bilateral Graves' disease. (Courtesy of
Antonella Boschi, M.D., Brussels, Belgium.)

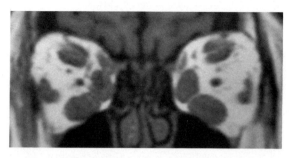

10–7A Coronal T1W image. All rectus muscles, and
particularly, the medial and inferior rectus muscles, are
enlarged bilaterally.

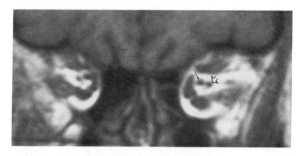

10–7B Coronal T1W image near the orbital apex. There
is no compression of the optic nerve (*arrow*) by the enlarged rectus muscles. Note the ophthalmic artery (*open
arrow*).

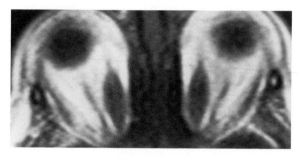

10–7C Axial T1W image. The enlarged bellies of both
medial rectus muscles, as well as the lack of involvement
of their tendons, are well visualized.

MRI of the Eye and Orbit,
by Patrick De Potter, Jerry A. Shields, and Carol L. Shields.
J. B. Lippincott Company, Philadelphia © 1995.

11

Vascular Tumors

PATRICK DE POTTER

CAROL DOLINSKAS

CAROL L. SHIELDS

JERRY A. SHIELDS

CAPILLARY HEMANGIOMA

Clinical and Pathological Features

Orbital capillary hemangioma occurs primarily in children during the first year of life and is usually apparent at birth. Capillary hemangioma often increases in size during the first 6 months of life, subsequently undergoing spontaneous involution when the child reaches the age of 2 to 3 years. If the mass involves the anterior orbital tissue, a bluish fluctuant mass is visible or palpable beneath the eyelid. Deeper involvement produces proptosis or displacement of the globe. The proptosis or eyelid fullness characteristically enlarges when the baby cries or strains.

Capillary hemangioma represents an abnormal growth of blood vessels dominated by varying degrees of endothelial proliferation. Microscopic examination reveals the capillary hemangioma to be composed of lobules of well-differentiated capillary endothelial cells and numerous capillaries separated by fibrous tissue septa. The most common location of a capillary hemangioma is the extraconal superior nasal quadrant. On computed tomography (CT), tumor margins may appear well defined or infiltrating, with extension to any orbital compartment and, in some cases, with intracranial extension via the optic canal or the superior orbital fissure. After administration of contrast agent, capillary hemangiomas enhance moderately to mark-

edly, depending on the degree of involution of the lesion.

MR Features

On magnetic resonance imaging (MRI), capillary hemangioma presents as a fairly well or poorly marginated lesion with homogeneous to heterogeneous low signal intensity on T1-weighted (T1W) images with respect to orbital fat, and a high signal intensity with respect to the extraocular muscles (Figs. 11–1, *A* through *C*; 11–2, *A* and *B*). On T2-weighted (T2W) images, the lesion has a high signal intensity with respect to fat and to the extraocular muscles [Figs. 11–1D and 11–2C (see Tables 10–1, 11–1)]. Multiple areas of hypointensity corresponding to flow voids may be seen within the lesion. These MR features can be shared by other ill-defined or well-circumscribed orbital lesions (Tables 10–1, 11–1, 11–2). However, the young age of the patient, the clinical presentation, and involution may help the ophthalmologist and radiologist in the differential diagnosis.

On T1W images that have been enhanced with gadolinium diethylenetriamine penta-acetic acid (Gd-DTPA), the capillary hemangioma may demonstrate diffuse heterogeneous or homogeneous enhancement [Figs. 11–1E and 11–2D (see Tables 10–1, 11–1)]. Enhancement of the tumor is best evaluated using fat-suppression techniques in order to separate the enhancement from the orbital fat.

TABLE 11-1 *MR Features of the Less Common Well-Circumscribed Orbital Lesions on Spin Echo Sequences*

| | Signal Intensity and Appearance with Respect to Orbital Fat | | Degree of Lesion Enhancement after Gd-DTPA |
	T1WI	T2WI	
Lymphoproliferative disorders	Hypo Homo	Iso/Hyper Homo	+ + + Homo
Capillary hemangioma	Hypo Homo/Hetero	Hyper Homo/Hetero	+ + + Homo/Hetero
Orbital varix	Hypo Homo/Hetero	Hyper Homo/Hetero	+ + + + Homo/Hetero
Thrombosed varix	Hypo/Iso/Hyper Hetero	Hypo/Iso/Hyper Hetero	− / + Hetero
Orbital metastasis from carcinoid, skin melanoma	Hypo Homo	Iso/Hyper Homo	+ / + + + Homo

T1WI, T1-weighted image; *T2WI*, T2-weighted image; *Gd-DTPA*, gadolinium ethylenetriamine penta-acetic acid; Hypo, hypointense; Iso, isointense; Hyper, hyperintense; Homo, homogeneous; Hetero, heterogeneous.

MR angiography helps to demonstrate the abnormal vascularity, and may suggest the arterial blood supply (Fig. 11–1, *F* and *G*). Conventional angiography may still be necessary if surgical removal is considered.

CAVERNOUS HEMANGIOMA

Clinical and Pathological Features

Cavernous hemangioma is one of the most common primary orbital tumors in adults, generally diagnosed in the fifth decade of life. Proptosis secondary to cavernous hemangioma is often slow in onset and clinical progression. The tumor is usually intraconal and may produce optic nerve compression, diplopia, and orbital pain.

On gross examination, cavernous hemangioma has a violaceous hue. Microscopic examination reveals that the tumor is composed of large, endothelium-lined, venous spaces separated by irregular fibrous connective tissue septa. Because of its stagnant circulation, intravascular thrombosis is often seen. CT scans typically show a well-circumscribed, rounded, intraconal mass that enhances homogeneously but to a variable degree after administration of contrast agent. The enhancement is progressive, with intratumoral accumulation of dye on later scans. Calcified phleboliths are occa-

sionally seen. Because of the lesion's slow growth pattern, adjacent bone remodeling may occur.

MR Features

On MRI, the cavernous hemangioma presents as a well-circumscribed, oval-to-round orbital mass located generally within the muscle cone. On T1W images, the lesion appears to have a homogeneous isointense to slightly hyperintense signal with respect to the extraocular muscles, and a hypointense signal relative to orbital fat (Figs. 11–3*A* and 11–4, *A* and *B*). On T2W images and gradient echo images, the lesion has a homogeneously high signal intensity with respect to fat and the extraocular muscles [Fig. 11–3*B* (see Table 11–2)]. Other differential diagnoses that can conceivably have identical MR characteristics most frequently include neurofibroma, neurilemoma, fibrous histiocytoma, and hemangiopericytoma (Table 11–2). Areas of signal void correspond to calcified phleboliths and may mimic vessels with high blood flow. Gradient echo images are most helpful in differentiating calcification from intratumoral vessels.

Immediately after Gd-DTPA administration, cavernous hemangioma demonstrates heterogeneous moderate enhancement (Fig. 11–3*C*). Delayed scans show increasing enhancement which appears even more homogeneous owing to the pooling of the contrast material within the tumor. Tumor enhancement is best evaluated on Gd-DT-

TABLE 11–2 *MR Features of the Most Frequent Well-Circumscribed Orbital Lesions on Spin Echo Sequences*

	Signal Intensity and Appearance with Respect to Orbital Fat		Degree of Lesion Enhancement after Gd-DTPA
	T1WI	*T2WI*	
Cavernous hemangioma	Hypo Homo/Hetero	Hyper Homo/Hetero	+ + + Hetero (early)/ Homo (late)
Neurofibroma	Hypo Hetero	Hyper Hetero	+/+ + + Hetero
Neurilemoma	Hypo Hetero	Hyper Hetero	+/+ + + Hetero
Fibrous histiocytoma	Hypo Hetero	Iso/Hyper Hetero	+ + + Hetero
Hemangiopericytoma	Hypo Homo	Hyper Homo	+ + + Homo

T1WI, T1-weighted image; *T2WI*, T2-weighted image; *Gd-DTPA*, gadolinium ethylenetriamine penta-acetic acid; *Hypo*, hypointense; *Iso*, isointense; *Hyper*, hyperintense; *Homo*, homogeneous; *Hetero*, heterogeneous.

PA–enhanced T1W images using fat-suppression techniques (Figs. 11–3*D* and 11–4*C*).

LYMPHANGIOMA

Clinical and Pathological Features

The orbit does not normally develop lymphatic channels, and there has been considerable controversy regarding the existence of orbital lymphangioma. Lymphangioma usually produces progressive proptosis in childhood. Superficial lesions involve the conjunctiva and are characterized by the presence of multiple, clear, and partially blood-filled cysts. Deep lesions typically present with sudden proptosis secondary to spontaneous or secondary hemorrhage into the vascular spaces, producing a large dark mass known as a chocolate cyst.

On histopathologic examination, lymphangioma is an unencapsulated, diffusely infiltrating lesion with diaphanous, serous-filled lymphatic channels, collagenous stromal network, and an accumulation of well-formed lymphoid aggregates. Features of new or old hemorrhage can be seen. Orbital CT shows a heterogeneous mass infiltrating the soft orbital tissues. The lesion is poorly defined, and enhancement after contrast administration is variable. Phleboliths may be demonstrable in some cases.

MR Features

A wide range of signal intensity, related to their internal architecture and cystic content, is found in orbital lymphangiomas evaluated by MRI. Lymphangioma appears as a unicystic or multicystic, homogeneous or nonhomogeneous mass with irregular margins. The tumor appears mildly hyperintense with respect to extraocular muscles and hypointense to orbital fat on T1W images and markedly hyperintense on T2W images [Fig. 11–5, *A* through *E* (see Table 8–1)]. This MR pattern is likely secondary to prominent lymphatic cystic channels containing clear fluid. The tendency of orbital lymphangiomas to cause recurrent hemorrhage makes them ideal for MRI, which is sensitive to hemorrhage at all phases (see Table 8–1). Acute hemorrhage in the lesion appears hypointense with respect to orbital fat on T1W images and markedly hypointense on T2W images owing to its high concentration of deoxyhemoglobin. As the hemorrhage ages, the tumor demonstrates a hyperintense signal on T1W and T2W images as a result of lysis of red blood cells with release of paramagnetic methemoglobin. A fluid level may be seen in the cystic portions of the tumor. The superior aspect of the cyst contains the methemoglobin released from the lysed erythrocytes and has a higher signal intensity than the dependent portion of the cyst, which contains the settled cellular elements of the hemorrhage with intracellular methemoglobin (Fig. 11–5, B and D). With further aging of the hemorrhage, the methemoglobin degrades into hemosiderin and ferritin, and the T1W and T2W hyperintensity gradually changes to hypointensity (see Table 8–1).

On Gd-DTPA–enhanced T1W images, the degree of enhancement of orbital lymphangioma is variable [Fig. 11–5, F and G (see Table 8–1)]. Without fat suppression, marked tumor enhancement may not be distinguishable from the high signal intensity of the orbital fat. So, as previously mentioned, postcontrast studies should be performed using fat-suppression techniques if possible to better delineate the extent of the lesion.

HEMANGIOPERICYTOMA

Clinical and Pathological Features

Hemangiopericytoma is an uncommon vascular tumor that originates from the pericytes and usually occurs in the head and neck. In the orbit, the tumor usually produces a progressive, unilateral proptosis. Its most common location is the superior part of the orbit. About one-third of hemangiopericytomas of the orbit will recur.

Microscopic examination reveals a lesion with a prominent vascular pattern of sinusoidal spaces between which are packed ovoid to spindle cells. The tumor is classified into sinusoidal, solid, or mixed patterns depending on the degree of vascularity between tumor cells. More than 50% of hemangiopericytomas of the orbit are completely benign. The benign tumors tend to have an increased number of sinusoidal spaces. Orbital CT scans demonstrate a well-circumscribed mass with homogeneous enhancement. When local invasion occurs, the margins may become indistinct.

MR Features

Based on the authors' experience, orbital hemangiopericytoma presents on MRI as a well-circumscribed mass with an isointense to slightly hyperintense signal with respect to the extraocular muscles and a hypointense signal with respect to orbital fat on T1W images (Fig. 11–6A). The tumor shows a variable signal on T2W images (Fig. 11–6B). On Gd-DTPA–enhanced T1W images, the tumor shows moderate and diffuse enhancement (Fig. 11–6C). Depending on the characteristics of

this tumor, it may be difficult on precontrast and Gd-DTPA–enhanced MR studies to differentiate orbital hemangiopericytoma from a cavernous hemangioma or other well-circumscribed orbital lesions (see Tables 11–1, 11–2).

ORBITAL VARIX

Clinical and Pathological Features

The classic presentation of an orbital varix is proptosis exacerbated by a change in head position or by a Valsalva maneuver. The patient experiences worsening of the "fullness" of the involved orbit when bending over or straining. Acute exacerbation of the proptosis with pain may sometimes be related to hemorrhage or thrombosis within the lesion. Most orbital varices involve the superior ophthalmic vein.

On histopathologic examination, the lesion is found to be composed of a single dominant venous space or a tangle of ectatic venous channels. Intraluminal organizing thrombosis can eventually calcify, forming phleboliths. In some cases, the orbital varix can only be seen on contrast-enhanced CT scans if the patient performs a Valsalva maneuver or if the patient is imaged prone in the coronal plane, as this position will also increase the venous pressure.

MR Features

Venous malformations are well delineated on MR studies, particularly when appropriate sequences to evaluate the blood flow (gradient echo scans) and clinical maneuvers (Valsalva maneuver) are used. On spin echo images, the high blood flow within the superior or inferior ophthalmic vein generally produces a signal void. An increase in size and changes in the configuration or course of the superior or inferior ophthalmic veins, as well as of connecting veins, can easily be detected on precontrast MR scans, with or without a Valsalva maneuver [Figs. 11–7, A through C; 11–8, A through C (see Table 11–1)]. A decrease in blood flow may produce a slight increase in signal intensity. On gradient echo images, the blood flow has a hyperintense signal.

The MR appearance of thrombosis of an orbital varix with sudden proptosis depends on the age of the thrombosis and the paramagnetic properties of the iron moiety of hemoglobin. Absence of signal void caused by lack of flow within a dilated orbital vein suggests the presence of thrombosis. Thrombosis of an orbital varix may produce a heterogeneous signal intensity. The hypointense signal on T1W images and the markedly hypointense signal on T2W images are related to the presence of deoxyhemoglobin. The increased signal intensity is produced by methemoglobin [Fig. 11–9, A through C (see Table 11–1)].

Venous malformations appear as multiple, irregular structures with low signal intensity (see Fig. 11–10, A and B).

On postcontrast MR studies, orbital varices show marked enhancement, particularly after the Valsalva maneuver and with fat-suppression techniques [Figs. 11–7D, 11–8D, and 11–10C (see Table 11–1)]. Thrombosed orbital varix demonstrates minimal or no enhancement (Fig. 11–9D).

BIBLIOGRAPHY

Bilaniuk LT, Zimmerman RA, Newton TH. Magnetic resonance imaging: Orbital pathology. In: Newton TH, Bilaniuk LT, eds. *Radiology of the Eye and Orbit.* New York: Raven Press; 1990, Chap 5.

Bond JB, Haik BG, Taveras JL, Francis BA, Numaguchi V, Mihara F, Gupta KL. Magnetic resonance imaging of orbital lymphangioma with and without gadolinium contrast enhancement. *Ophthalmology.* 1992; 99: 1318–1324.

Coll GE, Goldberg RA, Krauss H, Bateman BJ. Concomitant lymphangioma and arteriovenous malformation of the orbit. *Am J Ophthalmol.* 1991; 112:200–205.

Croxotto JO, Font RL. Hemangiopericytoma of the orbit. A clinicopathologic study of 30 cases. *Hum Pathol.* 1982; 13:210–218.

Davis KR, Hesselink JR, Dallow RL, Grove AS, Jr. CT and ultrasound in the diagnosis of cavernous hemangioma and lymphangioma of the orbit. *CT.* 1980; 4:98–104.

De Potter P, Flanders AE, Shields CL, Shields JA. Magnetic resonance imaging of orbital tumors. *Int Ophthalmol Clin.* 1993; 33:163–173.

Fox SA. Hemangiopericytoma of the orbit. *Am J Ophthalmol.* 1955; 40:786–789.

Haik BG, Jakobiec FA, Ellsworth RM, Jones IS. Capillary hemangioma of the lids and orbit: An analysis of the clinical features and therapeutic results in 101 cases. *Ophthalmology.* 1979; 86:760–792.

Harris GJ, Jakobiec FA. Cavernous hemangioma of the orbit: A clinicopathologic analysis of sixty-six cases. In: Jakobiec FA, ed. *Ocular and Adnexal Tumors.* Birmingham, AL: Aesculapius; 1977: 741–781.

Harris GJ, Sakol PJ, Bonavolonta G, De Conciliis C. An analysis of thirty cases of orbital lymphangioma. *Ophthalmology.* 1990; 97:1583–1592.

Hopper KD, Sherman JL, Boal DK, Eggli KD. CT and MR imaging of the pediatric orbit. *Radiographics.* 1992; 12:485–503.

Huckabee RE, Raila FA. MRI and CT comparison of an orbital cavernous lymphangioma. *Journal of the Mississippi State Medical Assocation.* 1991; 32(10):371–373.

Iliff WJ, Green WR. Orbital lymphangiomas. *Ophthalmology.* 1979; 86:914–929.

Jakobiec FA, Font RL. Vascular tumors and malformations. In: Spencer WH, Font RL, Green WR, Howes EL, Jakobiec FA, Zimmerman LE, eds. *Ophthalmic Pathology. An Atlas and Textbook.* Philadelphia; WB Saunders; 1986:2525–2554.

Lloyd GA. Pleboliths in the orbit. *Clin Radiol.* 1965; 16: 339–346.

Lloyd GA. Vascular anomalies in the orbit: CT and angiographic diagnosis. *Orbit.* 1982; 1:45–54.

Mafee MF, Putterman A, Valvassori GE, Campos M, Capek V. Orbital space-occupying lesions: Role of computed tomography and magnetic resonance imaging. *Radiol Clin North Am.* 1987; 25:529–559.

Mitchell DG, Burk DL, Vinitski S, Rifkin MD. The biophysical basis of tissue contrast in extracranial MR imaging. *AJR.* 1987; 149:831–837.

Orcutt JC, Wulc AE, Mills RP, Smith CF. Asymptomatic orbital cavernous hemangiomas. *Ophthalmology.* 1991; 98:1257–1260.

Rice CD, Kersten RC, Mrak RE. An orbital hemangiopericytoma recurrent after 33 years. *Arch Ophthalmol.* 1989; 107:552–556.

Roden DT, Savino PJ, Zimmerman RA. Magnetic resonance imaging in orbital diagnosis. *Radiol Clin North Am.* 1988; 26:535–545.

Rootman J, Graeb DA. Vascular lesions. In: Rootman J, ed. *Diseases of the Orbit.* Philadelphia: JB Lippincott; 1988:525–568.

Searl SS, Ni C. Hemangiopericytoma. *Int Ophthalmol Clin.* 1982; 22:141–162.

Shields JA. Vasculogenic tumors and malformations. In: Shields JA, ed. *Diagnosis and Management of Orbital Tumors.* Philadelphia: WB Saunders; 1989; 123–148.

Shields JA, Dolinskas C, Augsburger JJ, Shah HG, Shapiro ML. Demonstration of orbital varix with computed tomography and Valsalva maneuver. *Am J Ophthalmol.* 1984; 97:108–109.

Sklar EL, Quencer RM, Bryne SF, Sklar VE. Correlative study of computed tomography, ultrasonographic, and pathologic characteristics of cavernous versus capillary hemangiomas of the orbit. *J Clin Neuro-ophthalmol.* 1986; 6:14–21.

Slamovits TL, Gardner TA. Neuroimaging in neuro-ophthalmology. *Ophthalmology.* 1989; 96:555–568.

Sullivan JA, Harms SE. Surface coil MR imaging of orbital neoplasms. *AJNR.* 1986; 7:29–34.

Winter J, Centeno RS, Bentson JR. Maneuver to and diagnosis of orbital varix by computed tomography. *AJNR.* 1982; 3:39–40.

FIGURE 11-1 *Capillary Hemangioma*
A 3-month-old infant presented with a 3-week history of proptosis of the left eye.

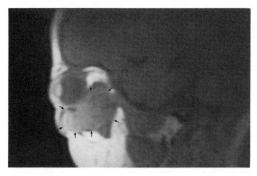

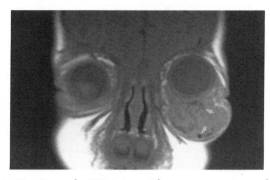

11-1A Sagittal T1W image. A large mass (*arrows*), which is slightly hyperintense in relation to the extraocular muscles, involves both the extraconal and intraconal spaces and displaces the optic nerve and globe superiorly.

11-1B Coronal T1W image. The tumor appears to be well-marginated and displaces the globe superiorly. It has an extraconal location in the anterior orbit. Signal voids within the tumor correspond to blood vessels (*arrows*).

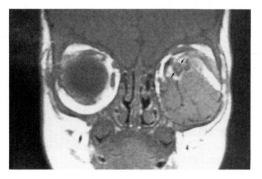

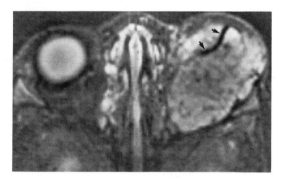

11-1C Coronal T1W image. More posteriorly, the mass demonstrates intraconal extension. The optic nerve is displaced superonasally (*arrows*).

11-1D Axial T2W image (inversion recovery). The mass has a hyperintense signal with respect to the extraocular muscles. A prominent vessel (*arrows*) is seen anteriorly.

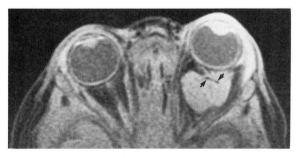

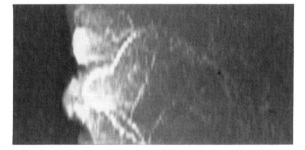

11-1E Fat-suppressed axial Gd-DTPA–enhanced T1W image at a higher level than in *D*. The tumor demonstrates diffuse enhancement. Note the signal void (*arrows*) produced by a vessel with high blood flow.

11-1F 2D time-of-flight MR angiography in the sagittal projection (see *A*). Marked increased vascularity with evidence of feeding and draining vessels is demonstrated.

(continued)

FIGURE 11-1 *Capillary Hemangioma* (continued)

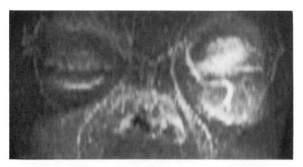

11-1G 2D time-of-flight MR angiography in the coronal projection (see *B*).

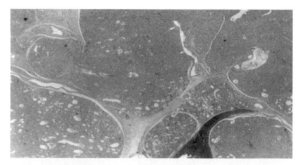

11-1H Low-power photomicrography shows the lobules of vascular tissue separated by connective tissue septa (hematoxylin-eosin ×40).

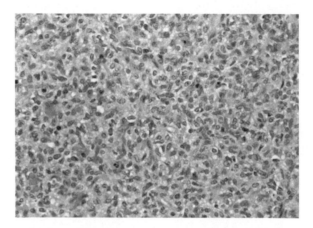

11-1I A higher power photomicrograph demonstrates a dense proliferation of well-differentiated endothelial cells. The lumina of capillaries are not apparent. The histopathologic features of this case may explain the relatively homogeneous signal intensity of the tumor (hematoxylin-eosin ×100).

FIGURE 11-2 *Capillary Hemangioma*
A 3-year-old boy presented with a soft tissue mass involving the left upper eyelid and
extending to the extracranial frontal and temporal regions.

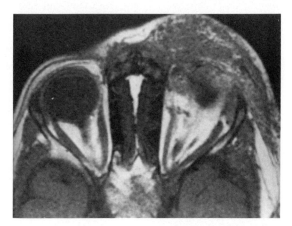

11-2A Axial T1W image. An irregularly marginated
mass with heterogeneously low signal intensity is located
in the left superior orbit and extends to the subcutaneous
tissues of the frontal and temporal regions. The mass
involves the left greater sphenoid wing and pterion.

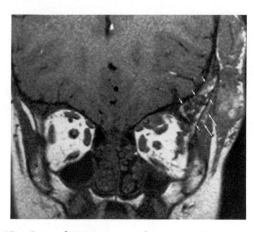

11-2B Coronal T1W image. The mass is located in the
superior aspect of the orbit and infiltrates and expands the
temporalis muscle (*long arrows*) and sphenoid wing (*short
arrows*).

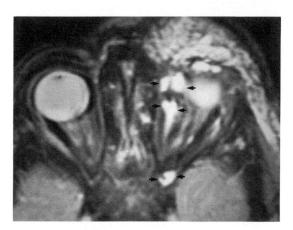

11-2C Axial T2W image. The multiloculated tumor
has a high signal intensity. The irregular intraorbital component of the lesion is well demonstrated as high-inten-
sity strands (*arrows*).

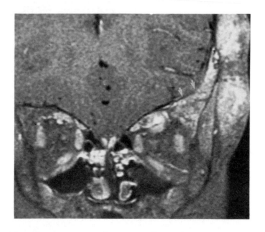

11-2D Fat-suppressed coronal Gd-DTPA–enhanced
T1W image at the same level as in *B*. The components of
the lesion in the orbit, the sphenoid wing, and the temporalis muscle show inhomogeneous enhancement. The
cortex of the greater sphenoid wing is eroded by the lesion
(*arrows*).

(continued)

FIGURE 11-2 *Capillary Hemangioma* (continued)

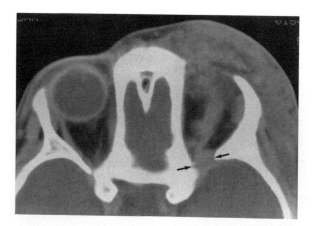

11-2E Axial contrast-enhanced CT scan. The poorly marginated mass has a heterogeneous density. The lesion extends into and expands the superior orbital fissure (*arrows*).

FIGURE 11–3 *Cavernous Hemangioma*

A 65-year-old man presented with a history of progressive horizontal diplopia.

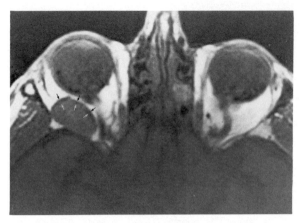

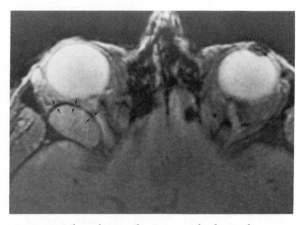

11–3A Axial T1W image. The well-defined oval mass in the temporal quadrant of the right orbit appears to be homogeneously isointense with respect to the extraocular muscles and hypointense with respect to orbit fat. The optic nerve is displaced medially. The tumor is surrounded by a hypointense capsule (*arrows*), accentuated by a chemical shift artifact. There is no bone destruction.

11–3B Axial gradient echo image. The lesion becomes homogeneously hyperintense with respect to the extraocular muscles and hypointense with respect to orbital fat. The hypointense capsule is increasingly discernible (*arrows*).

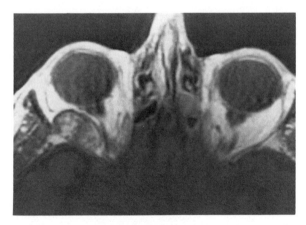

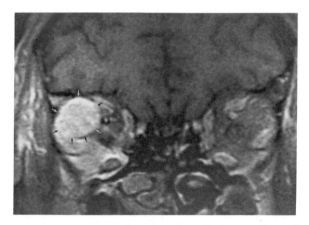

11–3C Axial Gd-DTPA–enhanced T1W image obtained 5 minutes after injection of contrast agent. The tumor demonstrates heterogeneous, patchy enhancement. The capsule does not show enhancement.

11–3D Fat-suppressed coronal Gd-DTPA–enhanced T1W image obtained 40 minutes after injection of contrast agent. The late pooling of the contrast agent within the large vascular spaces in the tumor (*arrows*) produces increasingly homogeneous enhancement.

(continued)

FIGURE 11–3 *Cavernous Hemangioma* (continued)

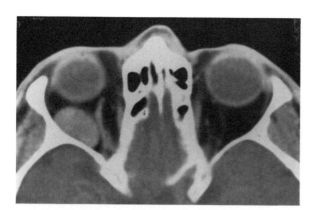

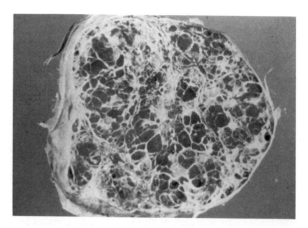

11–3E Axial contrast-enhanced CT scan. The tumor shows diffuse enhancement.

11–3F Low-power photomicrograph of the tumor shows dilated, congested venous channels, the intervening connective tissues creating septa, and the surrounding capsule.

FIGURE 11-4 *Cavernous Hemangioma*
A 38-year-old man presented with a history of intermittent episodes of blurry vision in the right eye.

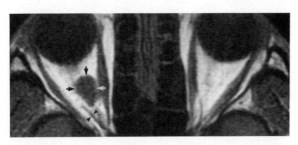

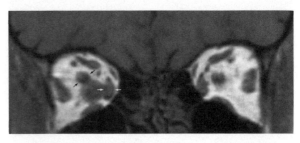

11-4A Axial T1W image. A well-defined intraconal mass (*arrows*) is located beneath the optic nerve. It has a homogeneous, low signal intensity that is isointense to the extraocular muscles. Note the ophthalmic artery (*arrowheads*). (From De Potter P, Flanders AE, Shields CL, Shields JA. Magnetic resonance imaging of orbital tumors. *Int Ophthalmol Clin.* 1993; 33:165.)

11-4B Coronal T1W image. The tumor abuts the optic nerve (*black arrows*) and the medial rectus muscle (*white arrows*).

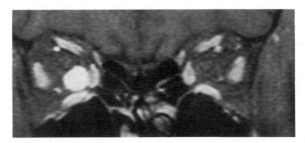

11-4C Fat-suppressed coronal Gd-DTPA–enhanced T1W image obtained 50 minutes after injection of contrast agent. The mass demonstrates late homogeneous and marked enhancement. (From De Potter P, Flanders AE, Shields CL, Shields JA. Magnetic resonance imaging of orbital tumors. *Int Ophthalmol Clin.* 1993; 33:165.)

FIGURE 11-5 *Hemorrhagic Lymphangioma*
A 2-year-old boy presented with a 3-week history of sudden swelling and bluish discoloration of the right upper eyelid after trauma.

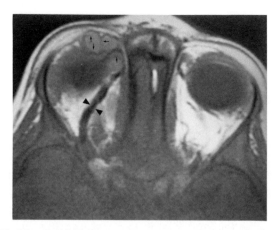

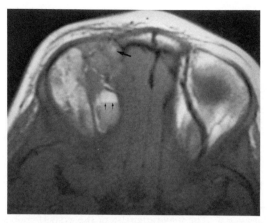

11-5A Axial T1W image. A multiloculated extraconal mass located anterior to the globe has a hyperintense signal compared to that of the extraocular muscles but hypointense signal with respect to orbital fat. This hyperintensity corresponds to blood mixed with fluid or a mixture of blood components. The surrounding septa (*arrows*) appear hypointense, and the superior ophthalmic vein (*arrowheads*) is dilated.

11-5B Axial T1W image at a higher level than in *A*. The lesion extends into the posterior orbit. The cysts appear to be increasingly heterogeneous in signal intensity. The most posterior lymphatic cyst demonstrates a fluid-fluid level. This appearance is explained by the release from lysed erythrocytes of methemoglobin into the superior portion of the cyst (*short arrows*) with resultant marked hyperintensity. The inferior portion of the cyst probably contains intact red blood cells and a mixture of intracellular methemoglobin and dioxyhemoglobin. Methemoglobin is also seen in the central core (*long arrow*) of the anterior medial cyst.

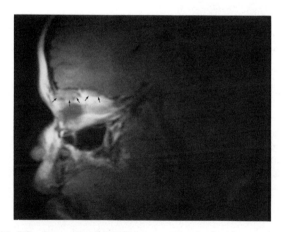

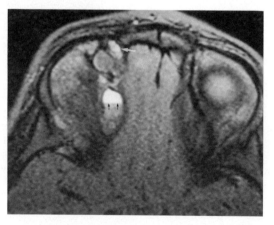

11-5C Parasagittal T1W image. The lesion (*arrows*) is mainly located anteriorly above the superior rectus muscle. The hemorrhagic lymphatic cyst is surrounded by a hypointense septum.

11-5D Axial T2W image at the same level as in *B*. The methemoglobin within the superior portion of the posterior hemorrhagic cyst (*black arrows*) and the central core of the anterior medial cyst (*white arrow*) remain markedly hyperintense. The rest of the lesion, which contains a mixture of blood components, remains moderately hyperintense to orbital fat.

(continued)

FIGURE 11–5 *Hemorrhagic Lymphangioma* (continued)

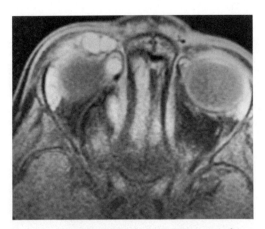

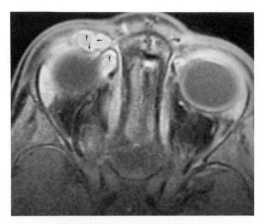

11–5E Fat-suppressed axial T1W image at the same level as in *A*. The hyperintensity of the cysts is increasingly pronounced.

11–5F Fat-suppressed axial Gd-DTPA–enhanced T1W image at the same level as in *E*. Enhancement mainly occurs in the surrounding septa (*arrows*), with minimal change in signal intensity within the cysts.

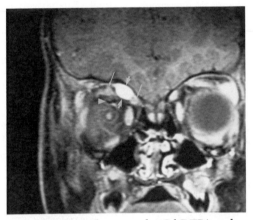

11–5G Fat-suppressed coronal Gd-DTPA–enhanced T1W image. The markedly hyperintense signal corresponds to the portion of the cyst containing methemoglobin (*short arrows*) and is surrounded by the superior rectus and superior oblique muscles (*long arrows*). Note the superior ophthalmic vein (*arrowhead*).

FIGURE 11–6 *Hemangiopericytoma*

A 63-year-old man presented with a 6-month history of proptosis of the right eye.

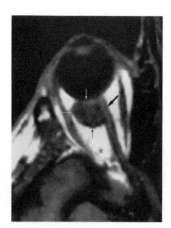

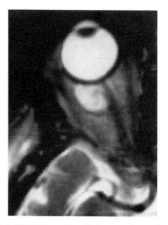

11–6A Axial T1W image. The intraconal, well-circumscribed tumor (*thin arrows*) that abuts the optic nerve (*thick arrow*) has an isointense signal with respect to the extraocular muscles and a hypointense signal with respect to orbital fat.

11–6B Axial T2W image. The tumor is hyperintense.

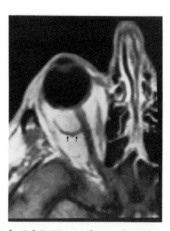

11–6C Axial Gd-DTPA–enhanced T1W image. The tumor demonstrates moderate homogeneous enhancement. Note the chemical shift artifact (*arrows*).

(continued)

FIGURE 11–6 *Hemangiopericytoma* (continued)

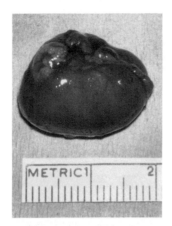

11–6D Photograph showing the resected, well-encapsulated tumor.

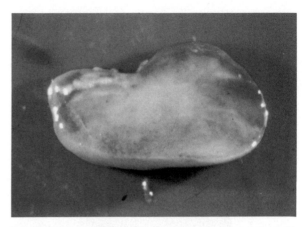

11–6E Gross photograph showing the resected, well-encapsulated tumor.

FIGURE 11-7 *Varix of Superior Ophthalmic Vein*

A 33-year-old woman presented with a 5-month history of intermittent proptosis of the left eye, which was more pronounced in face-down position.

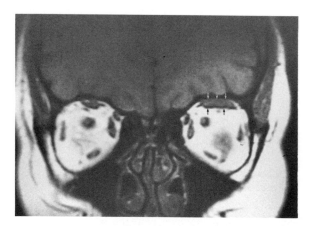

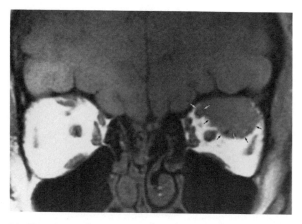

11-7A Coronal T1W image without a Valsalva maneuver. The curvilinear tissue (*white arrows*) juxtaposing the superior rectus-levator palpebrae complex has an isointense signal with respect to the extraocular muscles. The orbital roof remains intact. Note the chemical shift artifact (*black arrows*). (From Rao VM, Flanders AE, Tom BM, eds. *Orbit.* In: *MRI and CT Atlas of Correlative Imaging in Otolaryngology.* London: Martin Dunitz; 1992, chap 8, p 343.)

11-7B Coronal T1W image with a Valsalva maneuver. The mass enlarges massively (*black arrows*), filling the superior compartment of the orbit and displacing the superior rectus muscle medially (*white arrows*).

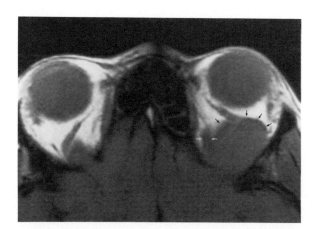

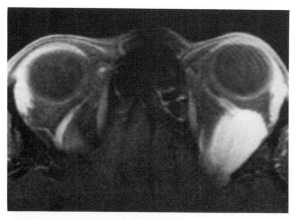

11-7C Axial T1W image with a Valsalva maneuver. The origin of the superior rectus muscle (*white arrows*), which almost blends with the orbital varix (*black arrows*), is displaced medially.

11-7D Fat-suppressed axial Gd-DTPA–enhanced T1W image with a Valsalva maneuver. The enlarged varix demonstrates marked enhancement. On this image, no brain involvement is identified.

(continued)

FIGURE 11-7 *Varix of Superior Ophthalmic Vein* (continued)

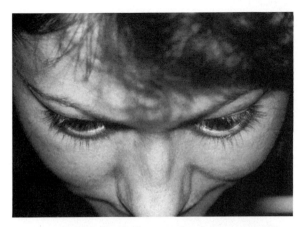

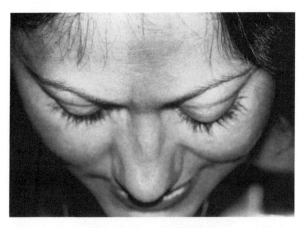

11-7E Clinical facial photograph of the same patient without the Valsalva maneuver.

11-7F Clinical facial photograph of the same patient with the Valsalva maneuver. Note the marked proptosis of the left eye.

FIGURE 11-8 *Varix of the Inferior Ophthalmic Vein*

A 59-year-old woman presented with a history of intermittent positional diplopia and discomfort in the right eye.

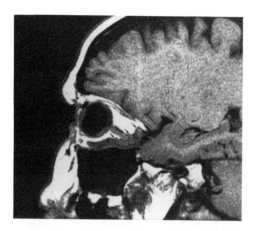

11-8A Sagittal T1W image with the Valsalva maneuver. An elongated mass (*arrows*), which is isointense with respect to the extraocular muscles, is located in the inferior orbit and extends to the orbital apex.

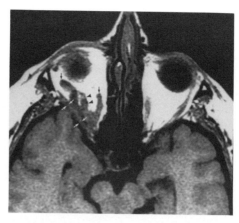

11-8B Axial T1W image with the Valsalva maneuver. The lesion, which is immediately adjacent to the lateral rectus muscle (*white arrows*), demonstrates fingerlike projections (*black arrows*) in the inferior intraconal space. The varix has a more heterogeneous appearance owing to its morphology and differences in the motion of blood within it. The posterior portion of the optic nerve sheath complex (*arrowheads*) is seen on this plane between the projections.

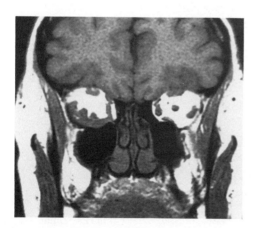

11-8C Coronal T1W image with the Valsalva maneuver. The inferior rectus muscle and optic nerve sheath complex cannot be distinguished from the varix.

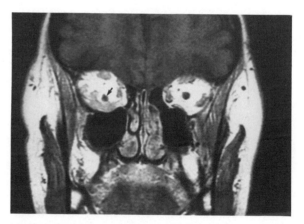

11-8D Coronal Gd-DTPA–enhanced T1W image with the Valsalva maneuver. The hypointense signal of the optic nerve sheath complex (*arrow*) is well visualized and can be differentiated from the enhancing varix.

FIGURE 11-9 *Thrombosed Varix of the Inferior Ophthalmic Vein*

A 63-year-old man presented with a history of sudden onset of vertical diplopia and proptosis of the right eye. A few days before the onset of ocular symptoms, he felt bulging of the right eye when bending down.

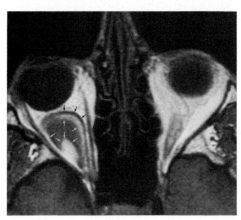

11-9A Axial T1W image. The well-circumscribed intraconal mass has a heterogeneous signal intensity pattern. The central core and the peripheral rim of hyperintense signal correspond to methemoglobin (*white arrows*). The more hypointense area within the lesion corresponds to deoxyhemoglobin. The hypointense demarcation line is the result of chemical shift artifact (*black arrows*).

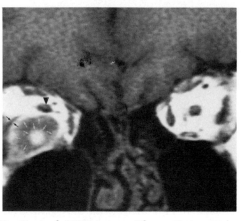

11-9B Coronal T1W image. The optic nerve (*arrowhead*) is displaced superiorly. The dilated inferior ophthalmic vein has a central and peripheral hyperintensity corresponding to methemoglobin (*white arrows*). The curvilinear black margin (*black arrows*) is the result of chemical shift artifact.

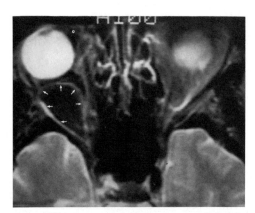

11-9C Axial T2W image. The contents of the thrombosed varix appear to be hypointense. The hyperintense peripheral rim and core demonstrated in *A* become hypointense as a result of the presence of intracellular methemoglobin. The hypointense midportion of the lesion in *A* becomes more hypointense owing to the presence of deoxyhemoglobin. The minimal hyperintense signal at the periphery likely represents the earliest extracellular methemoglobin (*arrows*).

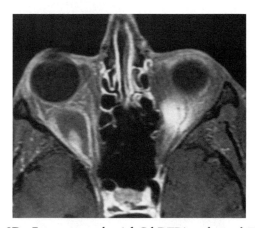

11-9D Fat-suppressed axial Gd-DTPA–enhanced T1W image. No enhancement is demonstrated, suggesting that a tumor is unlikely. The intensity pattern of the hemorrhage remains the same as on the non–fat-suppressed images.

(continued)

FIGURE 11–9 *Thrombosed Varix of the Inferior Ophthalmic Vein* (continued)

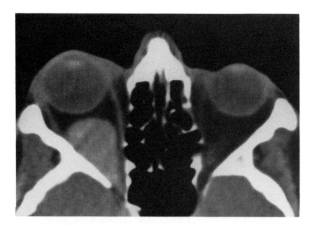

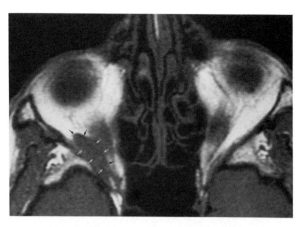

11–9E Nonenhanced axial CT scan. The thrombosed varix appears to be relatively homogeneous and simulates a cavernous hemangioma. No bone erosion or destruction is detected.

11–9F Axial T1W image obtained 5 months after the onset of symptoms. Marked resolution of the previous thrombosis is seen. Residual varix is likely present (*arrows*).

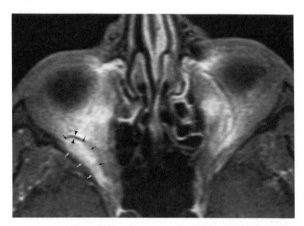

11–9G Fat-suppressed axial Gd-DTPA–enhanced T1W image. The residual varix (*arrows*) shows enhancement. The curvilinear hypointense signal is the result of chemical shift artifact (*arrowheads*).

FIGURE 11–10 *Venous Varicosities*
A 44-year-old woman presented with a vascular malformation in the left orbit. The lesion had a subconjunctival location and produced blepharoptosis.

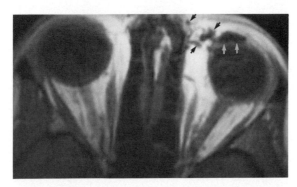

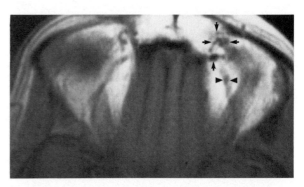

11–10A Axial T1W image. Multiple ovoid and curvilinear hypointense lesions (*black arrows*) are seen in the superomedial aspect of the left orbit. The low signal intensity corresponds to blood flow within the vessels. A larger vascular channel (*white arrows*) is adherent to the sclera anteriorly.

11–10B Axial T1W image at a higher level than in *A*. The dilated superior ophthalmic vein (*arrowheads*) drains the abnormal network of veins (*arrows*) that is located medially.

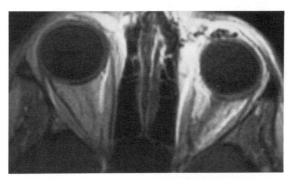

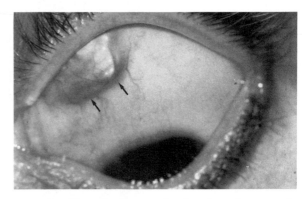

11–10C Fat-suppressed axial Gd-DTPA–enhanced T1W image at the same level as in *A*. The vascular dilated channels demonstrate heterogeneous enhancement. The slower-flowing vessels show enhancement, whereas those with more rapid flow produce signal voids.

11–10D Clinical photograph showing the vascular lesion (*arrows*) beneath the bulbar conjunctiva.

(continued)

FIGURE 11-10 *Venous Varicosities* (continued)

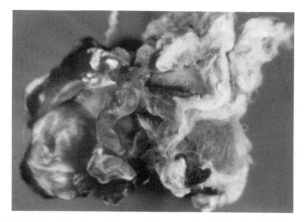

11-10E Gross specimen showing the dilated vascular network.

MRI of the Eye and Orbit,
by Patrick De Potter, Jerry A. Shields, and Carol L. Shields.
J. B. Lippincott Company, Philadelphia © 1995.

12
Peripheral Nerve Tumors

PATRICK DE POTTER

CAROL DOLINSKAS

JERRY A. SHIELDS

CAROL L. SHIELDS

NEURILEMOMA

Clinical and Pathological Features

Neurilemoma (schwannoma) is a benign, well-defined, slowly progressive tumor that arises from a peripheral nerve sheath. The orbital neurilemoma is a tumor of adulthood. The tumor is usually unilateral and solitary and produces proptosis and displacement of the globe. Although it generally does not cause pain, mild discomfort can sometimes occur.

Because the tumor is primarily composed of a proliferation of Schwann cells, some authorities prefer the term schwannoma. The classic histopathologic features of neurilemoma include solid cellular areas (Antoni A pattern) and areas of looser myxoid tissue having stellate or ovoid cells suspended in a mucinous background (Antoni B pattern). Immunohistochemical stains and electron microscopy may be helpful in differentiating neurilemoma from other neural tumors. Orbital computed tomography (CT) demonstrates a well-circumscribed, ovoid to fusiform, intraconal or extraconal mass. Molding or a defect in the orbital walls may be seen. With injection of contrast agent, mild enhancement of the tumor may be noted.

MR Features

On magnetic resonance imaging, isolated neurilemoma appears as a well-circumscribed, oval to elongated mass with the long axis of the lesion usually lying in an anteroposterior direction in the orbit. This ovoid to fusiform configuration of the tumor is suggestive of an expanding peripheral nerve tumor. Most commonly, the tumor has an extraconal location, and it can be associated with a defect in the orbital roof. Loss of the usual signal void between the mass and the brain indicates destruction or thinning of the orbital roof. Neurilemoma may demonstrate either homogeneity or heterogeneity in signal intensity, depending on the histologic features of the tumor. The lesion has an isointense to hyperintense signal intensity with respect to the extraocular muscles and a hypointense signal with respect to orbital fat on T1-weighted (T1W) images (Figs. 12–1*A* through *C*; 12–2*A*). On T2-weighted (T2W) images, the tumor demonstrates variable signal hyperintensity with respect to extraocular muscles and orbital fat. The myxoid portion of the tumor (Antoni B pattern) shows greater signal intensity on T2W images compared to the more cellular portion of the tumor (Antoni A pattern) (Fig. 12–1*D*). A very similar MR pattern can be seen with other circumscribed soft tissue orbital lesions such as cavernous hemangioma, neurofibroma, fibrous histiocytoma, and hemangiopericytoma (see Table 11–2).

On T1W images enhanced with gadolinium diethylenetriamine penta-acetic acid (Gd-DTPA), the orbital neurilemoma demonstrates a varying degree of enhancement within the mass depending on the histologic features of the tumor. The myxoid portion of the lesion usually enhances more than the cellular area of the tumor (Figs. 12–1, *E* through *G*; 12–2, *B* and *C*). Enhancement of the tumor is best delineated on contrast-enhanced scans when fat-suppression techniques are used (Figs. 12–1*G*, 12–2*C*).

NEUROFIBROMA

Clinical and Pathological Features

Neurofibroma is a benign tumor of the peripheral nerve sheath that is characterized histopathologically by a combined proliferation of Schwann cells, endoneural fibroblasts, and axons. Three types of neurofibroma occur in the orbit: plexiform, diffuse, and localized. Plexiform orbital neurofibroma, which has an early onset (first decade of life), is considered to be pathognomonic for neurofibromatosis. The diffuse orbital neurofibroma displays a more variable association with neurofibromatosis and clinically represents an intermediate lesion between the plexiform and localized types. Localized orbital neurofibroma tends to be seen in middle-aged patients and manifests as a solitary mass with a preponderance for the upper orbital quadrants. Occasionally, the tumor may cause pain, which is relieved by surgical excision of the lesion.

On histopathologic examination, plexiform neurofibroma is composed of interwoven bundles of axons, Schwann cells, and endoneural fibroblasts. The tumor is not encapsulated and insinuates throughout the orbital tissues. Orbital CT scans demonstrate contrast-enhancing irregular soft tissue infiltration with bony compensatory changes. Diffuse neurofibroma differs from plexiform neurofibroma only in the absence of the distinct perineural sheath in the latter. The localized neurofibroma is usually well encapsulated and contains loosely arranged, interlacing bundles of spindle cells and collagen fibrils within a mucoid matrix. On CT scan, it appears as a well-circumscribed, rounded-to-oval mass, usually with a homogeneous appearance.

MR Features

MR studies reveal isolated localized neurofibroma to be a well-circumscribed, oval to fusiform mass that is usually located outside of the muscle cone in the superior aspect of the orbit corresponding to the location of the frontal, supraorbital, or supratrochlear nerves. The elongated configuration of the tumor, with its long axis oriented anteriorly to posteriorly in the orbit, is also suggestive of peripheral nerve tumor. On T1W images, the tumor shows a homogeneous or heterogeneous isointense to slightly hyperintense signal with respect to the extraocular muscles and a hypointense signal with respect to orbital fat (Fig. 12–3, *A* and *B*). On T2W images, the tumor appears homogeneously or heterogeneously hyperintense with respect to extraocular muscles and orbital fat. The myxomatous portion of the tumor demonstrates a lower signal intensity on T1W images and a higher signal intensity on T2W images compared with the more cellular area of the tumor, or the portion containing more collagenous tissue (Fig. 12–3*C*). Expansion or destruction of the orbital bony walls may also be demonstrated. Other well-circumscribed orbital tumors may also share the same MR features (Table 11–2).

After Gd-DTPA administration, the localized neurofibroma shows heterogeneous enhancement. The mucoid matrix of the tumor demonstrates greater enhancement than does the cellular region or hyalinized core of the tumor (Fig. 12–3*D*). Fat-suppression techniques are most helpful in delineating the lesion.

Orbital plexiform neurofibroma appears on MRI as an ill-defined, irregular, orbital mass that can extend through the superior orbital fissure. The lesion demonstrates a heterogeneous hypointensity on T1W images and a high signal intensity on T2W images with respect to orbital fat. The associated bony thinning or erosion of the orbital walls may be clearly demonstrated by MR studies. On Gd-DTPA–enhanced T1W images, plexiform neurofibroma shows a variable degree of enhancement, which is better appreciated with fat-suppression techniques.

BIBLIOGRAPHY

Allman M, Frayer W, Hedges T. Orbital neurilemoma. *Ann Ophthalmol.* 1977; 9:1409–1413.

Armington WG, Bilaniuk LT. The radiologic evaluation of the orbit: Conal and intraconal lesions. *Semin Ultrasound, CT, MR.* 1988; 9:455–473.

Bilaniuk LT, Zimmerman RA, Newton TH. Magnetic resonance imaging: Orbital pathology. In: Newton TH, Bilaniuk LT, eds. *Radiology of the Eye and Orbit.* New York: Raven Press; 1990, chap 5.

Capps DH, Brodsky MC, Rice CD, Mrak RE, Glasier CM, Brown HH. Orbital intramuscular schwannoma. *Am J Ophthalmol.* 1990; 110:535–539.

De Potter P, Flanders AE, Shields CL, Shields JA. Magnetic resonance imaging of orbital tumors. *Int Ophthalmol.* 1993; 33:163–173.

De Potter P, Shields CL, Shields JA, Rao VM, Eagle RC, Trachtenberg WM. The CT and MRI features of an unusual case of isolated orbital neurofibroma. *Opthalmic Plast Reconstr Surg* 1992; 8:221–227.

Hopper KD, Sherman JL, Boal DK, Eggli KD. CT and MR imaging of the pediatric orbit. *Radiographics*. 1992; 12:485–503.

Jakobiec FA, Font RL. Peripheral nerve sheath tumors. In: Spencer WH, Font RL, Green WR, Howes EL, Jakobiec FA, Zimmerman LE, eds.: *Ophthalmic Pathology. An Atlas and Textbook*. Philadelphia: WB Saunders; 1986:2603–2632.

Kobrin JL, Blodi FC, Weingeist TA. Ocular and orbital manifestations of neurofibromatosis. *Surv Ophthalmol*. 1979; 24:45–51.

Konrad EA, Thiel HJ. Schwannoma of the orbit. *Ophthalmologica*. 1984; 188:118–127.

Krohel GB, Rosenberg PN, Wright JE, Smith RS. Localized orbital neurofibromas. *Am J Ophthalmol*. 1985; 100: 458–464.

Linder B, Campos M, Schafer M. CT and MRI of orbital abnormalities in neurofibromatosis and selected craniofacial anomalies. *Radiol Clin North Am*. 1987; 25: 787–802.

Mafee MF, Putterman A, Valvassori GE, Campos M, Capek V. Orbital space-occupying lesions: Role of computed tomography and magnetic resonance imaging. *Radiol Clin North Am*. 1987; 25: 529–559.

Mitchell DG, Burk DL, Vinitski S, Rifkin MD. The biophysical basis of tissue contrast in extracranial MR imaging. *AJR*. 1987; 149:831–837.

Rootman J, Goldberg C, Robertson W. Primary orbital schwannomas. *Br J Ophthalmol*. 1982; 66:194–204.

Rootman J, Robertson WD. Neurogenic tumors. In: Rootman J, ed. *Diseases of the Orbit*. Philadelphia: JB Lippincott; 1988:281–480.

Shields JA. Peripheral nerve tumors of the orbit. In: Shields JA, ed. *Diagnosis and Management of Orbital Tumors*. Philadelphia: WB Saunders; 1989:149–169.

Shields JA, Kapustiak J, Arbizo V, Augsburger JJ, Schnitzer RE. Orbital neurilemoma with extension through the superior orbital fissure. *Arch Ophthalmol*. 1986; 104:871–873.

Shields JA, Shields CL, Lieb WE, Eagle RC. Multiple orbital neurofibromas unassociated with von Recklinghausen's disease. *Arch Ophthalmol*. 1990; 108: 80–83.

Slamovits TL, Gardner TA. Neuroimaging in neuro-ophthalmology. *Ophthalmology*. 1989; 96:555–568.

Sullivan JA, Harms SE. Surface coil MR imaging of orbital neoplasms. *Am J Neuroradiol*. 1986; 7:29–34.

Wood JJ, Albert DM, Solt LC, Hu DN, Wang WJ. Neurofibromatosis of the eyeball and orbit. *Int Ophthalmol Clin*. 1982; 22:157–187.

Zimmerman RA, Bilaniuk LT, Metzger RA, Grossman RI, Schut L, Bruce DA. Computed tomography of orbital facial neurofibromatosis. *Radiology*. 1983; 146: 113–116.

FIGURE 12–1 *Isolated Orbital Neurilemoma*
A 54-year-old woman presented with a 4-month history of proptosis of the right eye associated with binocular diplopia and right orbital pain.

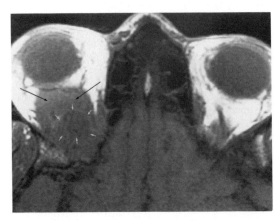

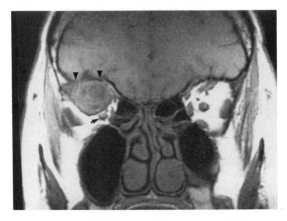

12–1A Axial T1W image. The tumor appears as a well-circumscribed, extraconal mass with heterogeneous low signal intensity. The posterior cystic portion (*white arrows*) of the lesion appears isointense, and the anterior portion slightly hyperintense, with respect to the extraocular muscles. The periphery of the posterior cystic component is composed of tissue demonstrating the Antoni A (cellular) pattern. The anterior portion (*black arrows*) is characterized by the Antoni B (myxomatous) loose pattern.

12–1B Coronal T1W image. The tumor still has a heterogeneous signal, primarily of low intensity. The right optic nerve (*arrow*) is displaced inferiorly. The mass has caused slight scalloping and thinning of the orbital roof (*arrowheads*). (From Orbit. In: Rao VM, Flanders AE, Tom BM, eds. *MRI and CT Atlas of Correlative Imaging in Otolaryngology*. London: Martin Dunitz; 1992, chap 8, p 344.)

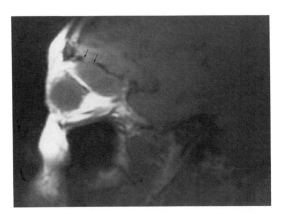

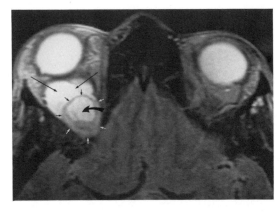

12–1C Sagittal T1W image. The loss of the usual signal void between the tumor and the brain (*arrows*) indicates thinning of the orbital roof. There is no sign of brain involvement.

12–1D Axial T2W image. The anterior portion (*long arrows*) of the tumor, which demonstrates an Antoni B pattern, becomes markedly hyperintense owing to the free water content of the mucinous degeneration. The posterior portion of the tumor shows a central core of moderate hyperintensity corresponding to the cyst (*curved arrow*) surrounded by a hypointense rim (*short arrows*) (Antoni A pattern with higher cellular content). Note the absence of tumor extension through the superior orbital fissure and the lack of brain involvement. (From Orbit. In: Rao VM, Flanders AE, Tom BM, eds. *MRI and CT Atlas of Correlative Imaging in Otolaryngology*. London: Martin Dunitz; 1992, chap 8, p 345.)

(continued)

FIGURE 12–1 *Isolated Orbital Neurilemoma* (continued)

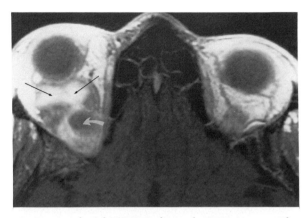

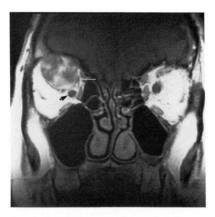

12–1E Axial Gd-DTPA–enhanced T1W image. The tumor shows heterogeneous enhancement. The portion with the Antoni B pattern (*black arrows*) enhances more markedly than does the posterior portion with Antoni A pattern. The cystic portion (*curved arrow*) does not enhance. The high signal of the orbital fat does not allow accurate delineation of the enhancing mass.

12–1F Coronal Gd-DTPA–enhanced T1W image. The superior rectus muscle (*white arrow*) and optic nerve (*black arrow*) are displaced inferonasally.

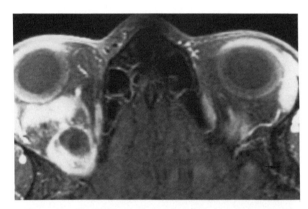

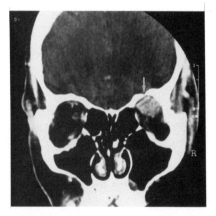

12–1G Fat-suppressed axial Gd-DTPA–enhanced T1W image. Delineation of the tumor is facilitated by suppression of the signal of the orbital fat. The enhancement of the tumor is more pronounced.

12–1H Coronal CT scan. The heterogeneity of the tumor is not well defined on CT. The thinning of the orbital roof (*arrow*) is confirmed.

(continued)

FIGURE 12-1 *Isolated Orbital Neurilemoma* (continued)

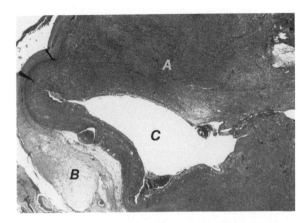

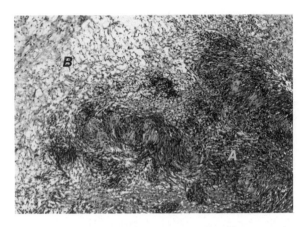

12-1I Low-power photomicrograph of the same tumor showing the collapsed cyst (*C*) surrounded by tissue with the Antoni A pattern (*A*). An area of Antoni B pattern (*B*) is also noted (hematoxylin-eosin, ×25).

12-1J Higher-power photomicrograph showing the Antoni (*A*) and (*B*) patterns within the tumor (hematoxylin-eosin, ×60).

FIGURE 12-2 *Isolated Orbital Neurilemoma of the Frontal Nerve*
A 57-year-old man developed progressive, painless proptosis of the left eye over a period of about 8 months.

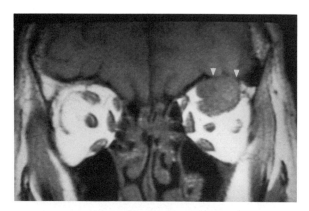

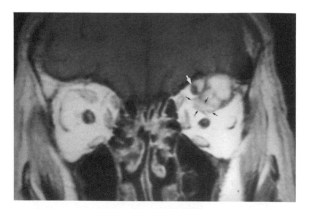

12-2A Coronal T1W image. The tumor is composed of multiple, circumscribed nodules of low signal intensity corresponding to mucinous material with pauci-cellularity. The tumor blends with the equally hypointense superior rectus and levator palpebrae superioris muscles. The tumor produces thinning of the orbital roof (*arrowheads*).

12-2B Coronal Gd-DTPA–enhanced T1W image. The lobules with the Antoni B pattern show marked enhancement. An eccentric, nonenhancing focus suggests collagenization within an Antoni A region (*white arrow*). The superior rectus and levator palpebrae superioris muscles are displaced inferonasally (*black arrows*).

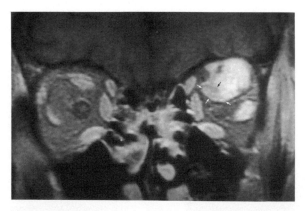

12-2C Fat-suppressed coronal Gd-DTPA–enhanced T1W image. The enhancement of the tumor is more pronounced than in the superior rectus and levator palpebrae superioris muscles (*arrows*).

FIGURE 12-3 *Isolated Neurofibroma*

A 35-year-old woman presented with a 7-mm proptosis of the left eye and a painful sensation of fullness in the left orbit. (From De Potter P, Shields CL, Shields JA, Rao VM, Eagle RC, Trachtenberg WM. The CT and MRI features of an unusual case of isolated orbital neurofibroma. *Ophthalm Plast Reconstr Surg.* 1992; 8:221-227.)

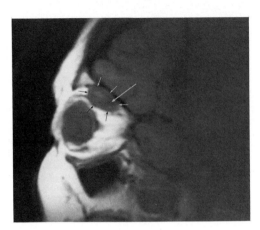

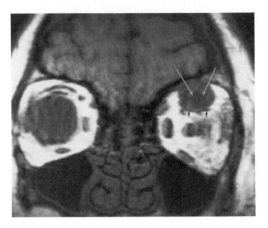

12-3A Sagittal T1W image. The extraconal, well-circumscribed tumor (*short arrows*) has a heterogeneous low signal intensity. The posterior portion (*long arrow*) of the lesion appears hypointense, and the anterior portion isointense, with respect to the extraocular muscles. The orbital roof appears to be intact on this plane.

12-3B Coronal T1W image. The superior rectus muscle (*black arrows*) is displaced downward by the tumor. The inferior portion of the tumor is hypointense and the superior portion is isointense with respect to the extraocular muscles. The hypointense region (*white arrows*) corresponds to the eccentric, hyalinized focus of dense collagen bundles (see Fig. 12–3*F*). The superior portion has undergone extensive myxomatous degeneration.

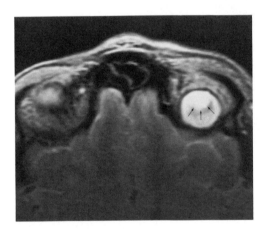

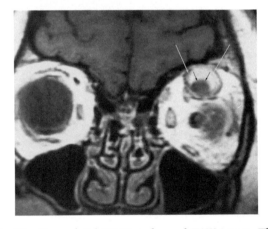

12-3C Axial T2W image. The mass has a heterogeneous hyperintensity with respect to the orbital fat. The myxomatous focus in the anterior portion (*arrows*) of the mass has a more hyperintense signal than does the posterior hyalinized focus.

12-3D Coronal Gd-DTPA–enhanced T1W image. The mass shows heterogeneous enhancement. The inferior hyalinized focus (*black arrows*) does not enhance, whereas the superior myxomatous portion (*white arrows*) shows marked enhancement.

(continued)

FIGURE 12–3 *Isolated Neurofibroma* (continued)

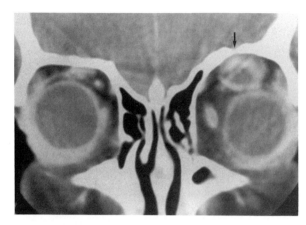

12–3E Coronal contrast-enhanced CT scan. The tumor is heterogeneous in density and is seen to have produced bone erosion (*arrow*).

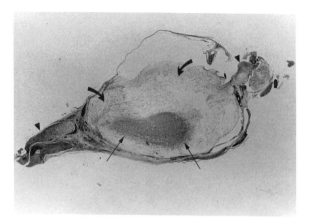

12–3F Low-power photomicrograph of the tumor showing the well-encapsulated, oval mass arising from and affixed to a peripheral nerve (*arrowheads*). The peripheral portion of the neurofibroma has undergone extensive myxomatous degeneration (*curved arrows*). A hyalinized focus of dense collagen bundles (*arrows*) correlates with the MR features.

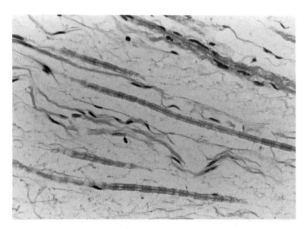

12–3G Photomicrograph of the peripheral portion of the tumor containing myelinated axons in a lucent acellular, myxomatous substance (hematoxylin-eosin, ×200).

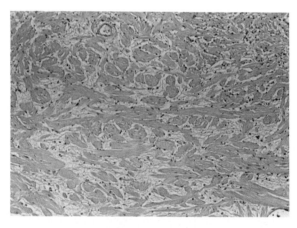

12–3H Photomicrograph of the eccentric area of hyalinization (hematoxylin-eosin, ×100).

MRI of the Eye and Orbit,
by Patrick De Potter, Jerry A. Shields, and Carol L. Shields.
J. B. Lippincott Company, Philadelphia © 1995.

13
Optic Nerve and Meningeal Tumors

PATRICK DE POTTER

CAROL L. SHIELDS

JERRY A. SHIELDS

JUVENILE PILOCYTIC ASTROCYTOMA

Clinical and Pathological Features

Juvenile pilocytic astrocytoma (JPA), also known as optic nerve glioma, is a tumor of low biologic potential that usually becomes apparent during the first decade of life and that has a female preponderance. Affected patients present with painless, progressive visual loss and proptosis, which initially occurs in an axial direction but can later assume a downward and outward direction. The tumor is usually unilateral. The incidence of JPA in children with neurofibromatosis who are 2 to 9 years of age may approach 3% to 10%. Conversely, approximately 50% of children with JPA may have neurofibromatosis. Bilateral JPA is pathognomonic of neurofibromatosis. Orbital JPA may be isolated, or it may be associated with involvement of the intracanalicular portion of the optic nerve. Posterior extension may be restricted to the chiasm or may involve the parachiasmal structures.

Histopathologic studies reveal that JPA is composed of well-differentiated astrocytes with elongated hairlike processes arranged in a parallel or intertwining pattern. A circumferential perineural pattern, termed perineural arachnoidal gliomatosis, with tumor extension into the arachnoid space is highly characteristic of JPA when associated with neurofibromatosis. In some cases, hyperplasia of the arachnoid over the surface of the tumor is noted. Factors that may account for enlargement of the tumor include deposition of mucin, arachnoidal hyperplasia, hemorrhage, and rarely, malignant transformation. There may be also a considerable sparing of the axonal component of the nerve. On computed tomography (CT), orbital JPA presents as an enlarged, fusiform, optic nerve mass with smooth, intact, dural margins. Characteristic kinking and low-density cystic areas are common. Calcification is not seen. After administration of contrast agent, the tumor shows uniform and intense enhancement. High-resolution axial and coronal CT scans are helpful in evaluating the optic canal and the parachiasmal region in order to define the extent of the tumor.

MR Features

The superior contrast resolution of magnetic resonance imaging (MRI) makes it the method of choice for evaluating the intraorbital and intracranial extent of JPA. Enlargement of the optic nerve may be tubular, fusiform, or lobulated. Kinks and buckling of the tumor may be present. On non–contrast-enhanced T1-weighted (T1W) images, the tumor usually has a low signal intensity that is isointense relative to the gray matter (Figs. 13–1A, 13–2, A through D). The signal intensity of the tumor shows greater variability on T2-weighted (T2W) images. Fusiform JPA demonstrates a relatively homogeneous high signal intensity on T2W images, whereas large lobulated tumors tend to show a more heterogeneous signal on T2W images

(Figs. 13–1B and 13–2E). The peripheral hyperintense portion surrounds a central linear core of lower signal intensity. In these cases, histopathologic examination has revealed a peripheral zone of perineural arachnoidal gliomatosis (a myxoid proliferation of glial cells intermixed with blood vessels) or arachnoidal hyperplasia surrounding a central core of optic nerve with a compact proliferation of glial cells. MR studies that show the double-intensity tubular thickening that is characteristic of perineural arachnoidal gliomatosis, along with elongation and downward kinking of the optic nerves in the orbit, are suggestive of JPA in patients with neurofibromatosis type 1.

Intracranial involvement is confirmed by enlargement of the chiasm and optic tracts, which present with low signal intensity on T1W images and high signal intensity on T2W images (Fig. 13–2D). In patients with neurofibromatosis type 1, foci of high signal intensity on T2W images may be seen in the cerebellar peduncles, globus pallidus, pons, midbrain, thalamus, and, less commonly, in the white matter (Fig. 13–2K).

After administration of gadolinium diethylenetriamine penta-acetic acid (Gd-DTPA), JPA usually shows variable enhancement (Figs. 13–1, C through F; 13–2, F and G). Fat-suppression techniques are most helpful in distinguishing the contrast enhancement of the tumor from the bright signal of the orbital fat. The enhancing tumor may expand the optic canal. In larger tumors, marked contrast enhancement is noted in the center of the mass. The nonenhancing peripheral portion of the tumor, which is hyperintense on T2W images, probably represents arachnoidal hyperplasia or an ectatic subarachnoid space around the nerve (Fig. 13–2, F and G). Perineural arachnoidal gliomatosis with reactive proliferation of the fibrovascular arachnoidal trabeculae will show enhancement after Gd-DTPA administration (Fig. 13–1, C and D). On postcontrast scans, the involvement of the optic nerve can be traced through the optic canal to the chiasm and optic tracts (Fig. 13–2, H through J).

MENINGIOMA OF THE OPTIC NERVE SHEATH

Clinical and Pathological Features

Meningioma of the optic nerve sheath is usually a unilateral, slowly growing, benign tumor that causes progressive unilateral visual loss with mild axial proptosis. Its incidence is highest in women and tends to be symptomatic between the ages of 30 to 50 years. Ophthalmoscopic examination may reveal optic disk swelling in early stages and optociliary shunt vessels with pallor of the optic disk in later stages. Meningioma may be multicentric, particularly in patients with neurofibromatosis.

On histopathologic examination, optic nerve sheath meningioma is believed to arise from the meningothelial cells of the arachnoid layer of the optic nerve sheath within the orbit or optic foramen. There are two histologic patterns of orbital meningioma: meningotheliomatous (syncytial) and transitional. Three radiologic patterns can be seen in optic nerve sheath meningioma: diffuse thickening, fusiform swelling, and globular enlargement. Central lucent areas are characteristically seen after administration of contrast agent and may help to identify the residual optic nerve with calcification ("railroad sign"). Foci of calcification can be seen within the tumor.

MR Features

MR studies are extremely valuable in detecting and evaluating the extent of optic nerve sheath meningioma. Intraorbital meningiomas have MR characteristics that are similar to those of intracranial meningiomas. Meningiomas present with appreciable variability in signal characteristics on noncontrast T1W and T2W images. Most meningiomas involving the optic nerve sheath appear isointense or hypointense to cortical gray matter on nonenhanced T1W images (Figs. 13–3, B and C; 13–4, A and B). In some cases, the tumor shows a lower signal intensity than the optic nerve and can easily be identified. On T2W images, the signal intensity of optic nerve sheath meningioma may be hypointense, isointense, or hyperintense to the gray matter (Fig. 13–4C). These T2 intensity scores have been correlated to histopathologic findings. Calcification within the tumor is characterized by a low signal intensity on T1W and T2W images and can be differentiated from the subarachnoid space, which shows a bright signal on T2W images (Fig. 13–3B). Small optic nerve sheath meningiomas may not be detected on noncontrast T1W images.

On Gd-DTPA–enhanced T1W images, optic nerve sheath meningiomas show marked enhancement surrounding the hypointense optic nerve. Fat-suppression techniques facilitate differentiation of the enhancing tumor from the hyperintense signal of the orbital fat on standard T1W images (Figs. 13–3, D and G; 13–4D). Intracranial extension of the meningioma is best evaluated on postcontrast T1W scans (Fig. 13–3, D, F through H).

OPTIC NEUROPATHIES

Clinical and Pathological Features

"Optic neuritis" is the general term used to describe optic nerve involvement as the result of inflammation, demyelination, or infection. Most patients with optic neuritis are younger than 50 years of age. Visual loss is the major symptom, and is often associated with pain. Optic neuritis may be idiopathic, or it may be associated with other diseases, such as multiple sclerosis. It may also be a manifestation of focal or systemic inflammatory or infectious diseases, such as syphilis, sarcoidosis, toxoplasmosis, or ilieocolitis. Optic neuritis can be caused by contiguous sinus diseases, encephalomyelitis, and meningitis. Lymphoproliferative and leukemic disorders, as well as inflammatory lesions such as tuberculosis and sarcoidosis, may also involve the anterior visual pathways.

Radiation-induced optic neuritis may ensue if the daily doses of radiotherapy exceed 200 cGy/day, to a total dose more than 4,500 cGy. On ophthalmoscopic examination, the optic disk initially appears swollen, subsequently becoming atrophied.

MR Features

On MR evaluation of intraorbital optic neuritis, T2W images and fat-suppressed, postcontrast T1W images are generally recommended. On these pulse sequences, the intensity of the optic nerve sheath complex is increased (Figs. 13–5; 13–6A; 13–7, B and C). In one series, 54% of the patients with optic neuritis and 100% of the patients with radiation-induced optic neuropathy showed enhancement of the optic nerves on Gd-DTPA–enhanced T1W images. The enhancement corresponds to the increased permeability of the blood–brain barrier in acute optic neuritis and radiation-induced optic neuropathy (Fig. 13–8, B and C). Suppression of orbital fat with short-inversion-time inversion-recovery (STIR) reduces the signal from Gd-DTPA. Lipid-suppressed chemical shift MR studies (chopper fat suppression) also increase the sensitivity and specificity for detection of optic neuritis without the constraints of sequence limitations or artifacts at fat and water interfaces with STIR imaging. About 50% of the patients with isolated, monosymptomatic optic neuritis have one to several brain lesions demonstrated by MRI (Fig. 13–6B). MRI appears to be useful in the detection of acute infarction of the optic nerve (Fig. 13–9, A and B).

MRI optimizes visualization of the extension of the infiltration of the optic nerve by inflammatory or lymphoproliferative disorders (Fig. 13–10, A through D). The enlarged perioptic subarachnoid space shows low signal intensity on T1W images and a high signal intensity on T2W images with respect to the optic nerve, and it does not enhance after Gd-DTPA administration (Fig. 13–2F). This can easily be differentiated from optic nerve tumor or infiltration that usually enhances.

INTRACRANIAL AND SECONDARY ORBITAL MENINGIOMA

Clinical and Pathological Features

The major sites of intracranial meningioma affecting the orbital and visual structures are the sphenoid ridge, suprasellar area, and olfactory groove. Meningiomas of the lateral third of the sphenoid ridge (greater wing) tend to be large and globular. En plaque meningioma has a propensity to involve the greater wing of the sphenoid. Meningiomas arising from the lateral portion of the sphenoid grow forward into the lateral aspects of the orbit, producing proptosis and swelling of the temporal fossa tissue. Meningioma arising from the medial portion gain access to the orbit through the superior or inferior orbital fissures, or through the optic canal, and produce early visual loss.

The histopathologic findings in both optic nerve sheath and secondary orbital meningiomas are quite similar. Sphenoid wing meningiomas characteristically produce hyperostosis of the bones at the orbital apex. These lesions are well defined and homogeneous and show uniform enhancement following infusion of contrast agent.

MR Features

The MR characteristics of optic nerve sheath meningioma and intracranial meningioma are similar. Tumor signals on nonenhanced T1W images are isointense or hypointense to the cortical gray matter (Figs. 13–11A and 13–12A). A moderately diverse signal intensity (hypointense, isointense, and hyperintense) is seen on T2W images (Fig. 13–12B).

The use of Gd-DTPA enhancement with fat-suppression technique is essential for delineating the orbital and cranial extent of the meningioma. Meningiomas that appear isointense to the cerebral cortex on T1W images can easily be identified after administration of contrast agent, and show marked enhancement (Figs. 13–11B and 13–12C). Peripheral enhancement can be seen in extra-axial calcified meningiomas (Fig. 13–11B). If the interface between the tumor and the brain is irregular, dural invasion should be suspected. Increased mottled signal intensity of the sphenoid medullary space may be attributable to its involvement by the intraosseous component of the meningioma (Fig. 13–11B).

BIBLIOGRAPHY

Aoki S, Barkovich AJ, Nishimura K, Kjos BO, Machida T, Cogen P, Edwards M, Norman D. Neurofibromatosis type 1 and 2: Cranial MR findings. *Radiology*. 1989; 172:527–534.

Azar-Kia B, Mafee MF, Horowitz SW, Fine M, Raofi B. CT and MRI of the optic nerve and sheath. *Semin Ultrasound, CT, MR*. 1988; 9:443–454.

Azar-Kia B, Naheedy MH, Elias DA, Mafee MF, Fine M. Optic nerve tumors: Role of magnetic resonance imaging and computed tomography. *Radiol Clin North Am*. 1987; 25:561–581.

Bilaniuk LT, Zimmerman RA, Newton TH. Magnetic resonance imaging: Orbital pathology. In: Newton TH, Bilaniuk LT, eds. *Radiology of the Eye and Orbit*. New York: Raven Press; 1990, Chap 5.

Bleeker GM. Orbital meningioma. *Orbit*. 1984; 3:3–17.

Bydder GM, Kingsley DPE, Brown J. Niendorf HP, Young IR. MR imaging of meningiomas including studies with and without gadolinium-DTPA. *J Comput Assist Tomogr*. 1985; 9:690–697.

Claveria LE, Sutton D, Tress BM. The radiological diagnosis of meningiomas. The impact of EMI scanning. *Br J Radiol*. 1977; 50:15–22.

Cohn EM. Optic nerve sheath meningioma. Neuroradiologic findings. *J Clin Neuro-ophthalmol*. 1983; 3:85–89.

De Potter P, Flanders AE, Shields CL, Shields JA. Magnetic resonance imaging of orbital tumors. *Int Ophthalmol Clin*. 1993; 33:163–173.

Elster AD, Challa VR, Gilbert TH, Richardson DN, Contento JC. Meningiomas: MR and histopathologic features. *Radiology*. 1989; 170:857–862.

Guy J, Mancuso A, Quisling RG, Beck R, Moster ML. Gadolinium-DTPA–enhanced magnetic resonance imaging in optic neuropathies. *Ophthalmology*. 1990; 97:592–600.

Guy J, Mao J, Bidgood D, Mancuso A, Quisling RG. Enhancement and demyelination of the intraorbital optic nerve. Fat suppression magnetic resonance imaging. *Ophthalmology*. 1992; 99:713–719.

Haik BG, Saint Louis L, Bierly J, Smith ME, Abramson DA, Ellsworth RM, Wall M. Magnetic resonance imaging in the evaluation of optic nerve glioma. *Ophthalmology*. 1987; 94:709–717.

Holman RE, Grimson BS, Drayer BP, Buckley EG, Brennan MW. Magnetic resonance imaging of optic gliomas. *Am J Ophthalmol*. 1985; 100:596–601.

Jacobs L, Munschauer FE, Kaba SE. Clinical and magnetic resonance imaging in optic neuritis. *Neurology*. 1991; 41:15–19.

Jakobiec FA, Depot MJ, Kennerdell JS, Shults WT, Anderson RL, Alper ME, Citrin CM, Housepian EM, Trokel SL. Combined clinical and computed tomographic diagnosis of orbital glioma and meningioma. *Ophthalmology*. 1984; 91:137–155.

Jakobiec FA, Font RL. Tumors of the optic nerve. In: Spencer WH, Font RL, Green WR, Howes EL, Jakobiec FA, Zimmerman LE, eds. *Ophthalmic Pathology. An Atlas and Textbook*. Philadelphia: WB Saunders; 1986:2633–2646.

Lee DH, Simon JH, Szumowski J, Feasby TE, Karlik SJ, Fox AJ, Pelz DM. Optic neuritis and orbital lesion: Lipid-suppressed chemical shift MR imaging. *Radiology*. 1991; 179:535–546.

Lexa FJ, Galetta SL, Yousem DM, Farber M, Oberholtzer JC, Atlas SW. Herpes Zoster ophthalmicus with orbital pseudotumor syndrome complicated by optic nerve infarction and cerebral granulomatous angiitis: MR pathologic correlation. *AJNR*. 1993; 14:185–190.

Marquardt MD, Zimmerman LE. Histology of meningiomas and gliomas of the optic nerve. *Hum Pathol*. 1982; 13:226–234.

Miller NR, ed. *Walsh and Hoyt's Clinical Neuro-Ophthalmology*. 4th ed. Baltimore: Williams & Wilkins; 1991:175–310.

Rootman J, Robertson WD. Neurogenic tumors. In: Rootman J, ed. *Diseases of the Orbit*. Philadelphia: JB Lippincott; 1988:281–480.

Seiff SR, Brodsky MC, MacDonald G, Berg BO, Howes EL, Hoyt WF. Orbital optic glioma in neurofibromatosis. Magnetic resonance diagnosis of perineural arachnoidal gliomatosis. *Arch Ophthalmol*. 1987; 105:1689–1692.

Shields JA. Optic nerve and meningeal tumors. In: Shields JA, ed. *Diagnosis and Management of Orbital Tumors*. Philadelphia; WB Saunders; 1989:170–191.

Sibony PA, Krauss HR, Kennerdell JS, Maroon JC, Slamovits TL. Optic nerve sheath meningioma. Clinical manifestations. *Ophthalmology*. 1984, 91: 1313–1326.

Spagnoli MV, Goldberg HI, Grossman RI, Bilaniuk LT, Hackney DB, Zimmerman RA. Intracranial meningiomas: High-field MR imaging. *Radiology*. 1986; 161:369–375.

Spencer WH. Diagnostic modalities and natural behavior of optic nerve gliomas. *Ophthalmology*. 1979; 86: 881–885.

Stern J, Jakobiec FA, Housepian EM. The architecture of optic nerve gliomas with and without neurofibromatosis. *Arch Ophthalmol*. 1980; 98:505–511.

Wright JE. Primary optic nerve meningiomas. Clinical presentation and management. *Ophthalmology*. 1977; 83:617–625.

Zimmerman CF, Schatz NJ, Glaser JS. Magnetic resonance imaging of radiation optic neuropathy. *Am J Ophthalmol*. 1990; 110:389–394.

FIGURE 13-1 *Bilateral Juvenile Pilocytic Astrocytoma*
A 21-month-old girl with neurofibromatosis type 1 presented with massive proptosis of the left eye.

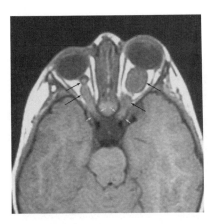

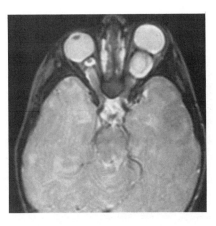

13-1A Axial T1W image. Both optic nerves are enlarged and show a signal that is isointense to the gray matter. The hypointense line surrounding both optic nerves corresponds to cerebrospinal fluid (CSF). Note the bilateral widening of the optic nerve canal (*white arrows*). The downward kinking of both gliomatous optic nerves (see *E* and *F*) explains the bilobulated appearance (*black arrows*) on axial planes.

13-1B Axial T2W image at the same level as in *A*. An area of hyperintense signal surrounds a central linear core of hypointense signal. The peripheral hyperintense signal may be related to the perineural arachnoidal gliomatosis and/or to CSF.

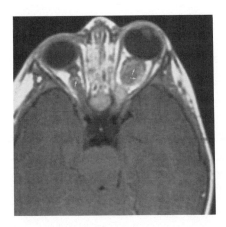

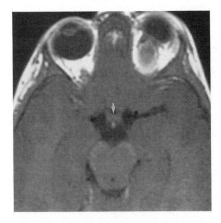

13-1C Axial Gd-DTPA–enhanced T1W image at the same level as in *A*. The peripheral portion of both enlarged optic nerves demonstrates minimal enhancement suggesting perineural arachnoidal gliomatosis (*arrows*).

13-1D Axial Gd-DTPA–enhanced T1W image at a higher level than in *A*. On this section, the chiasm appears normal (*arrow*).

(continued)

FIGURE 13-1 *Bilateral Juvenile Pilocytic Astrocytoma* (continued)

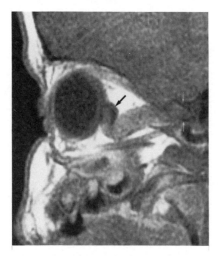

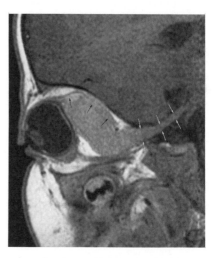

13-1E Sagittal Gd-DTPA–enhanced T1W image of the right orbit. The downward kinking of the enlarged optic nerve is clearly evident. Note the enlargement of the intracanalicular portion of the nerve (*white arrows*). The chiasm is not seen on this plane. The low signal intensity at the superior edge of the optic nerve (*black arrow*) corresponds to CSF in an ectatic subarachnoid space.

13-1F Sagittal Gd-DTPA–enhanced T1W image of the left orbit. The lobulated gliomatous left optic nerve is displacing the superior rectus muscle (*black arrows*) superiorly. The posterior intracanalicular and prechiasmal portion of the optic nerve (*white arrows*) does not show enhancement. The chiasm is not involved.

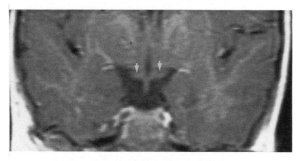

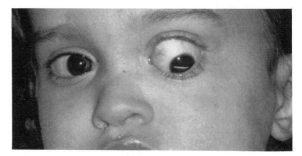

13-1G Coronal Gd-DTPA–enhanced T1W image. The optic tracts are normal (*arrows*).

13-1H Clinical photograph showing extensive proptosis of the left eye, which is displaced downward and outward from the pilocytic astrocytoma.

FIGURE 13–2 *Unilateral Juvenile Pilocytic Astrocytoma with Chiasmal Involvement*

A 3-month-old boy was found by his parents to have slight proptosis of the right eye. There was no family history of neurofibromatosis.

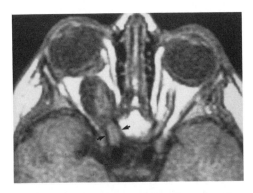

13–2A Axial T1W image. The enlarged right optic nerve sheath complex has a bilobulated appearance. In the posterior lobulated mass, an area of low signal intensity surrounds a central core of high signal intensity. The right optic canal is widened by the enlarged optic nerve (*arrows*).

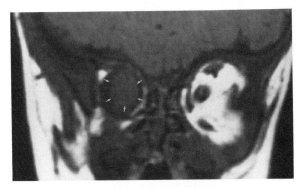

13–2B Coronal T1W image. In the right optic nerve sheath complex, a hypointense rim surrounds the central portion (*arrows*), which is isointense to the cortical gray matter.

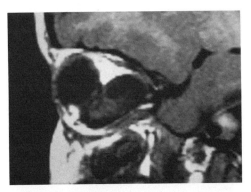

13–2C Sagittal T1W image of the right orbit. Note the downward kinking of the enlarged right optic nerve sheath complex.

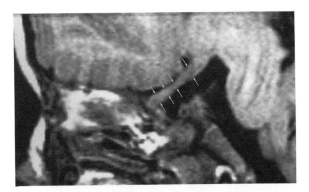

13–2D Parasagittal T1W image. The intracanalicular, intracranial portion of the right optic nerve and the chiasm are enlarged (*arrows*).

(continued)

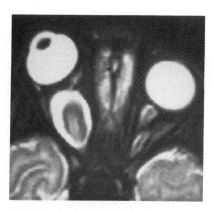

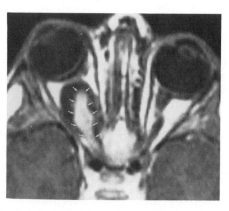

13–2E Axial T2W image. The hyperintense peripheral portion of the tumor surrounds the heterogeneous hypointense central core.

13–2F Axial Gd-DTPA–enhanced T1W image. The central portion of the mass shows enhancement (*arrows*). The nonenhancing peripheral portion, with its low signal intensity on T1W images and high signal intensity on T2W images, may represent arachnoidal hyperplasia and/or CSF.

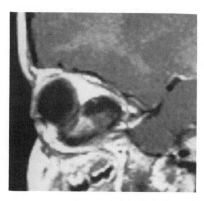

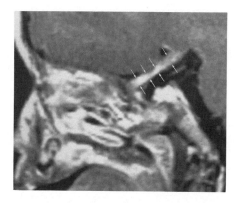

13–2G Sagittal Gd-DTPA–enhanced T1W image of the right orbit. On this section, the enhancement of the central portion of the tumor appears to be more heterogeneous.

13–2H Parasagittal Gd-DTPA–enhanced T1W image. The enhancing tumor (*arrows*) can be traced through the optic canal to the intracranial portion of the right optic nerve and chiasm.

(continued)

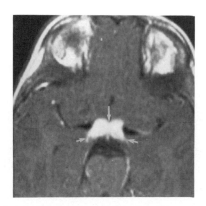

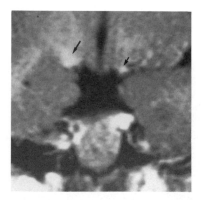

13-2I Axial Gd-DTPA–enhanced T1W image. Note the marked enhancement of the enlarged chiasm (*long arrow*) and the proximal portion of both optic tracts (*short arrows*).

13-2J Coronal Gd-DTPA–enhanced T1W image. The involvement of the right optic tract (*long arrow*), which is more pronounced than that of the left optic tract (*short arrow*), is clearly demonstrated after Gd-DTPA administration.

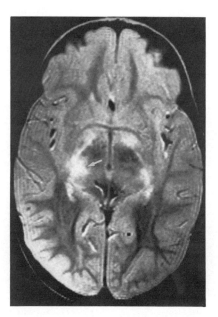

13-2K Axial proton-density weighted image. The tumor extends into the right lateral geniculate body (*arrow*).

FIGURE 13-3 *Optic Nerve Sheath Meningioma*

A 38-year-old woman presented with progressive, painless, decreased vision of the right eye. Fundus examination revealed significant optic disk swelling.

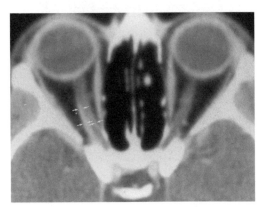

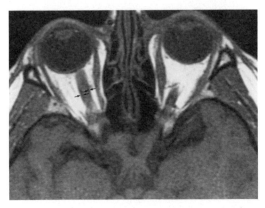

13-3A Axial contrast-enhanced CT scan. Linear calcification (*arrows*) surrounds the posterior portion of the enlarged right optic nerve sheath complex.

13-3B Axial T1W image. The right optic nerve sheath complex appears to be slightly enlarged in its orbital and intracranial portions. The chiasm is not involved. The perioptic calcification detected on CT shows a linear hypointense signal (*arrows*). This hypointense pattern is also seen on T2W images (not shown). The linear area of low signal intensity surrounding the left normal optic nerve sheath complex corresponds to CSF. Because of the slight tilt of the patient's head, the right intracanalicular portion of the optic nerve is not seen on this image.

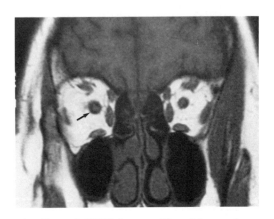

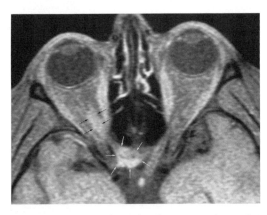

13-3C Coronal T1W image. The right optic nerve sheath complex (*arrow*) is enlarged.

13-3D Fat-suppressed axial Gd-DTPA–enhanced T1W image. The posterior orbital portion of the enlarged optic nerve sheath complex shows enhancement (*black arrows*). The enhancing tumor involving the tuberculum sellae (*white arrows*) expands at the intracranial opening of the right optic canal.

(continued)

FIGURE 13-3   *Optic Nerve Sheath Meningioma* (continued)

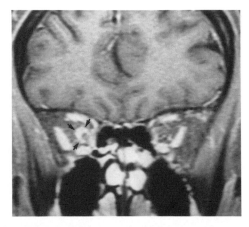

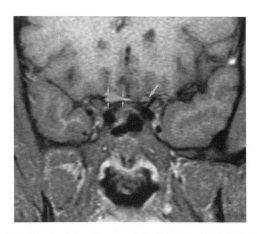

13-3E Fat-suppressed coronal Gd-DTPA–enhanced T1W image. The perioptic meningioma shows marked enhancement (*arrows*).

13-3F Fat-suppressed coronal Gd-DTPA–enhanced T1W image at a prechiasmal level. Note the enhancement of the planum sphenoidale (*short arrows*). The left optic nerve (*long arrow*) is normal.

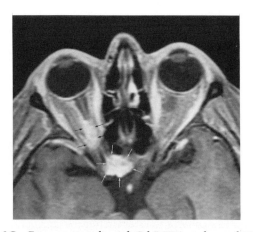

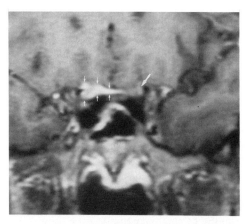

13-3G Fat-suppressed axial Gd-DTPA–enhanced T1W image obtained 10 months after the initial MRI studies. The orbital right optic nerve sheath complex (*black arrows*) and its intracranial portion with involvement of the tuberculum sellae (*white arrows*) have enlarged and show marked enhancement. The intracanalicular portion appears not to be involved on this plane.

13-3H Fat-suppressed coronal Gd-DTPA–enhanced T1W image at a prechiasmal level. The enhancing tumor (*short arrows*) is approaching the left, nonenhancing, intracranial optic nerve sheath complex (*long arrow*).

FIGURE 13-4 *Optic Nerve Sheath Meningioma*
A 38-year-old woman presented with progressive decreased vision of the right eye with color vision alteration and right optic disk swelling.

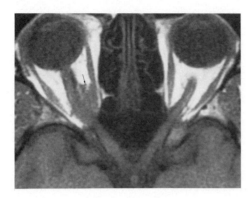

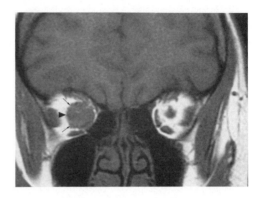

13-4A Axial T1W image. An oval-shaped mass (*arrow*) adjacent to the right optic nerve has a signal that is isointense to the optic nerve and the medial rectus muscle. The margins of the tumor cannot easily be identified.

13-4B Coronal T1W image. The mass (*arrows*) encircles the right optic nerve (*arrowhead*), but can be delineated from the medial rectus muscle, which is displaced nasally.

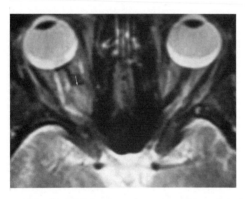

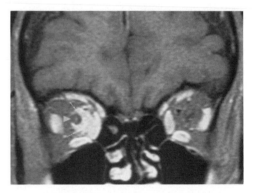

13-4C Axial T2W image. The tumor (*arrow*) is isointense to the cerebral gray matter.

13-4D Fat-suppressed coronal Gd-DTPA–enhanced T1W image. The tumor (*arrows*) encircling the right optic nerve (*arrowhead*) demonstrates marked enhancement.

FIGURE 13-5 *Unilateral Optic Neuritis*
A 49-year-old man with monosymptomatic acute optic neuritis without brain involvement. (Courtesy of Antonella Boschi, M.D., Brussels, Belgium.)

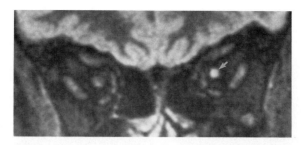

13-5 Coronal T2W image (inversion recovery). Note the increased signal of the left optic nerve (*arrow*) compared with the right optic nerve.

FIGURE 13-6 *Bilateral Optic Neuritis*

A 23-year-old man with multiple sclerosis. (Courtesy of Antonella Boschi, M.D., Brussels, Belgium.)

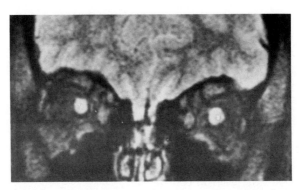

13-6A Coronal gradient echo image. The optic nerve sheath complex is enlarged with an increased signal bilaterally.

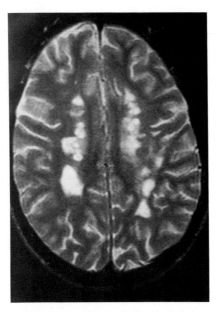

13-6B Axial T2W image. Multiple, well-defined foci of increased intensity in the periventricular white matter represent demyelinating plaques.

FIGURE 13-7 *Optic Neuritis*

A 10-year-old boy presented with left optic neuritis associated with left sphenoid sinusitis.

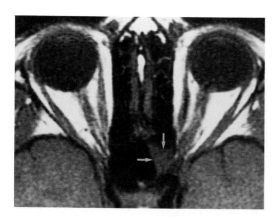

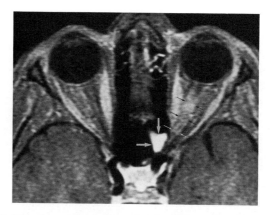

13-7A Axial T1W image. The left optic nerve sheath complex is diffusely enlarged. Note the opacification of the left sphenoid sinus with inflamed thickened mucosa (*arrows*).

13-7B Fat-suppressed axial Gd-DTPA–enhanced T1W image. The left optic nerve complex shows diffuse enhancement (*short arrows*). Note the enhancement of the sphenoid sinus mucosa (*arrows*).

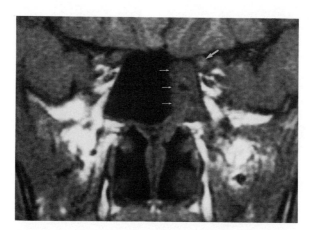

13-7C Fat-suppressed (incomplete) coronal Gd-DTPA–enhanced T1W image at the level of the optic canal. The enhancing left optic nerve (*large arrow*) is seen. Note the enhancement of the enflamed mucosa in the left sphenoid sinus (*thin arrows*).

FIGURE 13-8 *Radiation-Induced Optic Neuropathy*
A 45-year-old man with history of skin melanoma metastases to the brain received external radiotherapy to the brain 10 months before experiencing bilateral decreased vision.

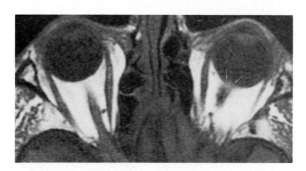

13-8A Axial T1W image. On this section, the optic disk swelling and peripapillary retinal thickening in the left eye (*arrows*) are well visualized.

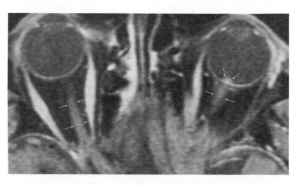

13-8B Fat-suppressed axial Gd-DTPA–enhanced T1W image. The optic nerve head in the left eye demonstrates marked enhancement, as does the retrobulbar portion of both optic nerve sheath complexes (*arrows*).

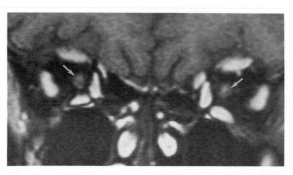

13-8C Fat-suppressed coronal Gd-DTPA–enhanced T1W image. Both intraorbital portions of the optic nerve show enhancement (*arrows*).

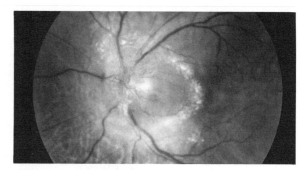

13-8D Fundus photograph of the left eye showing the optic disk swelling and the surrounding retinal edema and exudation.

FIGURE 13-9 Optic Nerve Infarction

A 41-year-old woman with a 5-day history of right periorbital pain subsequently developed herpes zoster ophthalmicus with orbital pseudotumor syndrome and cerebral granulomatous angiitis. (Courtesy of Frank J. Lexa, M.D., Philadelphia.) (From Lexa FJ, Galetta SL, Yousem DM, Farber M, Oberholtzer JC, Atlas SW. Herpes Zoster ophthalmicus with orbital pseudotumor syndrome complicated by optic nerve infarction and cerebral granulomatous angiitis: MR pathologic correlation. *AJNR.* 1993; 14:186.)

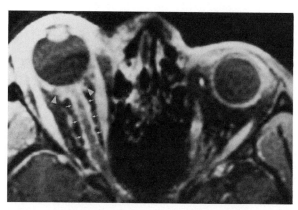 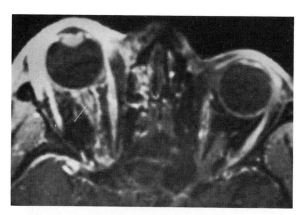

13-9A Fat-suppressed axial Gd-DTPA–enhanced T1W image. Peripheral enhancement of the right optic nerve sheath complex is demonstrated (*arrows*). Posterior scleritis is also documented (*arrowheads*).

13-9B Fat-suppressed axial Gd-DTPA–enhanced T1W image obtained using fat-saturation, gradient-recalled technique at a higher plane. Additional enhancement within the optic nerve (*arrow*) is detected in the distribution of the periaxial infarction.

FIGURE 13–10 *Sarcoid Retrobulbar Infiltrative Optic Neuropathy with Central Nervous System (CNS) Involvement*

A 37-year-old woman with a known history of sarcoidosis presented with rapid onset of blurred vision in the right eye and binocular diplopia. (Courtesy of Peter J. Savino, M.D., Philadelphia.)

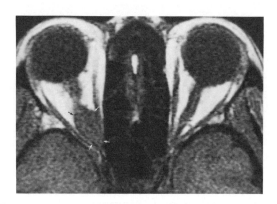

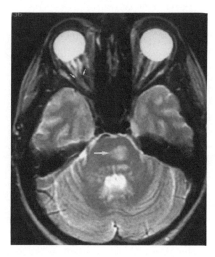

13–10A Axial T1-weighted image. There is abnormal enlargement of the right posterior intraorbital portion of the optic nerve sheath complex (*arrows*), which is isointense to the extraocular rectus muscles.

13–10B Axial T2W image. The inflammatory infiltration of the right optic nerve sheath complex demonstrates a low signal intensity (*short arrows*). Note the hyperintense focus, secondary to sarcoid vasculitis, that lies within the interpontine white matter (*long arrow*).

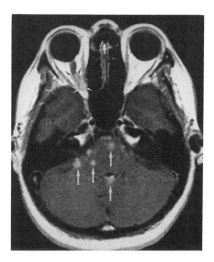

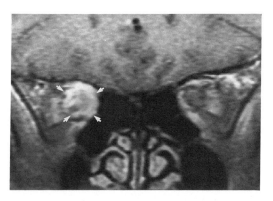

13–10C Fat-suppressed axial Gd-DTPA–enhanced T1W image at the level of the optic canal. The optic nerve and the surrounding meninges (*small arrows*) show marked enhancement. Multiple, focal, enhancing intracranial lesions (*large arrows*) at the level of the pontomedullary junction indicate inflammation along the Virchow-Robin spaces.

13–10D Fat-suppressed coronal Gd-DTPA–enhanced T1W image. The enhancing inflammatory mass (*arrows*) is seen at the orbital apex.

FIGURE 13–11 *Meningioma of the Sphenoid Wing*

A 54-year-old woman presented with minimal, painless proptosis of the left eye.

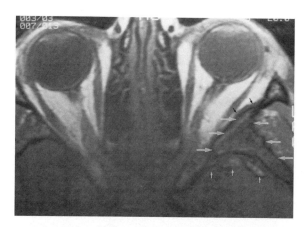

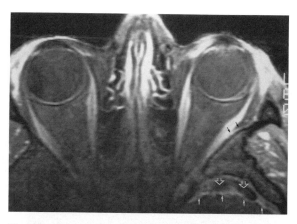

13–11A Axial T1W image. A meningioma of the left sphenoid wing shows an intraosseous and extraosseous component with extension into the orbit (*short black arrows*) and middle cranial fossa (*short white arrows*), as well as into the temporalis fossa. The left hyperostotic sphenoid wing (*long white arrows*) is relatively thicker and appears hyperintense compared with the hypointense signal of the right sphenoid wing.

13–11B Fat-suppressed axial Gd-DTPA–enhanced T1W image. The orbital (*black arrows*) and intracranial (*white arrows*) extension demonstrates peripheral enhancement. The intramedullary portion of the tumor in the left sphenoid bone shows mottled enhancement. The low signal intensity of the extra-axial mass along the anterior aspect of the middle cranial fossa is most likely attributable to dense calcification (*open arrows*).

FIGURE 13–12 *Meningioma of the Sphenoid Wing*
A 53-year-old woman noticed a progressive, painless decrease in vision in the right eye.
(Courtesy of Peter J. Savino, M.D., Philadelphia.)

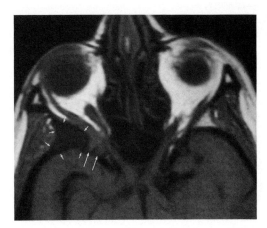

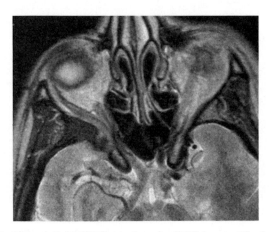

13–12A Axial T1W image. There is an abnormal decreased signal within the marrow space of the right sphenoid wing, as well as enlargement of the greater sphenoid wing secondary to hyperostosis (*short arrows*). Note the extension of the tumor through the superior portion of the superior orbital fissure (*long arrows*).

13–12B Axial T2W fast spin echo (FSE) image. The hyperostotic bone remains hypointense compared with the marrow space of the contralateral sphenoid wing.

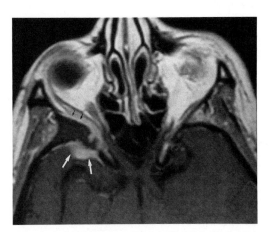

13–12C Axial Gd-DTPA–enhanced T1W image. There is a dura-based, enhancing lesion (*white arrows*) in the dura adjacent to the right sphenoid wing and anterior and anteromedial to the temporal lobe. Note the orbital involvement (*black arrows*).

MRI of the Eye and Orbit,
by Patrick De Potter, Jerry A. Shields, and Carol L. Shields.
J. B. Lippincott Company, Philadelphia © 1995.

14

Fibrous Tissue, Osseous, and Fibro-osseous Tumors

PATRICK DE POTTER

CAROL L. SHIELDS

JERRY A. SHIELDS

FIBROUS HISTIOCYTOMA

Clinical and Pathological Features

It is currently believed that fibrous histiocytoma is the most common mesenchymal tumor of the orbit in adults. Most tumors are well circumscribed, with involvement of the superior and nasal part of the orbit.

On histopathologic examination, fibrous histiocytoma shows a mixture of spindle-shaped fibroblasts and ovoid histiocytes. The typical architectural feature is the storiform pattern, wherein small bundles of cells tend to twist about a central focus. A moderate amount of collagen is deposited in the lesion. By comparison, malignant fibrous histiocytoma shows a greater degree of nuclear pleomorphism and increased mitotic activity. Locally aggressive and malignant fibrous histiocytomas usually have noncircumscribed, infiltrating margins. Orbital computed tomography (CT) demonstrates a well-circumscribed, round or irregular mass that may be impossible to differentiate from cavernous hemangioma, hemangiopericytoma, neurofibroma, or neurilemoma. Bone erosion can occur in recurrent or malignant fibrous histiocytoma.

MR Features

Based on the authors' limited experience, fibrous histiocytoma appears on magnetic resonance imaging (MRI) as a well-circumscribed, round or oval, orbital mass. On T1-weighted (T1W) images, the tumor usually shows a heterogeneous, iso-intense to hyperintense signal with respect to the extraocular muscles and a hypointense signal with respect to the orbital fat (Fig. 14–1A). On T2-weighted (T2W) images, the areas of decreased signal intensity seen on T1W images remain hypointense, and this feature is related to the presence of collagen found within the tumor (Fig. 14–1B). Other differential diagnoses that conceivably could have identical MR features include cavernous hemangioma, hemangiopericytoma, neurilemoma, neurofibroma, and other, less frequent, well-circumscribed orbital lesions (see Tables 11–1, 11–2).

After administration of gadolinium diethylenetriamine penta-acetic acid (Gd-DTPA), fibrous histiocytoma demonstrates heterogeneous enhancement (Fig. 14–1, C and D). The enhancement of the tumor may be difficult to differentiate from the signal of orbital fat unless fat-suppression techniques are used.

FIBROUS DYSPLASIA

Clinical and Pathological Features

Fibrous dysplasia develops almost exclusively in children during the first 2 decades of life. Most of the lesions occurring around the orbit are isolated lesions and are not part of the multifocal (polyostotic) fibrous dysplasia (Albright's syndrome). The patient characteristically presents with facial asymmetry, displacement of the globe, and proptosis. The symptoms and signs vary depending on the primary bones involved. Involvement of the sphenoid bone can produce optic nerve compression and atrophy.

Histopathologic study reveals the tumor to be composed of spicules of immature woven bone and osteoid within a matrix of cellular and vascularized fibrous stroma. Orbital CT scans demonstrate a lesion with a sclerotic, homogeneous, dense, ground-glass appearance. However, alternate areas of lucency and increased density can be observed.

MR Features

The orbital bones affected in fibrous dysplasia appear to be thickened on MR scans and to have a very low signal intensity on T1W and T2W images (Figs. 14–2, *A* and *B*; 12–3*A*). The less calcified tumor portion, composed of vascularized fibrous stroma, may not appear as hypointense as the bony lesion itself (Fig. 14–3*A*). No enhancement of the calcified portion of tumor is usually demonstrated on Gd-DTPA–enhanced T1W images. Depending upon its vascular component, the fibrous stroma may enhance (Figs. 14–2*C* and 14–3, *B* and *C*). MR studies allow evaluation of the extent of the lesion and the degree of displacement and compression at the orbital apex.

OSTEOSARCOMA

Clinical and Pathological Features

Periorbital osteogenic sarcoma typically arises in one of the sinuses, generally in younger individuals. The patient usually presents with a relatively rapid onset of painful, unilateral proptosis, along with periorbital numbness and soft tissue edema. The tumor generally occurs de novo, but may be seen in the context of chronic bone diseases (Paget's disease, fibrous dysplasia) or the inherited form of retinoblastoma, with or without prior orbital irradiation.

On histopathologic examination, the tumor shows a highly anaplastic spindle cell population with osteoid and neoplastic bone formation. Orbital CT scans demonstrate an irregular, invasive, and destructive tumor with lytic and sclerotic changes associated with focal areas of calcification.

MR Features

Replacement of the cortical bone and fat marrow by osteogenic sarcoma can be confirmed by MR studies. The tumor appears as an ill-defined mass

with a heterogeneous, isointense to hyperintense signal with respect to the extraocular muscles and gray matter and a hypointense signal with respect to orbital fat on T1W images (Fig. 14–4, *A* and *B*). The tumor shows heterogeneous hyperintensity with respect to extraocular muscles and orbital fat on T2W images. In cases of radiation-induced osteogenic sarcoma, the irradiated, regressed retinoblastoma shows a hyperintense signal on T1W images and a hypointense signal on T2W images with respect to the vitreous.

After Gd-DTPA administration, osteogenic sarcoma demonstrates heterogeneous enhancement. Orbital and cranial extension are well depicted on Gd-DTPA–enhanced T1W images, with or without fat suppression (Fig. 14–4, *C* through *F*).

ANEURYSMAL BONE CYST

Clinical and Pathological Features

The aneurysmal bone cyst of the orbit is an unusual nonneoplastic benign lesion that generally affects young adults. Most orbital aneurysmal bone cysts are located in the superior orbit. There is generally no history of trauma. The ocular signs and symptoms include pain, proptosis, diplopia, blurred vision, and a palpable mass.

Histopathologic studies indicate that aneurysmal bone cysts are composed of fibrous stroma with a large cystic space without endothelium. Reactive giant cells, histiocytes, and hemosiderin-laden macrophages, with both osteoid and bone formation, are present. Orbital CT scans show irregular expansion and destruction of bone associated with a mildly enhancing, loculated cystic mass.

MR Features

On MR scans, aneurysmal bone cysts of the orbit appear as multicystic, loculated masses associated with bone destruction and possible extension to the adjacent sinuses. These tumors have a heterogeneous signal intensity and fluid-fluid levels on both T1W and T2W images (Fig. 14–5*A*). The spectrum of signal intensities noted in the aneurysmal bone cyst reflects the various stages of evolution of the hemorrhagic content of cystic masses.

BIBLIOGRAPHY

De Potter P, Flanders AE, Shields CL, Shields JA. Magnetic resonance imaging of orbital tumors. *Int Clin Ophthalmol*. 1993; 33:163–173.

Donoso LA, Magargal LE, Eiferman RA. Fibrous dysplasia of the orbit with optic nerve decompression. *Ann Ophthalmol.* 1982; 14:80–83.

Font RL, Hidayat AA. Fibrous histiocytoma of the orbit. A clinicopathologic study of 150 cases. *Hum Pathol.* 1982; 13:199–209.

Hunter JV, Yokoyama C, Moseley IF, Wright JE. Aneurysmal bone cyst of the sphenoid with orbital involvement. *Br J Ophthalmol.* 1990; 74:505–508.

Jakobiec FA, Font RL. Mesenchymal tumors. In: Spencer WH, Font RL, Green WR, Howes EL, Jakobiec FA, Zimmerman LE, eds. *Ophthalmic Pathology. An Atlas and Textbook.* Philadelphia: WB Saunders; 1986:2554–2603.

Johnson TE, Bergin DJ, McCord CD. Aneurysmal bone cyst of the orbit. *Ophthalmology.* 1988; 95:86–89.

Klepach GL, Ho REM, Kelly JK. Aneurysmal bone cyst of the orbit. A case report. *J Clin Neuro Ophthalmol.* 1984; 4:49–52.

Mafee MF, Putterman A, Valvassori GE, Campos M, Capek V. Orbital space-occupying lesions: Role of computed tomography and magnetic resonance imaging. *Radiol Clin North Am.* 1987; 25:529–559.

Mitchell DG, Burk DL, Vinitski S, Rifkin MD. The biophysical basis of tissue contrast in extracranial MR imaging. *AJR.* 1987; 149:831–837.

Moore AT, Buncic JR, Munro IR. Fibrous dysplasia of the orbit in childhood. Clinical features and management. *Ophthalmology.* 1985; 92:12–20.

Moore RT. Fibrous dysplasia of the orbit. Review. *Surv Ophthalmol.* 1969; 13:321–334.

Mortada A. Orbital osteoma within the domain of ophthalmic surgery. *Can J Ophthalmol.* 1969; 68:258–265.

Patel BC, Sabir DI, Flaharty PM, Anderson RL. Aneurysmal bone cyst of the orbit and ethmoid sinus. *Arch Ophthalmol.* 1993; 111:586–587.

Rodrigues MM, Furgiuele FP, Weinreb S. Malignant fibrous histiocytoma of the orbit. *Arch Ophthalmol.* 1977; 95:2025–2028.

Ronner HJ, Jones IS. Aneurysmal bone cyst of the orbit: A review. *Ann Ophthalmol.* 1983; 15:626–629.

Rootman J, Lapointe JS. Mesenchymal tumors. In: Rootman J, ed. *Diseases of the Orbit.* Philadelphia: JB Lippincott; 1988:334–384.

Shields JA. Fibrous connective tissue tumors. In: Shields JA, ed. *Diagnosis and Management of Orbital Tumors.* Philadelphia: WB Saunders; 1989:192–204.

Shields JA. Osseous, fibro-osseous, and cartilaginous tumors. In: Shields JA, ed. *Diagnosis and Management of Orbital Tumors.* Philadelphia: WB Saunders; 1989:205–233.

FIGURE 14–1 *Fibrous Histiocytoma*
A 24-year-old woman presented with progressive proptosis of the left eye.

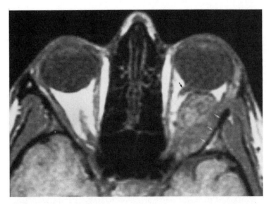

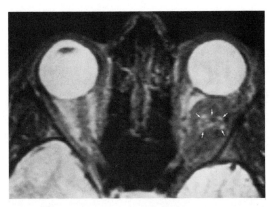

14–1A Axial T1W image. The well-defined intraconal mass appears with a heterogeneous hypointense signal that is isointense to slightly hyperintense to the extraocular muscles and hypointense to orbital fat. The posterior portion of the lateral rectus muscle cannot be identified on this plane. The optic nerve (*black arrow*) is displaced medially. The signal void of the sphenoid cortical bone (*white arrows*) is regular and is not affected by the tumor.

14–1B Axial T2W image. The collagen bundles areas remain hypointense compared to the hyperintense central portion (*arrows*) with its higher cellular content.

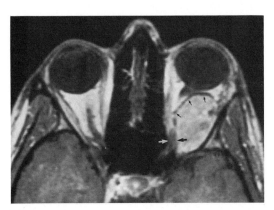

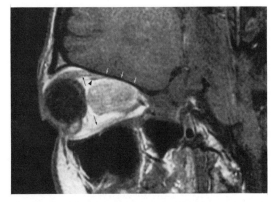

14–1C Axial Gd-DTPA–enhanced T1W image. The tumor demonstrates marked heterogeneous enhancement. The curvilinear hypointense signal corresponds to the tumor capsule (*small arrows*). The optic nerve (*large arrows*) is clearly evident at the orbital apex.

14–1D Parasagittal Gd-DTPA–enhanced T1W image. The tumor has an intraconal location between the superior and inferior rectus muscles (*black arrows*) and produces minimal indentation of the posterior pole of the globe. The linear, regular hypointensity of the cortical bone of the orbital roof indicates absence of bony involvement (*white arrows*). Note the superior ophthalmic vein (*arrowhead*).

FIGURE 14-2 *Fibrous Dysplasia*

A 38-year-old woman presented with progressive proptosis of the left eye associated with left facial asymmetry.

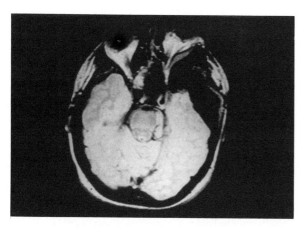

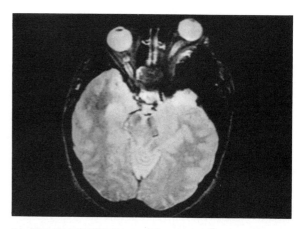

14-2A Axial T1W image. The posterolateral wall of the left orbit, the left posterior ethmoid and sphenoid sinuses, and the left middle cranial fossa are expanded and have a very low signal intensity.

14-2B Axial T2W image. The posterolateral wall of the left orbit and the left middle cranial fossa remain hypointense. The left posterior ethmoid and sphenoid sinuses show a slightly increased signal intensity, probably related to noncalcified fibrous stroma.

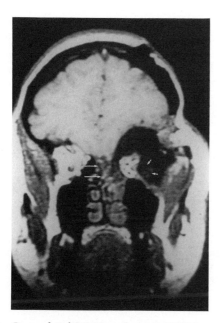

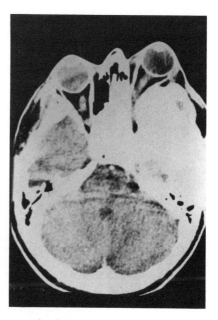

14-2C Coronal Gd-DTPA–enhanced T1W image. The immature bone does not enhance, but the fibrous stroma shows minimal enhancement (*short arrows*). Mild enhancement is seen in the left posterior superior ethmoid and sphenoid sinuses (*long arrows*).

14-2D Axial-enhanced CT. The bones of the left orbit and skull base are dense and thickened.

FIGURE 14-3 *Fibrous Dysplasia*
A 21-year-old woman presented with left orbital fibrous dysplasia and tuberous sclerosis.

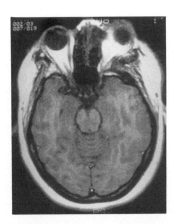

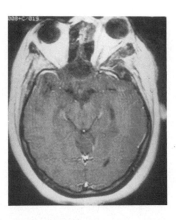

14-3A Axial T1W image. On this section, the posterolateral wall of the left orbit and the left middle cranial fossa are seen to be thickened, with a heterogenous signal intensity. The left anterior ethmoid sinus show increased signal intensity. The areas of low signal intensity correspond to immature bone. The intermediate signal areas probably represent fibrous stroma.

14-3B Axial Gd-DTPA–enhanced T1W image at the same level as in *A*. The lesion demonstrates mild heterogeneous enhancement.

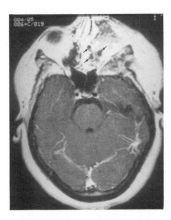

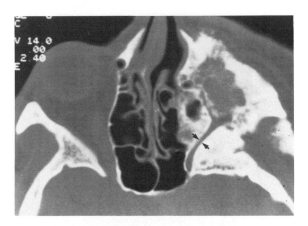

14-3C Axial Gd-DTPA–enhanced T1W image at a lower level than in *A*. The lesion involves the lateral wall of the left ethmoid sinus, the left sphenoid wing, and the orbital floor. The areas of low signal intensity correspond to air *(arrows)*.

14-3D Axial nonenhanced CT scan (bone window) at the same level as in *C*. Note the typical ground-glass appearance of the immature bone within a fibrous stroma. The left inferior orbital fissure is narrowed *(arrows)*.

FIGURE 14–4 *Osteogenic Sarcoma of the Sphenoid Wing*
An 11-year-old girl with bilateral familial retinoblastoma was successfully treated with external beam radiotherapy at the age of 11 months. Ten years later, she noticed swelling of the right temporal fossa.

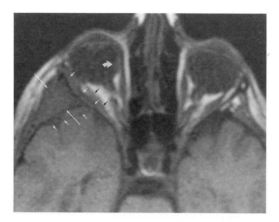

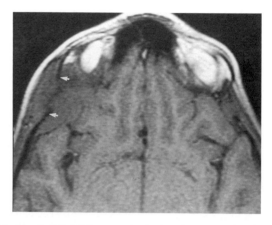

14–4A Axial T1W image. The greater wing of the right sphenoid and the lateral wall of the right orbit are replaced by a mass (*long white arrows*) with increased signal intensity that is isointense to the extraocular muscles. Intracranial and orbital extension of the tumor is evident (*short white arrows*). The lateral rectus muscle (*short black arrows*) is not involved. A slightly hyperintense mass with respect to the vitreous is seen at the equator nasally in the right eye and corresponds to the regressed retinoblastoma (*curved arrow*). The lens is absent in the left eye.

14–4B Axial T1W image at the level of the orbital roof. The subcutaneous and intracranial extra-axial extension of the tumor is well visualized. The linear signal void is missing owing to bone destruction by the tumor (*arrows*). The central portion of the tumor is slightly hypointense compared with the peripheral portion.

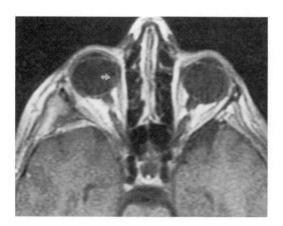

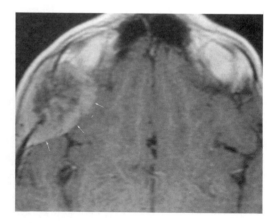

14–4C Axial Gd-DTPA–enhanced T1W image at the same level as in *A*. The mass, with its orbital and intracranial extension, shows marked heterogeneous enhancement. The regressed retinoblastoma in the right eye enhances minimally (*curved arrow*).

14–4D Axial Gd-DTPA–enhanced T1W image at the same level as in *B*. The central portion of the tumor remains hypointense. Brain involvement (*arrows*) is well documented after injection of contrast agent.

(continued)

FIGURE 14–4 *Osteogenic Sarcoma of the Sphenoid Wing* (continued)

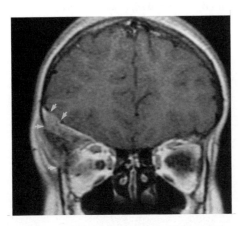

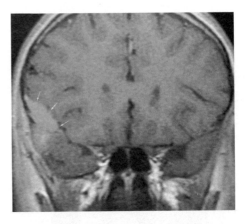

14–4E Coronal Gd-DTPA–enhanced T1W image. The destruction and replacement of the lateral orbital bone and orbital roof are clearly evident (*arrows*). Chemical shift artifact is seen around the extraocular muscles.

14–4F Coronal Gd-DTPA–enhanced T1W image at the level of the anterior temporal lobe. The intracranial, extra-axial extension of the tumor is well visualized (*arrows*).

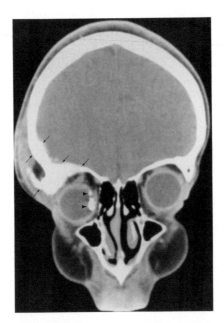

14–4G Coronal nonenhanced CT scan. The osteoblastic tumor (*arrows*) appears hyperdense, as does the right intraocular calcified regressed retinoblastoma (*arrowheads*).

FIGURE 14-5 *Aneurysmal Bone Cyst of the Orbit and Ethmoid Sinus*
An 11-month-old girl presented with a 2-week history of proptosis of the right eye, right facial swelling, and right epistaxis. (From Patel BC, Sabir DI, Flaharty PM, Anderson RL. Aneurysmal bone cyst of the orbit and ethmoid sinus. *Arch Ophthalmol.* 1993; 111:586–587. © 1993, American Medical Association.)

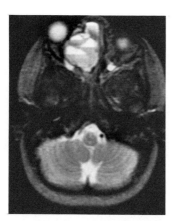

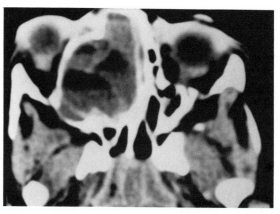

14-5A Axial T2W image. The orbital and ethmoidal mass shows multiple fluid-fluid levels. The superior portions of the cyst are hyperintense on both T1W (not shown) and T2W images and contain extracellular methemoglobin. The hypointense curvilinear signal on the temporal edge of the lesion corresponds to bone formation.

14-5B Axial nonenhanced CT. Note the hyperdense hyperostotic reactive bone surrounding the mass.

MRI of the Eye and Orbit,
by Patrick De Potter, Jerry A. Shields, and Carol L. Shields.
J. B. Lippincott Company, Philadelphia © 1995.

15

Myogenic Tumors

PATRICK DE POTTER

CAROL DOLINSKAS

JERRY A. SHIELDS

CAROL L. SHIELDS

RHABDOMYOSARCOMA

Clinical and Pathological Features

Rhabdomyosarcoma is a highly malignant neoplasm that is composed of cells with the histologic features of striated muscles in various stages of muscle embryogenesis. The average age at diagnosis is 8 years, and the tumor has a slight male preponderance. The characteristic clinical presentation is a rapid, progressive proptosis and displacement of the globe. The tumor is unilateral and, in some cases, may originate from the ethmoid sinus or nasal cavity. Often, the tumor is located anteriorly in the orbit. Orbital rhabdomyosarcoma may extend locally into the sinuses or nasal cavity. When the disease is advanced, lymph node involvement and lung metastasis can occur.

Rhabdomyosarcoma can be classified into four histologic types—pleomorphic, embryonal, alveolar, and botryoid—of which embryonal rhabdomyosarcoma is the most common variant affecting the orbit. The diagnostic histopathologic feature of the tumor is the presence of cross striations within the cytoplasm of the tumor cells. Orbital computed tomography (CT) demonstrates a moderately well-circumscribed but irregular orbital mass that may extend to the nasal cavity or surrounding sinuses.

MR Features

Like other orbital soft tissue tumors, orbital rhabdomyosarcoma appears on magnetic resonance imaging (MRI) studies as a relatively well-circumscribed, irregular orbital mass that may extend to involve the adjacent orbital bones and sinuses. The tumor has a homogeneous or heterogeneous isointense to hyperintense signal with respect to that of the extraocular muscles, and a hypointense signal with respect to that of the orbital fat on T1-weighted (T1W) images (Fig. 15–1, *A* through *C*). On T2-weighted (T2W) images, the lesion has a hyperintense signal with respect to that of the extraocular muscles and orbital fat (Fig. 15–1*D*). Orbital rhabdomyosarcoma may mimic other orbital lesions, and differentiation from rapidly growing capillary hemangioma or granulocytic sarcoma may be very difficult based solely on MR features of the lesions.

On T1W images enhanced with gadolinium diethylenetriamine penta-acetic acid (Gd-DTPA), orbital rhabdomyosarcoma demonstrates moderate to marked enhancement. However, in some cases, the tumor contains the highly vascular internal architecture seen in orbital capillary hemangioma. Delineation of an orbital rhabdomyosarcoma is best accomplished on contrast-enhanced T1W images with fat-suppression (Fig. 15–1, *E* and *F*).

BIBLIOGRAPHY

Armington WG, Bilaniuk LT. The radiologic evaluation of the orbit: Conal and intraconal lesions. *Semin Ultrasound, CT, MR.* 1988; 9:455–473.

Bilaniuk LT, Zimmerman RA, Newton TH. Magnetic resonance imaging: Orbital pathology. In: Newton TH, Bilaniuk LT, eds. *Radiology of the Eye and Orbit.* New York: Raven Press; 1990, Chap 5.

Hopper KD, Sherman JL, Boal DK, Eggli KD. CT and MR imaging of the pediatric orbit. *Radiographics.* 1992; 12:485–503.

Jakobiec FA, Font RL. Mesenchymal tumors. In: Spencer WH, Font RL, Green WR, Howes EL, Jakobiec FA, Zimmerman LE, eds. *Ophthalmic Pathology. An Atlas and Textbook.* Philadelphia: WB Saunders; 1986;2554–2603.

Jones IS, Reese AB, Kraut J. Orbital rhabdomyosarcoma. *Am J Ophthalmol.* 1966; 61:721–736.

Mafee MF, Putterman A, Valvassori GE, Campos M, Capek V. Orbital space-occupying lesions: Role of computed tomography and magnetic resonance imaging. *Radiol Clin North Am.* 1987; 25:529–559.

Mitchell DG, Burk DL, Vinitski S, Rifkin MD. The biophysical basis of tissue contrast in extracranial MR imaging. *AJR.* 1987; 149:831–837.

Nicholson DH, Green WR. Ocular tumors in children. In: Nelson LB, Calhoun JH, Harley RD, eds. *Pediatric Ophthalmology.* 3rd ed. Philadelphia: WB Saunders; 1991; 382–426.

Porterfield JF, Zimmerman LE. Rhabdomyosarcoma of the orbit. *Virchows Arch [A].* 1962; 335:329–344.

Rootman J, Lapointe JS. Mesenchymal tumors. In: Rootman J, ed. *Diseases of the Orbit.* Philadelphia: JB Lippincott; 1988;334–384.

Shields JA. Myogenic tumors. In: Shields JA, ed. *Diagnosis and Management of Orbital Tumors.* Philadelphia: WB Saunders; 1989:243–258.

Sullivan JA, Harms SE. Surface coil MR imaging of orbital neoplasms. *Am J Neuroradiol.* 1986; 7:29–34.

Vade A, Armstrong D. Orbital rhabdomyosarcoma in childhood. *Radiol Clin North Am.* 1987; 25:701–714.

FIGURE 15–1 *Orbital Rhabdomyosarcoma*
A 3-year-old boy presented with a 3-week history of rapidly progressive proptosis of the left eye. Histopathologic examination showed alveolar rhabdomyosarcoma. (Courtesy of G. Lueder, M.D. and H. D. McGowan, M.D., Toronto, Canada.)

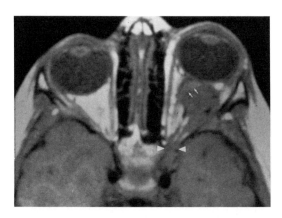

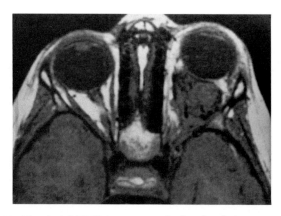

15–1A Axial T1W image. The tumor has a hypointense signal with respect to the orbital fat, but is isointense with respect to the extraocular muscles. The belly of the lateral rectus muscle is involved by the neoplastic lesion, which extends into the superior orbital fissure (*arrowheads*). The optic nerve sheath complex is displaced nasally (*arrows*).

15–1B Axial T1W image at a higher level than in *A*. Note the linear signal voids produced by vessels with high blood flow.

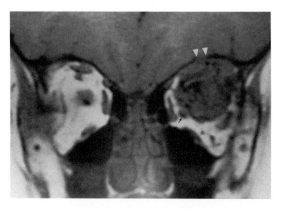

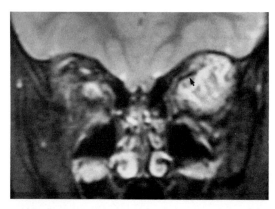

15–1C Coronal T1W image. The tumor displaces the optic nerve sheath complex (*arrow*) inferonasally. Orbital roof thinning (*arrowheads*) is suspected.

15–1D Coronal T2W image. The tumor has a heterogeneous hyperintense signal. Note the linear signal void produced by a vessel (*arrow*).

FIGURE 15-1 *Orbital Rhabdomyosarcoma* (continued)

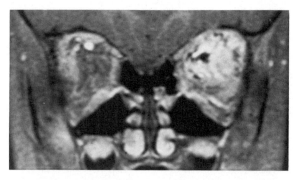

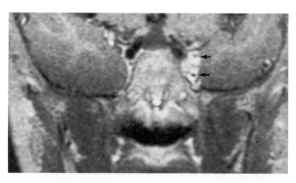

15-1E Fat-suppressed Gd-DTPA–enhanced coronal T1W image. The tumor demonstrates heterogeneous enhancement. Vessels with high blood flow remain hypointense.

15-1F Fat-suppressed Gd-DTPA–enhanced coronal T1W image at the level of the cavernous sinus. The left cavernous sinus is enlarged by the enhancing infiltrative mass *(arrows)*.

MRI of the Eye and Orbit,
by Patrick De Potter, Jerry A. Shields, and Carol L. Shields.
J. B. Lippincott Company, Philadelphia © 1995.

16

Tumors of the Lacrimal Gland

PATRICK DE POTTER

CAROL DOLINSKAS

CAROL L. SHIELDS

JERRY A. SHIELDS

PLEOMORPHIC ADENOMA

Clinical and Pathological Features

Although some variations exist from series to series, a recent review of lacrimal gland biopsies by Shields and coworkers showed that 78% of the lacrimal gland lesions were of nonepithelial origin and only 22% were primary epithelial neoplasms. The nonepithelial lesions included inflammation (64%) and lymphoid tumors (14%), whereas the epithelial lesions included dacryops (6%), pleomorphic adenoma (12%), and malignant epithelial tumors (4%).

Pleomorphic adenoma of the lacrimal gland (benign mixed tumor) is a tumor of adults that presents as a slow-growing mass. It produces a progressive, painless downward and inward displacement of the globe.

On gross examination, pleomorphic adenoma of the lacrimal gland appears as a grayish white, well-encapsulated, bosselated mass. On histopathologic examination, the tumor is found to be composed of epithelial elements (resembling ductal epithelium) and mesenchymal elements (spindle cells). Orbital computed tomography (CT) characteristically shows a dense, round-to-oval, well-circumscribed mass in the lacrimal gland region. Bone erosion or destruction usually is not found, but bone remodeling can be seen if the tumor is chronic.

MR Features

On magnetic resonance imaging (MRI), pleomorphic adenoma of the lacrimal gland (benign mixed tumor) presents as a well-circumscribed mass in the lacrimal gland fossa having a low signal intensity on T1-weighted (T1W) images and increased signal intensity on T2-weighted (T2W) images (Figs. 16–1, *A* through *C*; 16–2, *A* and *B*). Scalloping of the frontal bone may be seen. The anterior portion of the mass seems to end at or posterior to the orbital rim, suggesting that the lesion affects the orbital lobe of the lacrimal gland. After administration of gadolinium diethylenetriamine penta-acetic acid (Gd-DTPA), the tumor demonstrates moderate enhancement (Fig. 16–1*C*). Delineation of the pleomorphic adenoma of the lacrimal gland is best appreciated on fat-suppressed T1-weighted images.

ADENOID CYSTIC CARCINOMA

Clinical and Pathological Features

Adenoid cystic carcinoma is the most common primary malignant tumor involving the lacrimal gland. Unlike those with benign tumors of the lacrimal gland, patients with adenoid cystic carcinoma of the lacrimal gland present with pain, blepharoptosis, and motility disturbances. The duration of symptoms is shorter with malignant lacrimal gland tumors than with those that are benign. The accompanying pain has been attributed to the propensity of the tumor to invade perineurally, as well as into adjacent bone.

On histopathologic examination, adenoid cystic carcinoma consists of densely packed, hyperchromatic, small cells with scant cytoplasm. Five histologic patterns have been described: Swiss cheese (cribriform), sclerosing, basaloid (solid), comedocarcinomatous, and tubular (ductal). Orbital CT scans demonstrate a globular, rounded lesion, but with more irregular and serrated borders than are associated with pleomorphic adenoma. Destructive or sclerotic bony changes can be expected in 80% of cases. Because of the occurrence of bony abnormalities, CT scanning is the modality of choice for the evaluation of malignant lacrimal gland tumor.

MR Features

Based on the authors' limited experience, adenoid cystic carcinoma presents as an irregular, relatively well-defined, or infiltrative mass in the superolateral aspect of the orbit. The tumor shows a relatively heterogeneous hyperintense signal with respect to the extraocular muscles, and a hypointense signal with respect to the orbital fat on T1W images (Fig. 16–3, A and B). On T2W images, the lesion becomes heterogeneously hyperintense compared with the extraocular muscles and orbital fat (Fig. 16–3C). Calcifications within the tumor appear as hypointense areas on T1W and T2W images (Fig. 16–3, A and C). Destruction of the orbital roof and lateral orbital wall is evidenced by interruption of the low signal intensity of the cortical bone (Fig. 16–3B).

INFLAMMATORY LESIONS

Clinical and Pathological Features

Patients with a localized form of idiopathic orbital inflammation involving the lacrimal gland (dacryoadenitis) may present with acute or chronic symptoms of pain associated with swelling or drooping of the upper eyelid, protrusion or displacement of the globe, disturbance of extraocular motility, or diplopia. Chronic dacryoadenitis can follow acute dacryoadenitis, or it may present as an indolent, slightly tender, lacrimal mass. Because of its clinical presentation, dacryoadenitis may simulate primary epithelial tumor of the lacrimal gland.

As in the diffuse form of idiopathic orbital inflammation, the cellular response is a polymorphous inflammatory infiltrate consisting of lymphocytes, plasma cells, macrophages, eosinophils, and polymorphonuclear leukocytes. Tissue edema is often seen in the acute stage, and fibrosis is noted in the chronic stage. Unlike malignant epithelial tumors of the lacrimal gland, dacryoadenitis does not produce bone destruction. In its chronic form, scalloping of the lacrimal fossa may be seen.

MR Features

In the localized form of idiopathic orbital inflammation involving the lacrimal gland (dacryoadenitis), the lacrimal gland appears enlarged and relatively well circumscribed on MRI scans. However, the surrounding orbital tissue may be infiltrated. The inflammatory process usually appears isointense or slightly hypointense with respect to the extraocular muscles on T1W images (Figs. 16–4A and 16–5, A and B). On T2W images, the lesion shows variable signal intensity, depending on whether the disease is in its acute or chronic stage. In acute dacryoadenitis, which is often associated with tissue edema, the lesion shows an increased signal intensity with respect to the orbital fat. (Fig. 16–4, B through D). In the chronic form, which is usually associated with a greater degree of tissue fibrosis, the enlarged lacrimal gland shows a low signal intensity that is isointense to slightly hypointense to orbital fat (Fig. 16–5C). A reticular pattern in the surrounding orbital fat may be seen (Fig. 16–4A).

After Gd-DTPA injection, there is generally variable enhancement of the lesion. Marked enhancement is usually seen in the acute form of the disease. Minimal enhancement is often seen in the chronic or sclerosing type of idiopathic orbital inflammation (Fig. 16–5, D through F). Delineation of the inflammatory process is best accomplished with postcontrast studies using fat suppression.

BIBLIOGRAPHY

Armington WG, Bilaniuk LT. The radiologic evaluation of the orbit: Conal and intraconal lesions. *Semin Ultrasound, CT, MR.* 1988; 9:455–473.

Atlas SW, Grossman RI, Savino PJ, Sergott RC, Schatz NJ, Bosley TM, Hackney DB, Goldberg HI, Bilaniuk LT, Zimmerman RA. Surface coil MR of orbital pseudotumor. *AJNR.* 1987; 8:141–146.

Bilaniuk LT, Zimmerman RA, Newton TH. Magnetic resonance imaging: Orbital pathology. In: Newton TH, Bilaniuk LT, eds. *Radiology of the Eye and Orbit.* New York: Raven Press; 1990, Chap 5.

De Potter P, Flanders AE, Shields CL, Shields JA. Magnetic

resonance imaging of orbital tumors. *Int Ophthalmol Clin*. 1993; 33:163–173.

Font RL, Gamel JW. Epithelial tumors of the lacrimal gland: An analysis of 265 cases. In: Jakobiec FA, ed. *Ocular and Adnexal Tumors*. Birmingham, AL: Aseculapius; 1978:787–805.

Hopper KD, Sherman JL, Boal DK, Eggli KD. CT and MR imaging of the pediatric orbit. *Radiographics*. 1992; 12:485–503.

Jakobiec FA, Font RL. Lacrimal gland tumors. In: Spencer WH, Font RL, Green WR, Howes EL, Jakobiec FA, Zimmerman LE, eds. *Ophthalmic Pathology. An Atlas and Textbook*. Philadelphia: WB Saunders; 1986:2496–2525.

Jakobiec FA, Font RL. Noninfectious orbital inflammations. In: Spencer WH, Font RL, Green WR, Howes EL, Jakobiec FA, Zimmerman LE, eds. *Ophthalmic Pathology. An Atlas and Textbook*. Philadelphia: WB Saunders; 1986:2765–2812.

Jakobiec FA, Trokel SL, Abbott GF, Anderson R, Citrin CM, Alper MG. Combined clinical and computed tomographic diagnosis of primary lacrimal fossa lesions. *Am J Ophthalmol*. 1982; 94:785–807.

Kennerdell JS, Dresner SC. The nonspecific orbital inflammatory syndromes. *Surv Ophthalmol*. 1984; 29: 93–103.

Levine RA. Orbital and adnexal tumors. In: Peyman GA, Sanders DR, Goldberg MF, eds. *Principles and Practice of Ophthalmology*. Vol. 3. Philadelphia: WB Saunders; 1980:2199–2204.

Mafee MF, Haik BG. Lacrimal gland and fossa lesions: Role of computed tomography. *Radiol Clin North Am*. 1987; 25:767–780.

Mafee MF, Putterman A, Valvassori GE, Campos M, Capek V. Orbital space-occupying lesions: Role of computed tomography and magnetic resonance imaging. *Radiol Clin North Am*. 1987; 25:529–559.

Mitchell DG, Burk DL, Vinitski S, Rifkin MD. The biophysical basis of tissue contrast in extracranial MR imaging. *AJR*. 1987; 149:831–837.

Nugent RA, Rootman J, Robertson WD, Lapointe JS, Harrison PB. Acute orbital pseudotumors: Classification and CT features. *AJR*. 1981; 2:431–436.

Portis JM, Krohel GB, Steward WB. Calcifications in lesions of the fossa of the lacrimal gland. *Ophthalmic Plast Reconstr Surg*. 1985; 1:137–144.

Rootman J, Lapointe JS. Tumors of the lacrimal gland. In: Rootman J, ed. *Diseases of the Orbit*. Philadelphia: JB Lippincott; 1988:384–404.

Rootman J, Robertson W, Lapointe JS. Inflammatory diseases. In: Rootman J, ed. *Diseases of the Orbit*. Philadelphia; JB Lippincott; 1988:143–204.

Shields CL, Shields JA, Eagle RC, Rathmell JP. Clinicopathologic review of 142 cases of lacrimal gland lesions. *Ophthalmology*. 1989; 96:431–435.

Shields JA. Epithelial tumors of the lacrimal gland. In: Shields JA, ed. *Diagnosis and Management of Orbital Tumors*. Philadelphia: WB Saunders; 1989:259–274.

Shields JA. Inflammatory conditions that can simulate neoplasms. In: Shields JA, ed. *Diagnosis and Management of Orbital Tumors*. Philadelphia: WB Saunders; 1989:67–85.

Shields JA, Bakewell B, Augsburger JJ, Flanagan JC. Classification and incidence of space-occupying lesions of the orbit. A survey of 645 biopsies. *Arch Ophthalmol*. 1984; 120:1606–1611.

Slamovits TL, Gardner TA. Neuroimaging in neuro-ophthalmology. *Ophthalmology*. 1989; 96:555–568.

Sullivan JA, Harms SE. Surface coil MR imaging of orbital neoplasms. *AJNR*. 1986; 7:29–34.

Zimmerman LE, Sanders TE, Ackerman LV. Epithelial tumors of the lacrimal gland: Prognostic and therapeutic significance of histologic types. *Int Ophthalmol Clin*. 1962; 2:337–367.

FIGURE 16-1 *Pleomorphic Adenoma of the Lacrimal Gland*
A 46-year-old woman with progressive, painless swelling of the lateral portion of the right upper eyelid. The histologically proven pleomorphic adenoma of the lacrimal gland was excised completely, with no rupture of its capsule. (Courtesy of Angela Veloudios, M.D., Willingboro, NJ.)

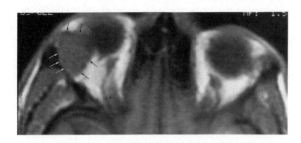

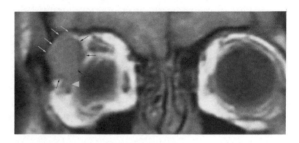

16-1A Axial T1W image. A well-circumscribed mass (*black arrows*) with low signal intensity, which is slightly hyperintense to the extraocular muscles, is seen to produce bone scalloping (*white arrows*) in the right lacrimal gland fossa.

16-1B Coronal T1W image. The tumor (*black arrows*) in the superolateral aspect of the right orbit has an extraconal location. Minimal bone deformation (*white arrows*) without bone destruction is seen. Note the lateral rectus muscle (*arrowhead*).

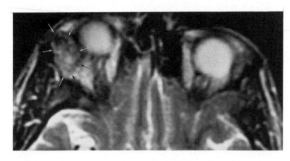

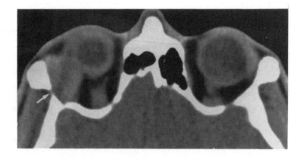

16-1C Axial T2W fast spin echo (FSE) image. The tumor (*arrows*) has a heterogeneous, hyperintense signal compared with the decreased signal of the normal left lacrimal gland.

16-1D Axial contrast-enhanced CT scan. Note the thinning of the bone in the lacrimal gland fossa (*arrow*).

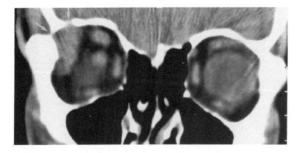

16-1E Coronal contrast-enhanced CT scan. Two areas of bone thinning (*arrows*) that had been suspected on MR scans are well documented.

FIGURE 16-2 *Recurrent Pleomorphic Adenoma of the Lacrimal Gland*
A 59-year-old man presented with recurrent pleomorphic adenoma of the right lacrimal gland after previous removal 10 years before by lateral orbitotomy. (Courtesy of Joseph C. Flanagan, M.D., Philadelphia, PA.)

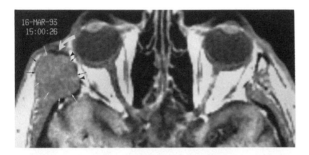

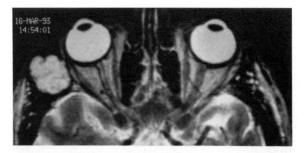

16-2A Axial T1W image. A relatively well-circumscribed mass (*arrows*) with a homogeneous low signal intensity is seen to involve the soft tissues lateral to the right orbit. It compresses but does not infiltrate the adjacent orbital fat and the lateral rectus muscle. There is no mass in the right lacrimal gland region. Note the bony defect (*arrowheads*) from the prior orbitotomy. The linear signal void (*curved arrow*) is produced by cortical bone.

16-2B Axial T2W fast spin echo (FSE) image. The lesion shows a relatively heterogeneous hyperintense signal.

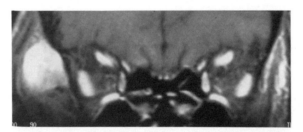

16-2C Fat-suppressed coronal Gd-DTPA–enhanced T1W image. The tumor shows relatively uniform enhancement in the temporal fossa and does not involve the temporalis muscle.

FIGURE 16-3 *Adenoid Cystic Carcinoma of the Lacrimal Gland*

A 50-year-old woman presented with a 6-month history of painful proptosis of the right eye. The histologically proven adenoid cystic carcinoma of the lacrimal gland was removed completely by lateral orbitotomy.

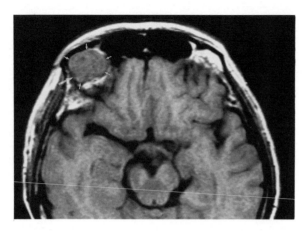

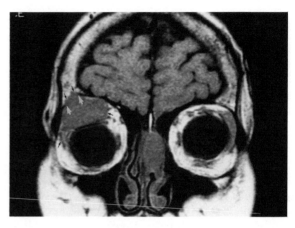

16-3A Axial T1W image. The enlarged right lacrimal gland (*small arrows*) has a heterogeneous low signal intensity that is isointense to the cerebral gray matter and slightly hyperintense to the extraocular muscles (not shown in this figure). Bony infiltration (*large arrow*) by the lesion is suspected.

16-3B Coronal T1W image. The neoplastic process (*black arrows*) infiltrates the extraconal orbital fat and the marrow space of the frontal bone. Note the loss of the signal void of the cortical margin of the frontal bone (*white arrows*). The right globe is compressed by the tumor.

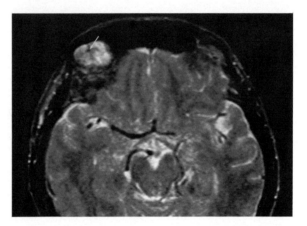

16-3C Axial T2W image. The tumor shows a heterogeneous, increased signal intensity. The focus of low signal intensity (seen as well on T1W images) probably corresponds to calcification (*arrow*).

FIGURE 16–4 *Acute Idiopathic Orbital Inflammation of the Lacrimal Gland (Dacryoadenitis)*

A 31-year-old woman presented with sudden onset of painful swelling of the left upper eyelid. A systemic work-up yielded normal results.

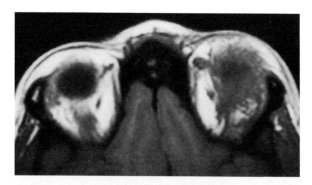

16–4A Axial T1W image. An ill-defined lesion located in the superolateral aspect of the left orbit has a low signal intensity that is isointense to the extraocular rectus muscles. The lesion infiltrates the lacrimal gland and the superior rectus muscle. The adjacent orbital fat has a reticular pattern.

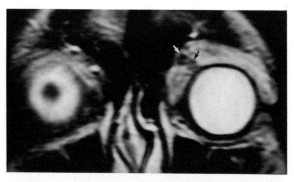

16–4B Coronal T2W image. The inflammatory process involves the lateral rectus, superior rectus, levator palpebrae superioris, and medial rectus muscles. The increased signal intensity on long TR/TE sequences is related to the presence of edema in the acute stage. The superior ophthalmic vein (*black arrow*) and the tendon of the superior oblique muscle (*white arrow*) are well demonstrated.

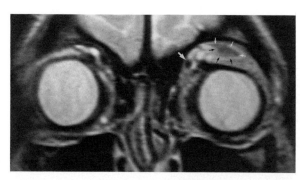

16–4C Coronal T2W image at a more posterior level than in *B*. The superior rectus and levator palpebrae superioris muscles are well visualized (*small arrows*). Note the tendon of the superior oblique muscle (*large arrow*).

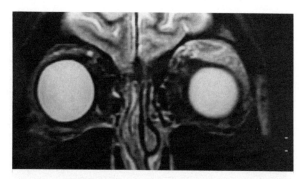

16–4D Coronal T2W image (inversion recovery) at the same level as in *C*. Note the decreased signal intensity of the orbital fat.

A 24-year-old woman presented with chronic left periorbital ache and mild proptosis of the left eye. No diplopia was documented. Incisional biopsy of the lacrimal gland tissue confirmed the diagnosis of chronic nongranulomatous inflammation of the lacrimal gland.

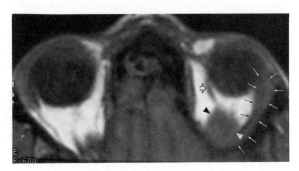

16–5A Axial T1W image. The left lacrimal gland is enlarged by the inflammatory tissue, which extends toward the posterior orbit and infiltrates the lateral rectus muscle (*arrows*). The mass has a decreased signal intensity, which is slightly hyperintense to the extraocular muscles. The superior rectus and levator palpebrae superioris muscles are also enlarged (*arrowheads*). Note the superior ophthalmic vein (*open arrow*).

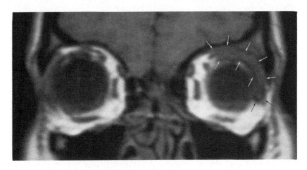

16–5B Coronal T1W image. The inflammatory process involves the left lacrimal gland, the superior muscle complex, and the lateral rectus muscle (*arrows*).

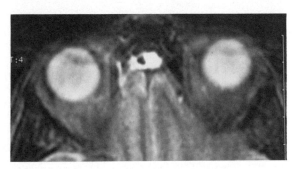

16–5C Axial T2W fast spin echo (FSE) image. The superolateral region of the left orbit shows a diffuse, decreased signal that is hypointense to the orbital fat and is related to tissue fibrosis.

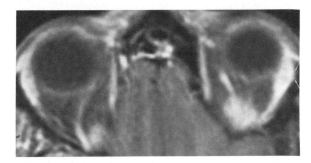

16–5D Fat-suppressed axial Gd-DTPA–enhanced T1W image at the level of the lacrimal gland. The left lacrimal gland and the superior rectus and levator palpebrae superioris muscles show diffuse, moderate enhancement. The mass has produced minimal irregularities of the bony cortex (*arrows*).

FIGURE 16–5 *Chronic Idiopathic Orbital Inflammation Involving the Lacrimal Gland* (continued)

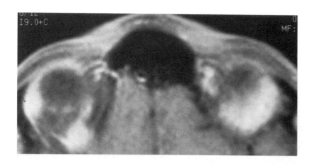 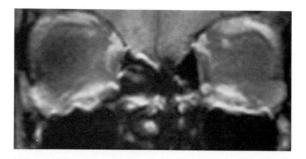

16–5E Fat-suppressed axial Gd-DTPA–enhanced T1W image at the level of the orbital roof.

16–5F Fat-suppressed coronal Gd-DTPA–enhanced T1W image. The superotemporal extraconal region of the left orbit shows diffuse enhancement.

MRI of the Eye and Orbit,
by Patrick De Potter, Jerry A. Shields, and Carol L. Shields.
J. B. Lippincott Company, Philadelphia © 1995.

17

Metastatic Tumors

PATRICK DE POTTER

CAROL DOLINSKAS

JERRY A. SHIELDS

CAROL L. SHIELDS

Clinical and Pathological Features

Tumors metastatic to the orbit are uncommon and occur less frequently than intraocular metastases. The diagnosis of orbital metastasis carries a poor prognosis for survival. The types of orbital metastatic tumors differ radically between adults and children. In adults, the breast and lung are the most common primary sites for carcinoma in women, whereas the prostate and lung are the most common sites for primary tumors in men. However, other primary carcinomas that have been reported to metastasize to the orbit include gastrointestinal carcinoma, carcinoid tumors, skin melanoma, renal cell carcinoma, seminoma, and others. In children, neuroblastoma, Ewing's sarcoma, and Wilm's tumor are the most common sources of orbital metastatic lesions.

The major clinical signs and symptoms relating to metastatic disease involving the orbit are rapid onset of proptosis and displacement secondary to the mass effect, as well as functional deficits caused by tumor infiltration and pressure effects. An interesting clinical variation occurring in patients with scirrhous breast carcinoma and gastric carcinoma that is metastatic to the orbit is the presence of enophthalmos rather than proptosis. This is related to the diffuse infiltration, cicatrization, and retraction of the orbital tissues by the scirrhous tumor.

On histopathologic examination, orbital metastases are often poorly differentiated, and the patho-logic findings are as varied as those of the primary neoplasm. Special immunohistochemical or tumor marking studies are helpful in establishing the correct diagnosis. Orbital computed tomography (CT) reveals an infiltrative or circumscribed mass that may be related to specific orbital structures, such as the lacrimal gland or the extraocular muscles. Bone destruction is often present, and osteoblastic changes may be seen with orbital metastasis from prostate carcinoma.

MR Features

Orbital metastases, such as those from metastatic breast or bronchogenic carcinoma, usually present on magnetic resonance imaging (MRI) as diffuse, infiltrating, nonencapsulated, orbital masses that often involve the extraocular muscles and, sometimes, the bony orbit. However, metastatic carcinoid, renal cell, or thyroid carcinoma and, in some cases, malignant melanoma, may present as a well-circumscribed orbital mass. Metastatic carcinoma usually has an isointense signal with respect to the extraocular muscles and a hypointense signal with respect to orbital fat on T1-weighted (T1W) images (Figs. 17–1, A, D, and E; 17–2, A and B; 17–3, A and B). On T2-weighted (T2W) images, the signal of the tumor is usually hyperintense with respect to that of the extraocular muscles and orbital fat (Figs. 17–1B and 17–2C). Hemorrhagic metastatic lesions, such as those seen with metastatic renal cell carcinoma, may appear with a heterogeneous hyperintense signal on T1W and T2W images. Metastatic prostatic carcinoma to the orbit produces osteoblastic changes that are well demonstrated on T1W images, with replacement of the high signal intensity of the normal fatty marrow and replacement of the signal void of cortical bone with the intermediate signal intensity of the sclerotic tumor. However, not all orbital metastatic lesions share the same MRI features. Orbital carcinoid metastasis can show a decreased signal intensity on T2W images (Fig. 17–3C). Because of the paramagnetic properties of melanin, metastatic melanoma to the orbit may show a slightly higher signal intensity on T1W images compared with that of other metastatic lesions (Fig. 17–2, A and B). MR features of orbital metastasis can be shared by other ill-defined or well-circumscribed orbital lesions (see Tables 10–1, 11–1, 11–2). Therefore, at times radiologic differentiation may be difficult.

Metastatic lesions usually demonstrate moderate to marked enhancement after administration of gadolinium diethylenetriamine penta-acetic acid (Gd-DTPA). Tumor enhancement and delineation are best appreciated on fat-suppressed, contrast-enhanced scans (Figs. 17–1, C, F, and G; 17–2D).

BIBLIOGRAPHY

Armington WG, Bilaniuk LT. The radiologic evaluation of the orbit: Conal and intraconal lesions. *Semin Ultrasound, CT, MR.* 1988; 9:455–473.

Bilaniuk LT, Zimmerman RA, Newton TH. Magnetic resonance imaging: Orbital pathology. In: Newton TH, Bilaniuk LT, eds. *Radiology of the Eye and Orbit.* New York: Raven Press; 1990, Chap 5.

Boldt HC, Nerad JA. Orbital metastases from prostate carcinoma. *Arch Ophthalmol.* 1988; 106:1403–1408.

Braffman BH, Bilaniuk LT, Eagle RC, Savino PJ, Hackney DB, Grossman RI, Goldberg HI, Zimmerman RA. MR imaging of a carcinoid tumor metastatic to the orbit. *J Comput Assist Tomogr.* 1987; 11:891–894.

De Potter P, Flanders AE, Shields CL, Shields JA. Magnetic resonance imaging of orbital tumors. *Int Ophthalmol Clin.* 1993; 33:163–173.

Ferry AP, Font RL. Carcinoma metastatic to the eye and orbit. A clinicopathologic study of 227 cases. *Arch Ophthalmol.* 1974; 92:276–286.

Freedman MI, Folk JC. Metastatic tumors to the eye and orbit. Patient survival and clinical characteristics. *Arch Ophthalmol.* 1987; 105:1215–1219.

Hopper KD, Sherman JL, Boal DK, Eggli KD. CT and MR imaging of the pediatric orbit. *Radiographics.* 1992; 12:485–503.

Jakobiec FA, Font RL. Metastasis tumors. In: Spencer WH, Font RL, Green WR, Howes EL, Jakobiec FA, Zimmerman LE, eds. *Ophthalmic Pathology. An Atlas and Textbook.* Philadelphia: WB Saunders; 1986:2749–2765.

Mafee MF, Putterman A, Valvassori GE, Campos M, Capek V. Orbital space-occupying lesions: Role of computed tomography and magnetic resonance imaging. *Radiol Clin North Am.* 1987; 25:529–559.

Mitchell DG, Burk DL, Vinitski S, Rifkin MD. The biophysical basis of tissue contrast in extracranial MR imaging. *AJR.* 1987; 149:831–837.

Peyster RG, Shapiro MD, Haik BG. Orbital metastasis: Role of magnetic resonance imaging and computed tomography. *Radiol Clin North Am.* 1987; 25:647–662.

Riddle PJ, Font RL, Zimmerman LE. Carcinoid tumors to the eye and orbit: A clinicopathologic study of 15 cases, with histochemical and electron microscopic observations. *Hum Pathol.* 1982; 13:459–469.

Rootman J, Ragaz J, Cline R, Lapointe JS. Orbital metastasis. In: Rootman J, ed. *Diseases of the Orbit.* Philadelphia: JB Lippincott; 1988:405–427.

Shields CL, Shields JA, Eagle RC, Peyster RG, Conner BE, Green HA. Orbital metastasis from a carcinoid tumor. *Arch Ophthalmol.* 1987; 105:968–971.

Shields CL, Shields JA, Peggs M. Tumors metastatic to the orbit. *Ophthalmol Plast Reconstr Surg.* 1988; 4:73–80.

Shields JA. Metastatic cancer to the orbit. In: Shields JA, ed. *Diagnosis and Management of Orbital Tumors.* Philadelphia: WB Saunders; 1989:291–315.

Shields JA, Bakewell B, Augsburger JJ, Flanagan JC. Classification and incidence of space-occupying lesions of the orbit. A survey of 645 biopsies. *Arch Ophthalmol.* 1984; 102:1606–1611.

Slamovits TL, Gardner TA. Neuroimaging in neuro-ophthalmology. *Ophthalmology.* 1989; 96:555–568.

Sullivan JA, Harms SE. Surface coil MR imaging of orbital neoplasms. *AJNR.* 1986; 7:29–34.

FIGURE 17–1 *Orbital Metastasis from Breast Carcinoma*
A 35-year-old woman with a history of metastatic breast carcinoma subsequently developed brain, choroidal, and left orbital metastases.

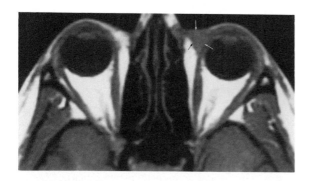

17–1A Axial T1W image. An ill-defined mass located at the medial canthus (*arrows*) shows an increased signal intensity that is slightly hyperintense to the extraocular muscles. The tendon of the medial rectus muscle is not involved.

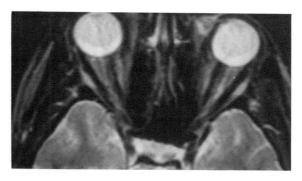

17–1B Axial T2W image. The mass becomes heterogeneously hyperintense with respect to the extraocular muscles and orbital fat.

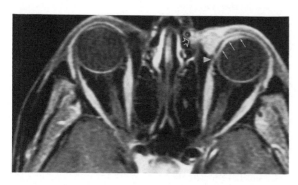

17–1C Fat-suppressed axial Gd-DTPA–enhanced T1W image. The lesion shows marked homogeneous enhancement. On this section, the hyperintense signal of the medial rectus muscle is well defined, with no involvement by the mass in its anterior portion (*arrowhead*). The enhancing ciliary body (*arrows*) appears to be thickened, suggesting uveal metastasis. The metastatic lesion erodes the medial orbital wall and extends into an anterior ethmoid air cell (*open arrow*) as also seen on nonenhanced scans.

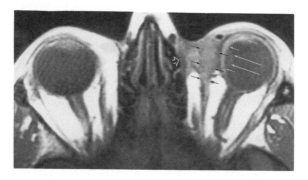

17–1D The patient refused systemic chemotherapy, presenting 1 month later with marked swelling of the medial canthus area and left upper eyelid. Fundus examination of the left eye disclosed a ciliochoroidal metastasis with secondary retinal detachment.

Axial T1W image. The infiltrative soft tissue mass appears to be enlarged and produces deformity of the left globe. The insertion and belly of the medial rectus muscle (*black arrows*) are involved by the tumor. The ciliary body and the choroid nasally are infiltrated by the hyperintense metastasis (*short white arrows*). An adjacent, less hyperintense, secondary retinal detachment is noted (*long white arrows*). The portion of the mass invading the ethmoid sinus has increased in size (*open arrow*).

(continued)

FIGURE 17-1 *Orbital Metastasis from Breast Carcinoma* (continued)

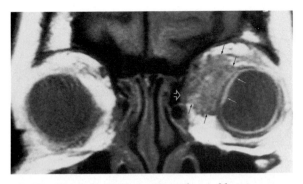 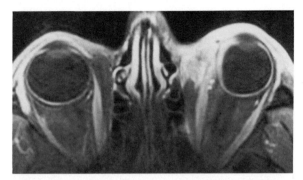

17-1E Coronal T1W image. The infiltrative mass (*black arrows*) has an extraconal and intraconal location. The sclera is not involved, but is deformed. The thickened, hyperintense choroid (*white arrows*) is well visualized. Note the extension of the lesion into the ethmoid sinus (*open arrow*).

17-1F Fat-suppressed axial Gd-DTPA–enhanced T1W image. The orbital mass demonstrates marked heterogeneous enhancement. The ciliochoroidal mass enhances homogeneously. The subretinal fluid does not show enhancement.

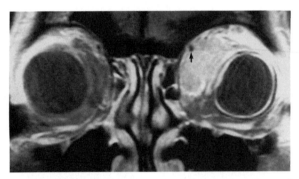

17-1G Fat-suppressed coronal Gd-DTPA–enhanced T1W image. The medial rectus muscle is not identified. The rounded, hypointense signal corresponds to the tendon of the superior oblique muscle (*arrow*).

FIGURE 17–2 *Orbital Metastasis from Skin Melanoma*
A 45-year-old man presented with rapid onset of proptosis of the left eye associated with conjunctival chemosis 1 month after the diagnosis of primary skin melanoma was established.

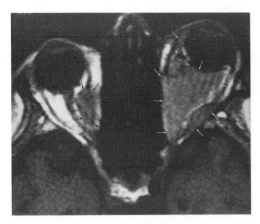

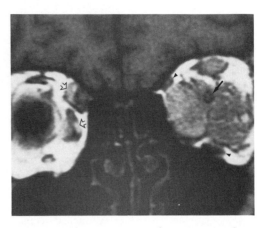

17–2A Axial T1W image. The left orbit is filled with an infiltrative mass (*white arrows*) occupying the intraconal and extraconal space. Because of its melanin content, the pigmented orbital mass, which infiltrates the medial and lateral rectus muscles, has a high signal intensity with respect to the extraocular muscles. In the right orbit, metastatic enlargement of the medial rectus muscle is seen (*black arrows*).

17–2B Coronal T1W image. The metastatic lesion in the left orbit encircles the optic nerve (*arrow*). The superior oblique and inferior rectus muscles (*arrowheads*) are not involved. In the right orbit, the superior oblique and medial rectus muscles have been infiltrated by tumor (*open arrows*).

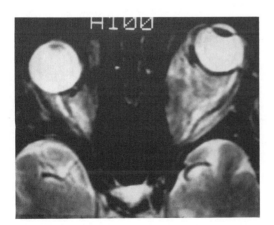

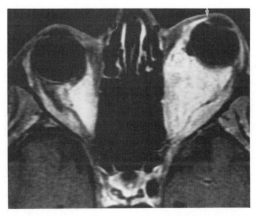

17–2C Axial T2W image. Bilateral orbital metastases demonstrate a heterogeneous, hyperintense signal.

17–2D Fat-suppressed axial Gd-DTPA–enhanced T1W image. Diffuse enhancement is seen to fill most of the left orbit and to involve the medial half of the right orbit. The tumor's infiltration of the left medial rectus muscle is identifiable up to its anterior scleral extension (*arrow*) (as seen in *E*).

(continued)

FIGURE 17-2 *Orbital Metastasis from Skin Melanoma* (continued)

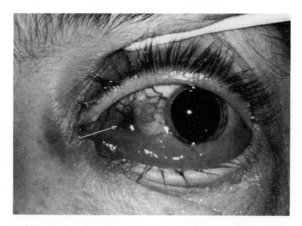

17-2E Clinical photograph showing the pigmented scleral area nasally (*arrow*) corresponding to the insertion of the medial rectus muscle, which is infiltrated with melanocytes. Note the conjunctival chemosis secondary to orbital compression by the metastatic process.

FIGURE 17–3 *Orbital Carcinoid Metastasis*

A 73-year-old woman presented with slowly progressive proptosis of the right eye. Seven years prior to the ocular symptoms, she was diagnosed with carcinoid of the ileum, which was completely excised. Excisional biopsy of the orbital mass confirmed the diagnosis of carcinoid metastasis. No other systemic metastasis was found. (From Shields CL, Shields JA, Eagle RC, Peyster RG, Conner BE, Green HA. Orbital metastasis from a carcinoid tumor. *Arch Ophthalmol.* 1987; 105:968–971. © 1987, American Medical Association.)

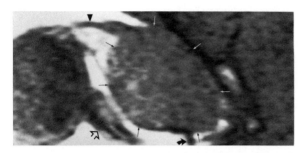

17–3A Sagittal T1W image. A well-circumscribed mass (*thin arrows*) with a heterogeneous hypointense signal is seen to be infiltrating the superior rectus muscle. The emergence of the tendon of the superior rectus muscle is seen anteriorly (*arrowhead*). The optic nerve sheath complex (*open arrow*) is displaced inferiorly. The orbital roof appears to be intact. Note the ophthalmic artery (*curved arrow*).

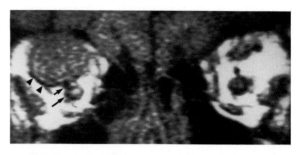

17–3B Coronal T1W image. The ophthalmic artery (*short arrow*) is located between the tumor and the optic nerve sheath complex (*long arrow*). Note the chemical shift artifact (*arrowheads*).

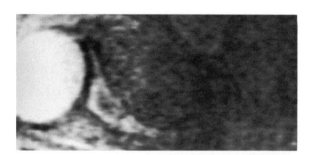

17–3C Sagittal T2W image. The tumor remains hypointense and is less conspicuous than in the T1W image because of the loss of contrast from the orbital fat.

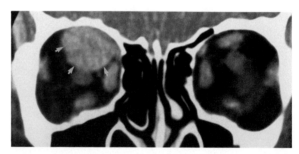

17–3D Coronal contrast-enhanced CT scan. The mass (*arrows*) does not produce bone destruction or erosion.

MRI of the Eye and Orbit,
by Patrick De Potter, Jerry A. Shields, and Carol L. Shields.
J. B. Lippincott Company, Philadelphia © 1995.

18

Lymphoproliferative and Histiocytic Disorders

PATRICK DE POTTER

CAROL DOLINSKAS

CAROL L. SHIELDS

JERRY A. SHIELDS

LYMPHOPROLIFERATIVE DISORDERS

Clinical and Pathological Features

Lymphoproliferative disorders represent a group of lesions whose basic unifying histopathologic feature is a densely cellular infiltrate consisting mostly of small lymphocytes. The lymphoproliferative disorders include benign, atypical, and malignant lymphomatous lesions, usually of the non-Hodgkin's variety. Clinically, the orbital manifestations of these lymphoproliferative disorders are quite similar and are characterized by an insidious, indolent course. Because of their tendency to involve the superior and anterior portions of the orbit, the lesions often can be palpated, and conjunctival involvement can be seen as a pink subepithelial conjunctival infiltrate. Orbital lymphoid tumors also have a predilection for involving the lacrimal gland; in these cases, the lesions can be palpated at the orbital rim.

On histopathologic examination, benign lymphoid hyperplasia is characterized by scant fibrous stroma surrounding hyperplastic abnormal lymphoid tissue. The individual cells are small, dark lymphocytes without significant mitotic activity. The germinal centers contain mitotically active, large, and irregularly shaped blastic cells. In atypical lymphoid hyperplasia, the nuclei are larger but the mitotic activity is sparse or absent. There may be remnants of small or abortive follicles. Malignant non-Hodgkin's lymphoma is characterized by an increased number of anaplastic cells with large nuclei, a greater degree of nuclear pleomorphism, and prominent nucleoli.

Orbital computed tomography (CT) demonstrates a fairly well-defined, solid, orbital mass that tends to mold itself to the adjacent globe and orbital bones. Lymphoid tumors are usually homogeneous masses of high density that have sharp margins. Lacrimal gland involvement is common. Orbital bony involvement is relatively rare. Both benign and malignant lymphomatous processes have similar features on CT.

MR Features

Compared with other ill-defined or relatively well-circumscribed orbital lesions, lymphoproliferative disorders present with nonspecific MR features (see Tables 10–1, 11–1, 11–2). The lymphoid tumor appears as a solid, poorly circumscribed, infiltrative orbital lesion that tends to insinuate and infiltrate itself into the potential fascial spaces and around the globe and optic nerve. The mass tends to mold to the globe, without indenting it, and to the orbital walls without usually producing bone destruction or erosion. The lymphoid tissues usually have an isointense to hyperintense signal with respect to the extraocular muscles and a hypointense signal with respect to orbital fat on T1-weighted (T1W) images (Figs. 18–1A and 18–3, A through C). The tumor may show minimal to marked hyperintensity with respect to extraocular muscles and orbital fat on T2-weighted (T2W) images (Fig. 18–3D). These MR features are probably related to the amount of extracellular water in these lesions, as well as to their cellular density.

After administration of gadolinium diethylene-triamine penta-acetic acid (Gd-DTPA), lymphoid tumors demonstrate moderate to marked enhancement on T1W images (Figs. 18–1, B and C; 18–2, A through C; 18–3, E and F). This enhancement is better delineated on fat-suppressed scans. Based on the authors' experience, MRI does not provide sufficient tissue specificity to allow reliable differentiation among benign reactive lymphoid hyperplasia, atypical lymphoid hyperplasia, and malignant lymphoma and among benign and malignant lymphoproliferative disorders and idiopathic orbital pseudotumor (see Table 10–1). Delineation and extent of the lymphoproliferative process are best evaluated on Gd-DTPA–enhanced, fat-suppressed images.

EOSINOPHILIC GRANULOMA

Clinical and Pathological Features

Eosinophilic granuloma (Langerhans' cell histiocytosis) is generally a solitary osseous lesion when it occurs in the orbital region. Orbital involvement has a distinct predilection for the superotemporal orbital rim. The patient typically develops a rapidly progressive, tender swelling of the superotemporal aspect of the orbit, along with cutaneous erythema. Orbital soft tissue involvement without an obvious bone defect is uncommon. Children and teenagers are most commonly affected.

Histopathologic examination reveals that eosinophilic granuloma is composed of large histiocytes and multinucleated giant cells with scattered eosinophils. Hemorrhage is frequent within the tumor because of the scant stroma and rich vascularity. Electron microscopy reveals distinctive cytoplasmic granules or inclusions referred to as Birbeck granules in the mononucleated histiocytes. Orbital CT scans demonstrate focal bone lysis with predominant involvement of the frontal or zygomatic bones. The intraosseous lesion usually has an irregular contour with possible marginal hyperostosis. The soft tissue mass may extend into the temporal fossa and brain.

MR Features

Based on the authors' limited experience with MR studies of this lesion, eosinophilic granuloma appears as a solid, relatively well-defined, orbital mass located in the superotemporal aspect of the orbit. The tumor shows a heterogeneous hyperintense signal with respect to the brain and the extraocular muscles on T1W images (Fig. 18–4, A and B). On T2W images, the mass becomes hyperintense to the orbital fat and brain (Fig. 18–4, C and D). Destruction of the orbital roof and lateral orbital wall, with extension through the skull and into the temporal fossa, is easily demonstrated on MR scans (Fig. 18–4, A through E).

After administration of Gd-DTPA, with or without fat suppression, eosinophilic granuloma demonstrates heterogeneous marked enhancement on T1W images (Fig. 18–4E). Cerebral involvement can also be easily documented on postcontrast images.

BIBLIOGRAPHY

Armington WG, Bilaniuk LT. The radiologic evaluation of the orbit: Conal and intraconal lesions. *Semin Ultrasound, CT, MR.* 1988; 9:455–473.

Bilaniuk LT, Zimmerman RA, Newton TH. Magnetic resonance imaging: Orbital pathology. In: Newton TH, Bilaniuk LT, eds. *Radiology of the Eye and Orbit.* New York: Raven Press; 1990, Chap 5.

De Potter P, Flanders AE, Shields CL, Shields JA. Magnetic resonance imaging of orbital tumors. *Int Ophthalmol Clin.* 1993; 33:163–173.

Ellis JH, Banks PM, Campbell J, Liesegang TJ. Lymphoid tumors of the ocular adnexa. *Ophthalmology.* 1985; 92:1311–1324.

Flanders AE, Espinosa GA, Markiewicz DA, Howell DD. Orbital lymphoma: Role of CT and MRI. *Radiol Clin North Am.* 1987; 25:601–614.

Jakobiec FA, Font RL. Leukemic and histiocytic disorders. In: Spencer WH, Font RL, Green WR, Howes EL, Jakobiec FA, Zimmerman LE, eds. *Ophthalmic Pathology. An Atlas and Textbook.* Philadelphia: WB Saunders; 1986:2712–2736.

Jakobiec FA, Font RL. Lymphoid tumors. In: Spencer WH, Font RL, Green WR, Howes EL, Jakobiec FA, Zimmerman LE, eds. *Ophthalmic Pathology. An Atlas and Textbook.* Philadelphia: WB Saunders; 1986:2663–2711.

Jakobiec FA, Trokel SL, Aron-Rosa D, Iwamoto T, Doyon D. Localized eosinophilic granuloma (Langerhans' cell histiocytosis) of the frontal orbital bone. *Arch Ophthalmol.* 1980; 98:1814–1820.

Knowles DM, Jakobiec FA. Ocular adnexal lymphoid neoplasms: Clinical, histopathologic, electron microscopic, and immunologic characteristics. *Hum Pathol.* 1982; 13:148–162.

Mafee MF, Putterman A, Valvassori GE, Campos M, Capek V. Orbital space-occupying lesions: Role of computed tomography and magnetic resonance imaging. *Radiol Clin North Am.* 1987; 25:529–559.

Mitchell DG, Burk DL, Vinitski S, Rifkin MD. The biophysical basis of tissue contrast in extracranial MR imaging. *AJR.* 1987; 149:831–837.

Moore AT, Pritchard J, Taylor DSI. Histiocytosis X: An ophthalmological review. *Br J Ophthalmol.* 1985; 69:7–14.

Peyster RG, Shapiro MD, Haik BG. Orbital metastasis: Role of magnetic resonance imaging and computed tomography. *Radiol Clin North Am.* 1987; 25: 647–662.

Rootman J, Robertson W, Lapointe JS, White V. Lymphoproliferative and leukemic lesions. In: Rootman J, ed. *Diseases of the Orbit.* Philadelphia: JB Lippincott; 1988:205–240.

Shields JA. Histiocytic tumors and pseudotumors. In: Shields JA, ed. *Diagnosis and Management of Orbital Tumors.* Philadelphia: WB Saunders; 1989:378–388.

Shields JA. Lymphoid tumors and leukemia. In: Shields JA, ed. *Diagnosis and Management of Orbital Tumors.* Philadelphia: WB Saunders; 1989:316–340.

Shields JA, Bakewell B, Augsburger JJ, Flanagan JC. Classification and incidence of space-occupying lesions of the orbit. A survey of 645 biopsies. *Arch Ophthalmol.* 1984; 102:1606–1611.

Sullivan JA, Harms SE. Surface coil MR imaging of orbital neoplasms. *AJNR.* 1986; 7:29–34.

Yeo JH, Jakobiec FA, Abbott GF, Trokel SL. Combined clinical and tomographic diagnosis of orbital lymphoid tumors. *Am J Ophthalmol.* 1982; 94:235–245.

Yuh WTC, Flickinger FW, Willekes CL, Sato Y, Nerad JA. Intraorbital tumor as the initial symptom of childhood acute lymphoblastic leukemia. Magnetic resonance imaging findings. *Clin Imaging.* 1990; 14: 120–122.

Zimmerman LE, Font RL. Ophthalmoscopic manifestations of granulocytic sarcoma (myeloid sarcoma or chloroma). *Am J Ophthalmol.* 1975; 80:975–990.

FIGURE 18-1 *Orbital Benign Reactive Lymphoid Hyperplasia*

A 38-year-old man presented with progressive painless swelling of the left upper eyelid and proptosis of the left eye. The immunoglobulin light chain profile of the B-cell type infiltrate appeared polyclonal.

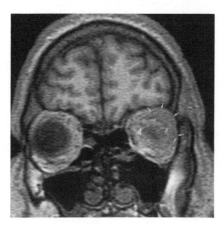

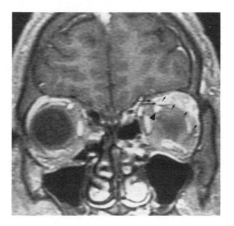

18-1A Fat-suppressed coronal T1W image. An ill-defined mass (*arrows*) with decreased signal intensity infiltrates the left lacrimal gland and is barely discernible from the surrounding orbital tissues. Note the superior ophthalmic vein (*arrowhead*).

18-1B Fat-suppressed coronal Gd-DTPA–enhanced T1W image. The mass shows marked heterogeneous enhancement (*short arrows*). The superior rectus and levator palpebrae superioris muscles are clearly evident (*long arrows*). Note the enhancement of the superior ophthalmic vein (*arrowhead*).

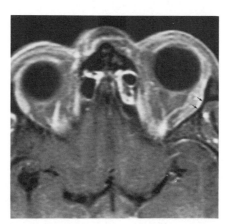

18-1C Fat-suppressed axial Gd-DTPA–enhanced T1W image. The enlarged left lacrimal gland produces bone molding (*arrows*), but the regular curvilinear signal void indicates absence of bone destruction or thinning.

FIGURE 18-2 *Atypical Lymphoid Hyperplasia (Predominantly T-lymphocyte)*
A 55-year-old man with a two-month history of recurrent swelling of the right periorbital area, diplopia, and right afferent pupillary defect. CT studies showed a focal enhancing mass in the region of the right orbital apex. Incisional biopsy confirmed the diagnosis of atypical lymphoid hyperplasia with predominantly T-lymphocytes infiltrate. (Courtesy of Marlon Maus, M.D., Philadelphia.)

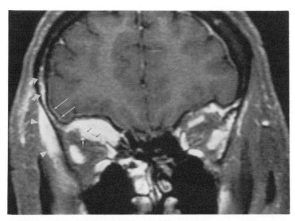

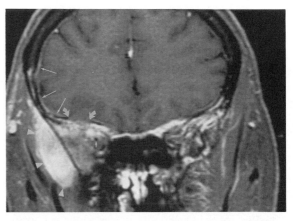

18-2A Fat-suppressed coronal Gd-DTPA–enhanced T1W image. An extraconal markedly-enhancing mass displaces the superior rectus and superior levator palpebrae muscles inferiorly (*black arrows*) in the right orbit. The enhancing infiltrative process extends into the right temporalis muscle (*arrowheads*). There is meningeal enhancement (*long white arrows*) along the right temporal convexity. Enhancement of the marrow space (*curved arrows*) suggests bone marrow replacement by the lymphoid tissue. Note the superior ophthalmic vein (*short white arrow*).

18-2B Fat-suppressed coronal Gd-DTPA–enhanced T1W image at a more posterior level than *A*. Enhancing lymphoid infiltrate extends to the right orbital apex. The signal void corresponds to the ophthalmic artery (*short white arrow*). Note the massive temporal fossa involvement (*arrowheads*) and meningeal infiltration (*long white arrows*). Bony destruction of the orbital roof is indicated by the loss of signal void (*curved arrows*).

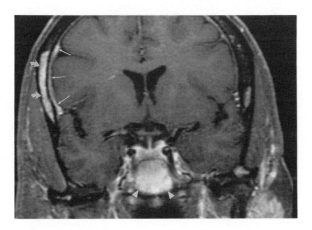

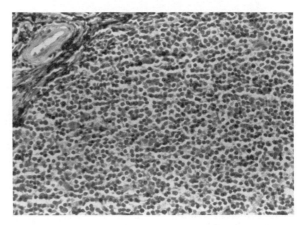

18-2C Fat-suppressed coronal Gd-DTPA–enhanced T1W image at the level of the chiasm. The enhancement of the diploic space (*curved arrows*), right meninges (*arrows*), and clivus (*arrowheads*) is well demonstrated.

18-2D Orbital biopsy specimen showing monomorphic population of well-differentiated lymphocytes (hematoxylin-eosin ×100).

FIGURE 18-3 *Orbital Malignant Lymphoma*
An 80-year-old man presented with ptosis of the left upper eyelid associated with soft tissue swelling. An incisional biopsy confirmed the diagnosis of lymphocytic lymphoma of intermediate differentiation.

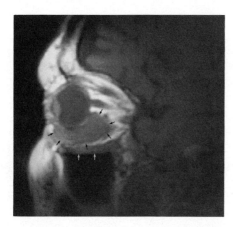

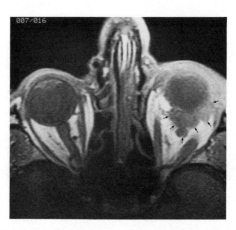

18–3A Sagittal T1W image. A soft tissue mass with low signal intensity, which is isointense to the extraocular muscles, is located within the inferior intraconal and extraconal space of the left orbit (*black arrows*). The mass engulfs the inferior rectus muscle, which is not identified anteriorly. Note the thickened mucosa of the sinus maxillary roof (*white arrows*).

18–3B Axial T1W image. The mass (*arrows*) is molding to the posterior pole of the left eye without invasion into the globe.

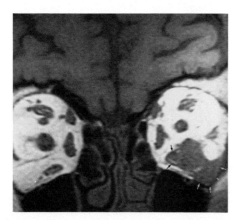

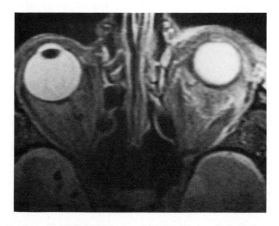

18–3C Coronal T1W image. There is extraconal extension of the lesion in the inferolateral aspect of the left orbit (*white arrows*). The inferior rectus muscle (*black arrows*) is barely identified. There is no gross invasion or destruction of the left zygoma.

18–3D Axial T2W image. The lesion is slightly hyperintense to the orbital fat.

FIGURE 18-3 *Orbital Malignant Lymphoma* (continued)

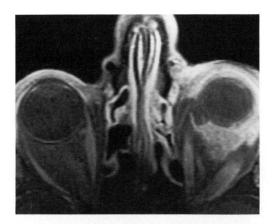

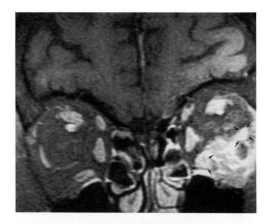

18-3E Fat-suppressed axial Gd-DTPA–enhanced T1W image. The mass demonstrates marked homogeneous enhancement. The insertion of the lateral rectus muscle is engulfed by the enhancing tumor. This was not appreciated on precontrast images.

18-3F Fat-suppressed coronal Gd-DTPA–enhanced T1W image. The inferior and lateral rectus muscles (*arrows*) are identified and are seen to be displaced by the infiltrative process.

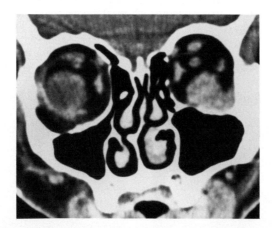

18-3G Coronal nonenhanced CT scan. The mass appears isodense to the inferior rectus muscle. No bone destruction or erosion is seen.

FIGURE 18-4 *Orbital Eosinophilic Granuloma*

A 7-year-old boy presented with a 4-week history of swelling of the left upper eyelid. Ten days later, the swelling became extensive and nonresponsive to antibiotics. Incisional biopsy showed histiocytes with Touton's cells.

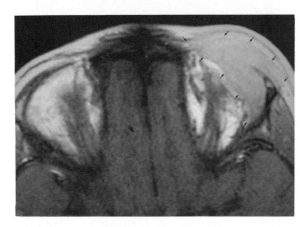

18-4A Axial T1W image. The soft tissue mass (*arrows*), which has an epicenter in the superolateral aspect of the left orbit, has infiltrated the subcutaneous tissues. The mass is hyperintense to the superior rectus muscle and hypointense to the orbital fat. On this section, the lateral orbital wall does not appear to be involved.

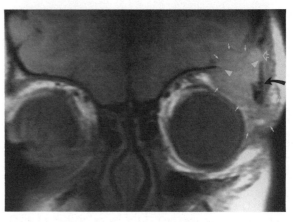

18-4B Coronal T1W image. The absence of continuity of the curvilinear signal void (*arrowheads*) indicates destruction of the orbital roof by the infiltrative process. The mass (*arrows*) is seen to infiltrate the temporal fossa. The frontal bone is also destroyed laterally (*open arrow*). The left lacrimal gland is not identified. The irregular signal void (*curved arrow*) at the lateral margin of the lesion represents residual frontal bone (also seen in *D* through *F*).

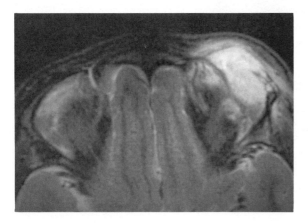

18-4C Axial T2W fast spin echo (FSE) image. The lesion is hyperintense.

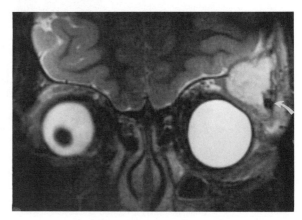

18-4D Coronal T2W fast spin echo (FSE) image. This section clearly demonstrates that the brain parenchyma is not involved by the lesion.

FIGURE 18-4 *Orbital Eosinophilic Granuloma* (continued)

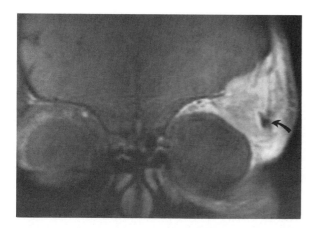

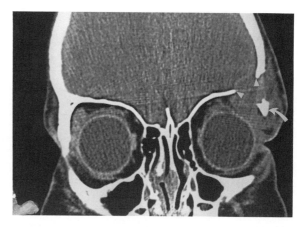

18-4E Fat-suppressed coronal Gd-DTPA–enhanced T1W image. The lesion demonstrates marked and slightly heterogeneous enhancement. The brain parenchyma does not show enhancement. Note a remaining fragment of frontal bone (*curved arrow*).

18-4F Coronal nonenhanced CT scan. The destruction of the frontal bone (*arrowheads*) reflects that seen on MRI. The tumor appears isodense to the brain.

MRI of the Eye and Orbit,
by Patrick De Potter, Jerry A. Shields, and Carol L. Shields.
J. B. Lippincott Company, Philadelphia © 1995.

19

Secondary Orbital Tumors

PATRICK DE POTTER

JERRY A. SHIELDS

CAROL L. SHIELDS

ORBITAL TUMORS OF EYELID ORIGIN

Clinical and Pathological Features

Among the primary tumors of the skin and adnexa that may invade the orbit, basal cell carcinoma, sebaceous cell carcinoma, and squamous cell carcinoma are the most common. Orbital extension of eyelid tumors usually results from long-delayed presentation, incomplete excision with subsequent multiple recurrences, or very aggressive growth of the lesion. Because of its malignant behavior, which can masquerade as chronic inflammation, sebaceous gland carcinoma has a higher tendency to invade the orbit than the others mentioned. The patient with orbital invasion has a history of a neglected or incompletely excised eyelid lesion. The patient may experience progressive discomfort associated with gradual restriction of ocular motility, induration of the subcutaneous tissues, and fixation of the globe. Perineural involvement is associated with pain.

On histopathologic examination, the tumor shows features of the primary eyelid tumor. However, sebaceous cell carcinoma may be misdiagnosed as basal or squamous cell carcinoma. Orbital computed tomography (CT) usually reveals a solid infiltrative mass arising from the eyelid region and extending deep into the orbit. Bone window settings are helpful in determining the extent of bony involvement.

MR Features

Like other malignant orbital tumors, primary eyelid carcinoma invading the orbit demonstrates, on magnetic resonance imaging (MRI), a low signal intensity on T1-weighted (T1W) images and a low to high signal intensity on T2-weighted (T2W) images with respect to orbital fat (Fig. 19–1, *A* through *C*). The role of MR studies is to define the extent of the lesion prior to surgical exploration. Secondary brain invasion by the tumor can easily be detected by MRI.

After administration of gadolinium diethylenetriamine penta-acetic acid (Gd-DTPA), the orbital component of the primary eyelid carcinoma demonstrates marked enhancement (Fig. 19–1, *D* and *E*). Fat-suppression techniques are recommended for better delineation of the orbital extension of the eyelid tumor.

ORBITAL TUMORS OF CONJUNCTIVAL ORIGIN

Clinical and Pathological Features

Squamous cell carcinoma and malignant melanoma are the two most important neoplasms of the conjunctiva that may secondarily invade the orbit. Orbital invasion is usually a part of either advanced disease and delayed presentation or multiple recurrences following incomplete excision. Lesions arising in the fornices or caruncle have an increased tendency to infiltrate the anterior orbital tissues. The orbital symptoms and signs include a palpable anterior orbital mass, displacement of the globe, oculomotor palsies, and fixation of the globe. Despite several reports, it is very difficult to estimate accurately the frequency with which tumors of conjunctival origin invade the orbit.

On histopathologic study, the rare mucoepidermoid squamous cell carcinoma of the conjunctiva has a much more aggressive behavior and may infiltrate the orbit. Most malignant melanomas of the conjunctiva that invade the orbit are loosely cohesive epithelioid cell tumors. Orbital CT scans usually show a solid mass with infiltrative features located adjacent to the globe.

MR Features

MR scans play a critical role in the preoperative staging of conjunctival malignant lesions in patients who have clinical signs of orbital invasion. Because of its high soft tissue definition, MRI is particularly helpful in choosing among the possible routes for biopsy and in planning surgical or radiation therapy.

Orbital invasion of malignant melanoma is characterized by an ill-defined, solid mass with a heterogeneous hyperintense signal with respect to the extraocular muscles, and a hypointense signal with respect to orbital fat on T1W images (Fig. 19–2 A). The melanin content of the tumor may explain these MR features. On T2W images, the tumor shows a hyperintense signal compared with that of orbital fat (Fig. 19–2B).

Marked heterogeneous enhancement of the orbital extension is shown on Gd-DTPA–enhanced T1W images (Fig. 19–2C). Bone destruction, with extension to the adjacent sinuses, is best evaluated on contrast-enhanced images using fat-suppression techniques.

ORBITAL TUMORS OF INTRAOCULAR ORIGIN

Clinical and Pathological Features

The two most important intraocular lesions that may extend transsclerally into the orbital soft tissues are malignant melanoma of the posterior uvea in adults and retinoblastoma in children.

Posterior choroidal melanomas gain access to the retrobulbar orbit via emissarial channels or, less often, via the optic nerve. A long delay in the clinical recognition of uveal melanoma usually explains the extraocular extension of the intraocular tumor.

However, in rare cases, an aggressive uveal melanoma may develop early extraocular extension. In these cases, the patient develops progressive proptosis, glaucoma, and, sometimes, pain. Another form of orbital involvement from uveal melanoma is as orbital recurrence after previous removal of the eye. The interval between orbital recurrence and prior enucleation varies from months to years. Orbital recurrence can appear as a visible, palpable mass in the anophthalmic socket with displacement of the prosthesis and the orbital ball implant.

Histopathologic studies indicate that most cases of uveal melanoma extending into the orbit are of mixed or epithelioid cell types. Orbital CT scans demonstrate an intraocular mass and a relatively well-circumscribed, solid orbital mass. In cases in which the eye was removed, a solid orbital mass is seen to displace the ball implant on CT.

Extraocular extension of retinoblastoma into the orbit may also occur through the optic nerve or through scleral emissaria. The presence of tumor cells beyond the lamina cribrosa carries a poor prognosis and indicates the need for additional therapy. Orbital invasion of retinoblastoma should be suspected in a child with leukocoria and proptosis or displacement of the affected eye. However, most cases of orbital retinoblastoma represent orbital recurrence after enucleation of the eye containing retinoblastoma. In this situation, the child presents with displacement or protrusion of the prosthetic eye. In contrast to orbital recurrent uveal melanoma, the interval between enucleation and orbital recurrent retinoblastoma is usually a few months. Retinoblastoma that invades the orbit is usually poorly differentiated, with loosely cohesive retinoblastoma cells. Orbital CT studies demonstrate an irregular but relatively well-delineated soft tissue mass that often does not contain calcification. Necrotic retinoblastoma can manifest as orbital cellulitis and may simulate orbital invasion, but CT scans reveal anterior orbital soft tissue swelling without a solid component.

MR Features

Extraocular extension of uveal melanoma usually appears on MR scans as a well-circumscribed area with a signal that is isointense to the extraocular muscles and hypointense to orbital fat on T1W (Figs. 19–3A and 19–4A). On T2W images, these lesions have a hyperintense signal with respect to that of orbital fat and extraocular muscles (Figs. 19–3B and 19–4B). Based on the authors' experience, the extraocular extension shows the same signal intensity as the primary uveal melanoma on both T1W and T2W images. This low signal intensity on T1W and T2W images is mainly related to the paramagnetic properties of melanin within the intraocular and extraocular mass. However, tumor necrosis or hemorrhage can be seen in the tumor (Fig. 19–4, *A* and *B*).

After Gd-DTPA administration, extraocular extension of choroidal melanoma shows minimal to moderate heterogeneous enhancement (Figs. 19–3*C* and 19–4*C*). In the authors' experience, ultrasonography appears to be as accurate as MRI in detecting extraocular extension. However, MRI provides more information in delineating significant extraocular extension for the planned surgical approach.

ORBITAL TUMORS OF SINUS ORIGIN

Clinical and Pathological Features

Epithelial tumors may extend into the orbit from the paranasal sinuses by direct erosion through the thin bones separating the sinuses from the orbit or through osseous fissures and foramina. About 80% of malignant tumors involving the sinuses are carcinomas, whereas 20% are sarcomas. The most common origin of sinus carcinoma is the maxillary sinus. Because carcinomas produce symptoms related to their location and extent, nasal stuffiness, epistaxis, and dysphagia may be seen, along with progressive proptosis, displacement of the globe, and oculomotor palsies.

On histopathologic examination, these tumors present with features of sinus carcinoma and have the tendency to be poorly differentiated and unencapsulated. Approximately 90% of sinus carcinomas are squamous cell carcinomas. Adenocarcinoma accounts for about 7% of the epithelial neoplasms involving the sinuses. Orbital CT scans show a primary tumor with irregular margins and high density. CT studies help to delineate the extent of sinus carcinoma invasion of the orbit. Bone destruction and erosion are often seen.

MR Features

The major role of MR studies in secondary orbital tumors is to delineate the extent of the infiltrative tumor process within the orbit, the sinuses, and the brain. These malignant neoplasms are fairly cellular and usually show a low signal intensity on T1W images and an increased signal intensity on T2W images with respect to orbital fat (Figs. 19–5, *A* and *B*; 19–6*A*). The bony wall of the orbit can be evaluated if orbital invasion is suspected. The lack of signal void produced by the orbital walls between the tumor and the orbital tissue or the brain indi-

cates either thinning or destruction of the bone. The presence of bone erosion, expansion, hyperostosis, and bone marrow infiltration can be demonstrated by MRI (Figs. 19–5, *B* through *E*, and 19–6*D*).

After Gd-DTPA administration, the tumor usually shows moderate to marked enhancement. Fat-suppression techniques are useful in differentiating tumor margins from orbital fat (Figs. 19–5, *C* through *E*; 19–6, *B* through *D*).

BIBLIOGRAPHY

Bilaniuk LT, Zimmerman RA, Newton TH. Magnetic resonance imaging: Orbital pathology. In: Newton TH, Bilaniuk LT, eds. *Radiology of the Eye and Orbit*. New York: Raven Press; 1990, Chap 5.

Conley JJ. Sinus tumors invading the orbit. *Trans Am Acad Ophthalmol Otolaryngol*. 1966; 70:615–619.

De Potter P, Shields JA, Shields CL, Santos R. Modified enucleation via lateral orbitotomy for choroidal melanoma with orbital extension: A report of two cases. *Ophthalm Plast Reconstr Surg*. 1992; 8:109–113.

Ellsworth RM. Orbital retinoblastoma. *Trans Am Ophthalmol Soc*. 1974; 72:79–88.

Iliff W, Marback R, Green WR. Invasive squamous cell carcinoma of the conjunctiva. *Arch Ophthalmol*. 1975; 93:119–122.

Jakobiec FA, Font RL. Secondary tumors, mucoceles, and metastatic tumors. In: Spencer WH, Font RL, Green WR, Howes EL, Jakobiec FA, Zimmerman LE, eds. *Ophthalmic Pathology. An Atlas and Textbook*. Philadelphia: WB Saunders; 1986:2737–2765.

Johnson LN, Krohel GB, Yeon EB, Parnes SM. Sinus tumors invading the orbit. *Ophthalmology*. 1984; 91:209–217.

Mohan H, Sen D, Gupta D. Orbital affection in nasal and paranasal neoplasms. *Acta Ophthalmol*. 1969; 47:289–294.

Plotsky D, Quinn G, Eagle RC, Shields JA, Granowetter L. Congenital retinoblastoma: A case report. *J Pediatr Ophthalmol Strabismus*. 1987; 24:120–123.

Rao NA, Font RL. Mucoepidermoid carcinoma of the conjunctiva. *Cancer*. 1976; 38:1699–1709.

Rootman J. Secondary tumors of the orbit. In: Rootman J, ed. *Diseases of the Orbit*. Philadelphia: JB Lippincott; 1988:427–480.

Rootman J, Ellsworth RM, Hofbauer J, Kitchen D. Orbital extension of retinoblastoma: A clinicopathologic study. *Can J Ophthalmol*. 1978; 13:72–80.

Shields CL, Shields JA, Yarian DL, Augsburger JJ. Intracranial extension of choroidal melanoma via the optic nerve. *Br J Ophthalmol*. 1987; 71:172–176.

Shields JA. Secondary orbital tumors. In: Shields JA, ed. *Diagnosis and Management of Orbital Tumors*. Philadelphia: WB Saunders; 1989:341–377.

Shields JA, Bakewell B, Augsburger JJ, Flanagan JC. Classification and incidence of space-occupying lesions of the orbit. A survey of 645 biopsies. *Arch Ophthalmol.* 1984; 120:1606–1611.

Shields JA, Shields CL. Massive orbital extension of posterior uveal melanoma. *Ophthalm Plast Reconstr Surg.* 1991; 7:238–251.

Shields JA, Shields CL. Posterior uveal melanoma: Clinical and pathologic features. In: Shields JA, Shields CL, eds. *Intraocular Tumors. A Textbook and Atlas.* Philadelphia: WB Saunders; 1992:117–136.

Shields JA, Shields CL. Retinoblastoma: Clinical and pathologic features. In: Shields JA, Shields CL, eds. *Intraocular Tumors. A Textbook and Atlas.* Philadelphia: WB Saunders; 1992:305–332.

Shields JA, Shields CL, Suvarnamani C, Schroeder RP, De Potter P. Retinoblastoma manifesting as orbital cellulitis. *Am J Ophthalmol.* 1991; 112:442–449.

Wilbur AC, Dobben GD, Linder B. Paraorbital and tumor-like conditions: Role of CT and MRI. *Radiol Clin North Am.* 1987; 25:631–646.

FIGURE 19–1 *Squamous Cell Carcinoma of the Eyelid with Orbital Invasion*
A 69-year-old man was diagnosed as having a large invasive squamous cell carcinoma that was subsequently removed from the right upper eyelid and eyebrow. One month post excision, he presented with massive swelling and chemosis of the right upper eyelid, at which time a right orbital mass was palpated.

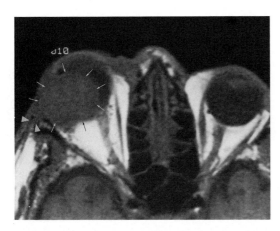

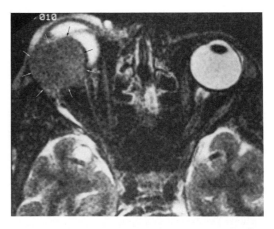

19–1A Axial T1W image. The orbital tumor (*arrows*) that overlies the right globe appears ill defined and has a low signal intensity, which is slightly hyperintense to the vitreous. The neoplastic process infiltrates the eyelid and the right zygoma (*arrowheads*).

19–1B Axial T2W image (inversion recovery). The orbital component (*arrows*) shows a low signal intensity compared with that of the eyelid tumor and the vitreous.

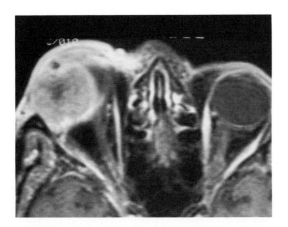

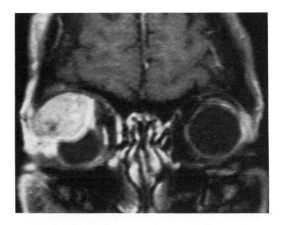

19–1C Fat-suppressed axial Gd-DTPA–enhanced T1W image. Both the eyelid and the orbital components demonstrate marked heterogeneous enhancement.

19–1D Fat-suppressed coronal Gd-DTPA–enhanced T1W image. The right frontal sinus and the globe are not involved by the tumor.

(continued)

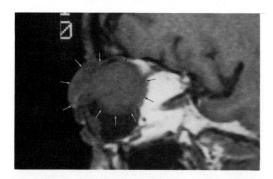

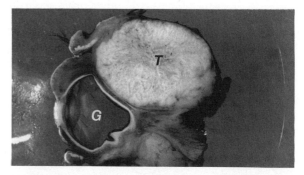

19–1E   Parasagittal T1W image. The well-defined orbital tumor shows a slightly hyperintense signal with respect to the extraocular muscles. The lesion (*arrows*) infiltrates anteriorly the upper eyelid and produces marked indentation of the right globe without intraocular extension. The orbital roof appears to be intact.

19–1F   Photograph of the exenteration specimen showing the well-circumscribed orbital tumor (*T*) indenting the globe (*G*).

FIGURE 19–2 *Malignant Melanoma of the Conjunctiva with Orbital and Lid Invasion*

A 79-year-old woman presented with recurrent malignant melanoma of the conjunctiva arising from primary acquired melanosis of the conjunctiva that had been treated with multiple excisional biopsies and cryotherapy.

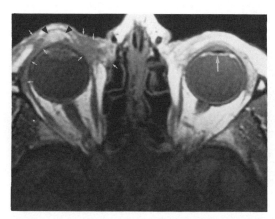

19–2A Axial T1W image. An infiltrative lesion of the conjunctiva (*small arrows*) with increased signal intensity overlies the right globe and extends into the medial canthus and the insertion of the horizontal rectus muscles. The lesion shows a heterogeneous hyperintense signal with respect to the extraocular muscles. The nodule palpated in the upper eyelid (*arrowheads*) shows an increased signal intensity due to its melanin content. The globe and the bony orbit are intact. There is no evidence of retrobulbar extension. Note the posterior chamber intraocular lens (*large arrow*) in the left eye.

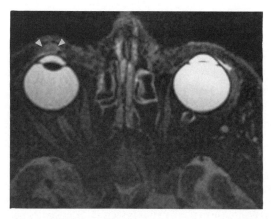

19–2B Axial T2W image (inversion recovery). The tumor is difficult to visualize except for the upper eyelid nodule (*arrowheads*), which remains slightly hyperintense.

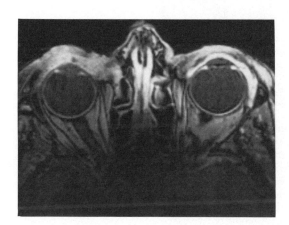

19–2C Fat-suppressed axial Gd-DTPA–enhanced T1W image. The infiltrative tumor shows marked heterogeneous enhancement.

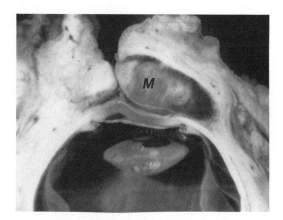

19–2D Exenteration specimen showing the oval nodule of invasive malignant melanoma (*M*) in the substantia propria of the central portion of the upper eyelid. Foci of invasive malignant melanoma were found in the forniceal conjunctiva and extended into the temporal aspect of the orbit.

FIGURE 19–3 *Massive Orbital Extension of Posterior Uveal Melanoma*
A 61-year-old woman was found to have a small choroidal melanoma in the posterior pole of the right eye. Ultrasonography revealed a well-circumscribed orbital mass that appeared to be in direct continuity with the intraocular tumor.

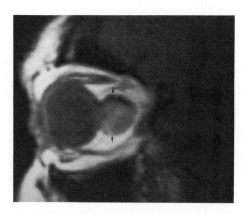

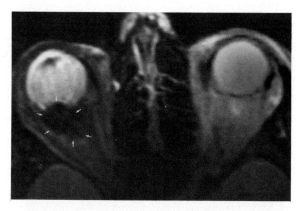

19–3A Sagittal T1W image. An intraocular mass that is hyperintense to the vitreous is seen at the posterior pole of the right eye. The contiguous, massive, well-circumscribed, extraocular extension of the lesion (*arrows*) shows a heterogeneous hyperintense signal.

19–3B Axial T2W image. The intraocular and extraocular tumor (*arrows*) becomes hypointense to the vitreous.

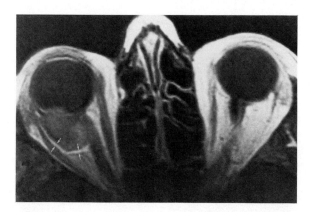

19–3C Axial Gd-DTPA–enhanced T1W image. The choroidal melanoma and its extraocular extension demonstrate minimal, heterogeneous enhancement. The extraocular component is surrounded by a thin, enhancing capsule (*arrows*). The optic nerve is displaced medially. (From De Potter P, Shields JA, Shields CL, Santos R. Modified enucleation via lateral orbitotomy for choroidal melanoma with orbital extension: A report of two cases. *Ophthalm Plast Reconstr Surg.* 1992; 8:111.)

(continued)

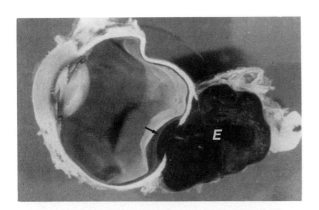

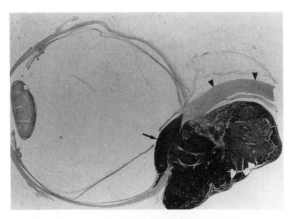

19–3D A surgical specimen, obtained at the time of modified enucleation, shows the markedly pigmented extraocular extension (*E*) of the posterior choroidal melanoma (*arrow*) against the optic nerve. (From De Potter P, Shields JA, Shields CL, Santos R. Modified enucleation via lateral orbitotomy for choroidal melanoma with orbital extension: A report of two cases. *Ophthalm Plast Reconstr Surg.* 1992; 8:112.)

19–3E Low-power photomicrograph showing the posterior choroidal melanoma (*arrow*) extending through the sclera and the massive orbital component of the tumor. Note the long section of the optic nerve (*arrowheads*).

FIGURE 19–4 *Recurrent Uveal Melanoma with Extraocular Extension*
A 65-year-old woman presented with recurrent ciliochoroidal melanoma of the right eye after tumor resection and hemorrhagic retinal detachment. She subsequently developed an enlarging, firm mass in the upper inner quadrant of the right orbit with displacement of the globe.

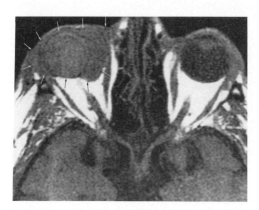

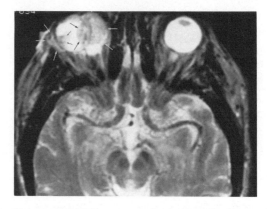

19–4A Axial T1W image. The right globe has an increased signal intensity due to the vitreous hemorrhage and recurrent uveal melanoma. The extraocular component of the tumor (*arrows*) appears to be isointense to the intraocular portion, involves the insertion of the lateral and medial rectus muscles, and extends to the intraconal space.

19–4B Axial T2W image. Both the intraocular (*black arrows*) and extraocular (*white arrows*) areas of the tumor become hypointense with respect to the hemorrhagic vitreous. The posterior portion of the nasal orbital component shows a high signal intensity, which is probably related to tumor necrosis.

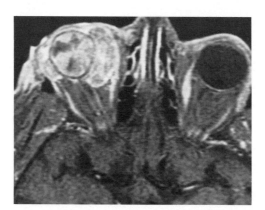

19–4C Fat-suppressed axial Gd-DTPA–enhanced T1W image. The recurrent intraocular uveal melanoma is well identified by its marked enhancement compared with the nonenhancing hemorrhagic vitreous. The extraocular components show marked heterogeneous enhancement.

(continued)

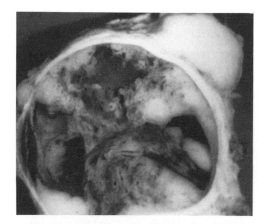

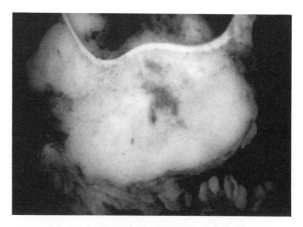

19–4D   Photograph of the grossly sectioned eye showing mainly the intraocular tumor recurrence filling the vitreous cavity.

19–4E   Photograph of the grossly sectioned eye showing mainly the nasal extraocular tumor extension.

FIGURE 19–5 *Squamous Cell Carcinoma of the Maxillary Sinus with Invasion of the Orbit*

A 64-year-old man presented with progressive, painful, right periorbital swelling and proptosis associated with diplopia and upward displacement of the right globe.

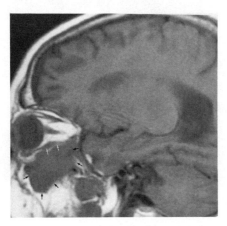

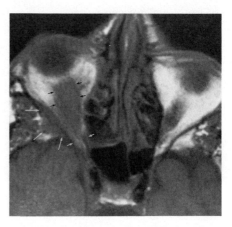

19–5A Sagittal T1W image. The hypointense infiltrative tumor (*black arrows*) originates from the right maxillary sinus and has destroyed the orbital floor. The inferior rectus muscle (*white arrows*) is displaced superiorly by the orbital component of the tumor.

19–5B Axial T1W image. The inferior rectus muscle is surrounded by the infiltrative tumor (*short arrows*), which extends posteriorly through the superior orbital fissure. Note the erosion of the lateral orbital wall with infiltration of the marrow space (*long arrows*) of the sphenoid bone.

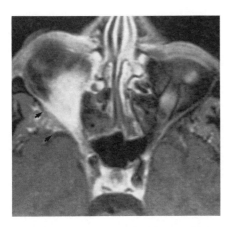

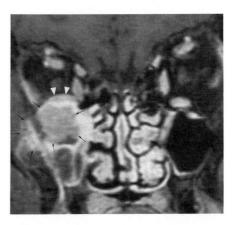

19–5C Fat-suppressed axial Gd-DTPA–enhanced T1W image. The tumor demonstrates marked homogeneous enhancement surrounding the inferior rectus muscle. Loss of the signal void (*arrows*) between the mass and the medullary space of the right sphenoid bone indicates infiltration of the bone by the tumor, as seen in *B* and confirmed after administration of contrast agent.

19–5D Fat-suppressed coronal Gd-DTPA–enhanced T1W image. The inferior rectus muscle (*arrowheads*) is displaced by the enhancing infiltrative lesion (*arrows*), which fills the superior space of the maxillary sinus and involves the lateral wall of the maxillary sinus. There is enhancement of the mucosal lining of the maxillary sinus. Fluid collection along the inferior part of the sinus shows decreased signal intensity.

(continued)

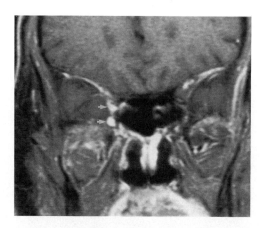

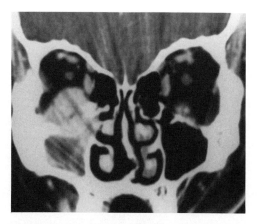

19–5E Fat-suppressed coronal Gd-DTPA–enhanced T1W image at the level of the superior orbital fissure. Note the enhancement of the right cavernous sinus, as well as the perineural spread of the tumor (*arrows*).

19–5F Coronal contrast-enhanced CT scan. The soft tissue mass is destroying the orbital floor. The inferior rectus muscle is not identified.

FIGURE 19–6 *Primary Mucosal Malignant Melanoma of the Paranasal Sinuses with Orbital Invasion*

An 80-year-old man presented with epistaxis and was diagnosed as having primary malignant melanoma of the right nasal cavity, maxillary sinus, ethmoidal sinus, and frontal sinus with orbital invasion.

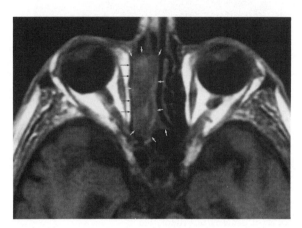

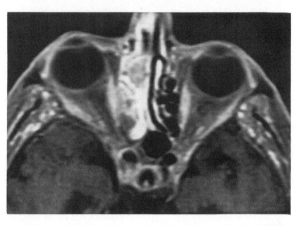

19-6A Axial T1W image. The right ethmoidal sinus is filled with a heterogenous mass (*white arrows*) of high signal intensity that is slightly more hyperintense than the extraocular muscles. On this level, the continuity of the signal void of the right medial orbital wall (*black arrows*) indicates its integrity from tumor invasion.

19-6B Fat-suppressed axial Gd-DTPA–enhanced T1W image. The tumor demonstrates marked heterogeneous enhancement.

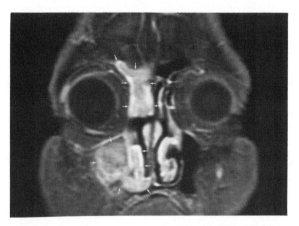

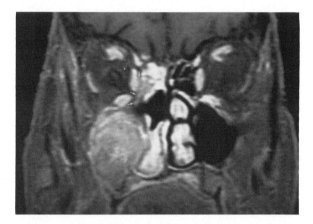

19-6C Fat-suppressed coronal Gd-DTPA–enhanced T1W image at the level of the globe. On this level, the enhancing tumor (*arrows*) is seen to invade the right maxillary sinus, right nasal cavity, right ethmoidal sinus, and right frontal sinus.

19-6D Fat-suppressed coronal Gd-DTPA–enhanced T1W image at a retrobulbar level. The right orbital invasion (*arrows*) through the eroded medial orbital wall is detected in the inferonasal aspect of the retro-orbital space.

Part Four | Miscellaneous Disorders

MRI of the Eye and Orbit,
by Patrick De Potter, Jerry A. Shields, and Carol L. Shields.
J. B. Lippincott Company, Philadelphia © 1995.

20

Anophthalmic Socket

PATRICK DE POTTER

CAROL L. SHIELDS

JERRY A. SHIELDS

NONINTEGRATED IMPLANT

General Considerations

Orbital implants are used to occupy the orbital space after enucleation of the eye. They are classified as integrated or nonintegrated and buried or nonburied. Until recently, a simple sphere made of silicone or polymethylmethacrylate was generally used as a nonintegrated, buried implant after enucleation or evisceration. The complications associated with the nonintegrated, buried implant include implant extrusion, implant migration, and infection. Moreover, the final motility of the prosthesis has been generally limited owing to the lack of coupling of the implant to the prosthesis.

Orbital computed tomography (CT) has shown utility in assessing implant migration, orbital inflammation, or orbital recurrence of retinoblastoma or uveal malignant melanoma. On CT scanning, the conventional polymethylmethacrylate sphere appears to be as dense as the mature bone.

MR Features

On precontrast and postcontrast magnetic resonance imaging (MRI), the polymethylmethacrylate sphere shows a low signal intensity owing to the chemical composition of the ball. The high tissue definition afforded by MR scans allows for evaluation of the anatomic position of the sphere in the muscle cone and for diagnostic exclusion of orbital

recurrence of malignant intraocular orbital tumors (Figs. 20–1, *A* and *B*; 20–2, *A* through *C*).

T1-weighted (T1W) images enhanced by administration of gadolinium diethylenetriamine penta-acetic acid (Gd-DTPA) with fat-suppression technique are most helpful in evaluating the extraocular muscles if secondary implantation with a hydroxyapatite orbital implant is being considered (Figs. 20–1, *C* and *D*; 20–2D).

INTEGRATED IMPLANT

General Considerations

The recently introduced coralline-derived hydroxyapatite sphere for ophthalmic surgery is composed primarily of calcium phosphate and has been used successfully in the past for orthopedic, maxillofacial, and orthognathic surgery (Fig. 20–3, *A* and *B*). The hydroxyapatite orbital implant, as an integrated buried orbital implant, is associated with few complications and provides excellent prosthetic motility. Once the implant has become permeated with fibrovascular tissue, a peg can be placed in the implant and attached to an indentation in the posterior portion of the prosthesis. Rare cases of orbital cellulitis, implant extrusion, or implant migration have been reported. The lack of blind passages or cul-de-sacs in this porous material allows ingrowth of vascularized fibrous connective tissue and, therefore, successful integration. The fibrovascularity is most extensive near the precut scleral windows, which are designed for rectus muscle attachment, and at the posterior position of the sphere. The documentation of fibrovascular tissue within the hydroxyapatite orbital implant by imaging studies is advised prior to proceeding with drilling of the sphere and peg placement.

The use of conventional imaging studies for the evaluation of hydroxyapatite orbital implants has been limited owing to the density of the calcified sphere. Because of the dramatic sound attenuation produced by the hydroxyapatite material, the presence of blood flow cannot be detected by A- and B-mode ultrasonography or by color Doppler imaging. The density of the hydroxyapatite sphere, which is similar to that of mature bone, does not allow detection of fibrovascular tissue on contrast-enhanced CT studies (Fig. 20–3C). The limited tissue specificity of technetium-99m bone scans precludes high-resolution visualization of the intraocular structures and localization of the fibrovascular tissue within the ball implant (Fig. 20–3D).

MR Features

Based on the authors' experience, the integrated hydroxyapatite orbital implant, made of a complex internal porous network filled with fibrovascular tissue and extracellular water, exhibits an intermediate heterogeneous signal, which is isointense to hyperintense to the extraocular muscles and hypointense to orbital fat on T1W images (Figs. 20–4A, 20–5A, 20–6, 20–7A, 20–8A, and 20–9A). The signal of the hydroxyapatite sphere appears heterogeneously hyperintense to the extraocular muscles and orbital fat on T2-weighted (T2W) images (Figs. 20–4B and 20–7B). All extraocular muscles that are surgically reattached to the wrapped hydroxyapatite orbital implant at the time of enucleation are clearly identified on T1W and T2W images.

After Gd-DTPA administration, the integrated hydroxyapatite implant demonstrates a pattern of enhancement that is consistent with the presence of fibrovascular ingrowth. Postcontrast T1W images reveal that the enhancement is initially most notable in the peripheral portions of the sphere, and is variable in intensity and location within the sphere. The enhancement may be localized (Figs. 20–5, B and C; 20–6, 20–7C) or diffuse and heterogeneous (Fig. 20–8B) or diffuse and homogeneous (Fig. 20–9B), and may be seen as early as 5 months after implantation of the hydroxyapatite ball implant. There is no definitive correlation between the extent of enhancement of the hydroxyapatite sphere and the time interval since implantation.

The presence of enhancing fibrovascular tissue within the hydroxyapatite implant is best evaluated on fat-suppressed Gd-DTpA–enhanced T1W image and constitutes our guide for drilling.

BIBLIOGRAPHY

De Potter P, Shields CL, Shields JA, Flanders AE, Rao VM. Role of magnetic resonance imaging in the evaluation of the hydroxyapatite implant. *Ophthalmology.* 1992; 99:824–830.

De Potter P, Shields CL, Shields JA, Singh AD. Use of hydroxyapatite ocular implant in the pediatric population. *Arch Ophthalmol.* 1994; 112:208–212.

Perry AC. Advances in enucleation. *Ophthalmol Clin North Am.* 1991; 4:173–182.

Rosner M, Edward DP, Tso MON. Foreign-body giant-cell reaction to the hydroxyapatite orbital implant. *Arch Ophthalmol.* 1992; 110:173.

Sartoris DJ, Gershuni DH, Akeson WH, Holmes RE, Resnik D. Coralline hydroxyapatite bone graft substitutes: Preliminary report of radiographic evaluation. *Radiology.* 1986; 159:133–137.

Shields CL, Shields JA, De Potter P. Hydroxyapatite orbital implant after enucleation. Experience with initial 100 consecutive cases. *Arch Ophthalmol.* 1992; 110:333–338.

Shields CL, Shields JA, De Potter P, Singh AD. Problems with hydroxyapatite implant. Experience with 250 consecutive cases. *Br J Ophthalmol.* 1994; 78:702–706.

Shields CL, Shields JA, Eagle RC, De Potter P. Histopathologic evidence of fibrovascular ingrowth four weeks after placement of the hydroxyapatite orbital implant. *Am J Ophthalmol.* 1991; 111:363–366.

Shields JA, Shields CL, De Potter P. Hydroxyapatite orbital implant after enucleation. Experience with 200 cases. *Mayo Clin Proc.* 1993; 68:1191–1195.

FIGURE 20-1 *Anophthalmic Socket with Polymethylmethacrylate Sphere*
A 20–year-old woman underwent enucleation of the left eye as a young child for unilateral sporadic retinoblastoma. MR studies were performed in order to evaluate the extraocular muscles before secondary implantation of a hydroxyapatite implant.

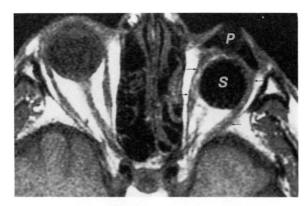

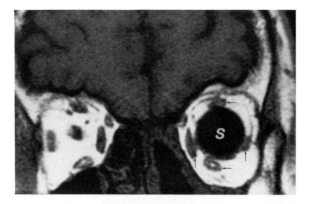

20-1A Axial T1W image. The nonintegrated buried ball implant shows a very low signal intensity (*S*). The lateral and medial rectus muscles (*arrows*) are seen to wrap around the sphere, which is well centered in the anophthalmic socket. The curvilinear signal void crescent corresponds to the overlying prosthesis (*P*). The left orbital cavity is smaller than that on the right.

20-1B Coronal T1W image. All four rectus muscles (*arrows*) are well visualized around the sphere (*S*). No signs of orbital tumor recurrence are detected.

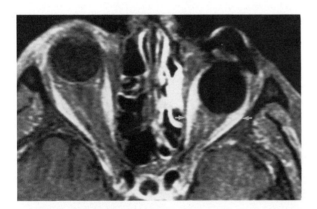

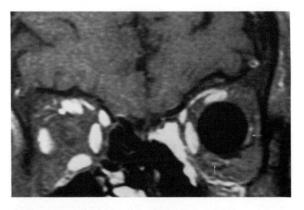

20-1C Fat-suppressed axial Gd-DTPA–enhanced T1W image. Note the marked enhancement of the lateral and medial rectus muscles (*arrows*).

20-1D Fat-suppressed coronal Gd-DTPA–enhanced T1W image. On this plane, the bellies of the left medial rectus, superior oblique, superior rectus, and levator palpebrae superioris muscles enhance markedly. The lateral and inferior rectus muscles show minimal enhancement at their insertion (*arrows*).

FIGURE 20-2 *Anophthalmic Socket with Migration of the Polymethylacrylate Sphere*

A 50-year-old man who underwent enucleation of the left eye following trauma was experiencing discomfort in the left anophthalmic socket.

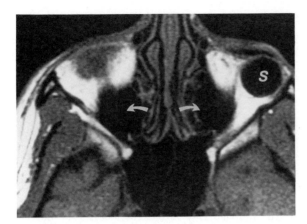

20-2A Axial T1W image at the level of the orbital floor. The polymethylmethacrylate sphere (S) is displaced inferolaterally. Note the signal void produced by the maxillary sinus (*curved arrows*) on both sides of the nasal cavity.

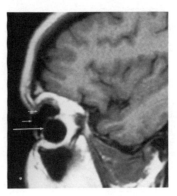

20-2B Parasagittal T1W image. The remodelled prosthesis in the superior fornix (*short arrows*) overhangs the polymethylmethacrylate sphere (*arrow*).

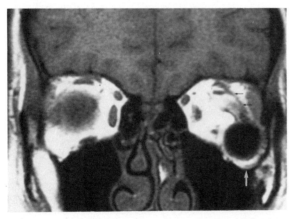

20-2C Coronal T1W image. The polymethylmethacrylate sphere has an extraconal location. An intermuscular membrane (*black arrows*) courses vertically between the superior rectus and lateral rectus muscles. Note the bowing of the orbital floor (*white arrow*).

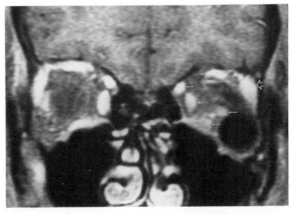

20-2D Fat-suppressed coronal Gd-DTPA–enhanced T1W image. The orbital lobe of the left lacrimal gland (*open arrow*) shows marked enhancement, as do the extraocular rectus muscles (*arrows*).

FIGURE 20–3 *Evaluation of a Hydroxyapatite Implant*
(From De Potter P, Shields CL, Shields JA, Flanders AE, Rao VM. Role of magnetic resonance imaging in the evaluation of the hydroxyapatite implant. *Ophthalmology.* 1992; 99:824–830. © 1992, American Academy of Ophthalmology.)

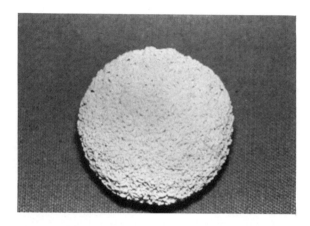

20–3A Hydroxyapatite ball sphere.

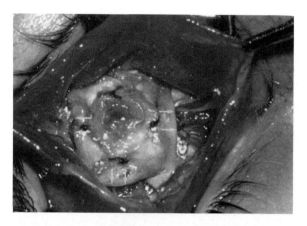

20–3B Photograph showing placement of the scleralized hydroxyapatite implant in the anophthalmic socket. The rectus muscles are attached through scleral windows at their anatomic insertion (*arrows*).

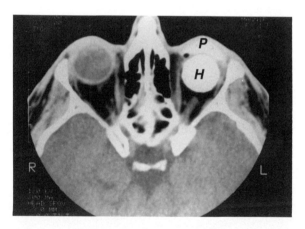

20–3C Axial-enhanced CT scan obtained 6 months after insertion of the implant. The hydroxyapatite ball sphere (*H*) in the left socket has the same density as cortical bone. The presence of fibrovascular tissue cannot be confirmed. The overlying prosthesis (*P*) is hyperdense. The opposite eye is normal.

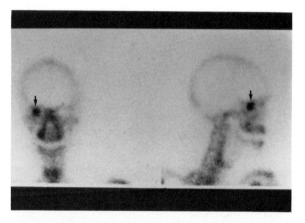

20–3D Technetium-99m bone imaging of the head and neck of a patient who underwent surgical implantation of a hydroxyapatite implant 6 months previously. Diffuse, nonspecific, high uptake of the radioisotope in the right orbit (*arrows*) is seen on the anterior and right lateral projections. (Courtesy of Dr. Arthur C. Perry, San Diego, CA.)

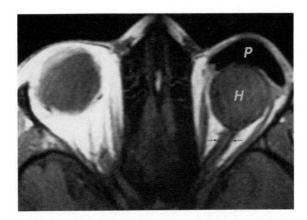

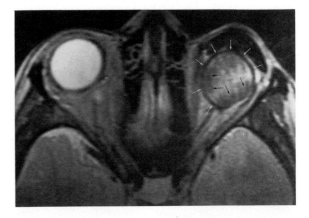

20-4A Axial T1W image. The hydroxyapatite sphere (*H*) shows a slightly increased signal with respect to the vitreous. The horizontal rectus muscles are well identified. The stump of the optic nerve sheath complex (*arrows*) is seen posterior to the sphere. The signal void crescent corresponds to the prosthesis (*P*).

20-4B Axial T2W image. The hydroxyapatite implant becomes heterogeneously hyperintense. The areas of increased signal intensity correspond to accumulation of extracellular free water. The hypointense areas correspond to fibrovascular tissue (*black arrows*). The implant is surrounded by a hypointense linear signal (*white arrows*) that corresponds to the sclera that was wrapping the implant before surgery.

FIGURE 20-5 *Hydroxyapatite Sphere Implanted 3 Months Previously after Enucleation of the Left Eye for Treatment of Unilateral Sporadic Retinoblastoma in a 3-Year-Old Child*

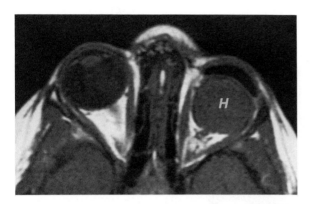

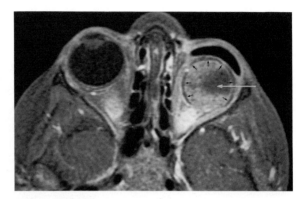

20-5A Axial T1W image. The hydroxyapatite sphere (*H*) appears to be slightly hyperintense to the vitreous. The medial and lateral rectus muscles are attached anteriorly.

20-5B Fat-suppressed axial Gd-DTPA–enhanced T1W image. Marked homogeneous enhancement is seen in the anterior, nasal, and posterior portions of the sphere. No enhancing fibrovascular tissue is detected in the temporal portion of the sphere (*white arrow*). The wrapping sclera (*black arrows*) shows a decreased signal intensity.

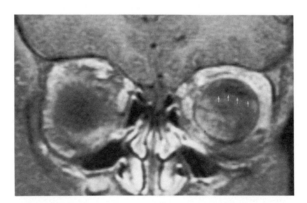

20-5C Fat-suppressed coronal Gd-DTPA–enhanced T1W image. The superior portion of the sphere is not vascularized (*arrows*).

FIGURE 20–6 *Hydroxyapatite Sphere Implanted for 6 Months in the Right Orbit of a 55-Year-Old Man*

Axial precontrast (*top*) and post–Gd-DTPA injection (*bottom*) T1W images. The presence of fibrovascular tissue is suspected in the anterior portion of the hydroxyapatite sphere. After contrast administration, the fibrovascular ingrowth (*arrows*) is well delineated at the anterior aspect of the sphere, at the insertion of the medial rectus muscle through the scleral window, and at the posterior portion.

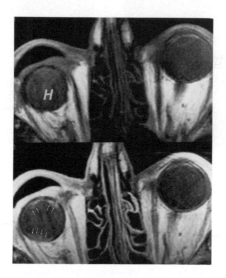

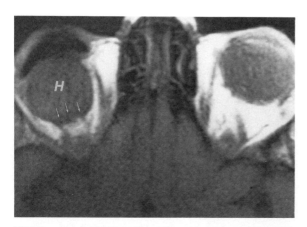

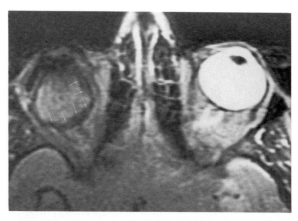

20–7A Axial T1W image. The posterior portion (*arrows*) of the sphere (*H*) appears to be slightly hypointense compared with the central portion.

20–7B Axial T2W image. The central portion of the sphere becomes hyperintense, which corresponds to the presence of extracellular free water. The posterior and nasal portions of the sphere (*arrows*) remain hypointense owing to the presence of fibrovascular tissue.

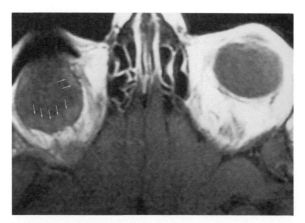

20–7C Axial Gd-DTPA–enhanced T1W image. The hypointense fibrovascularized areas seen on T2W images show homogeneous enhancement (*arrows*).

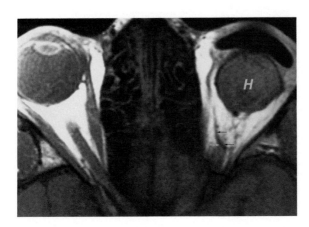

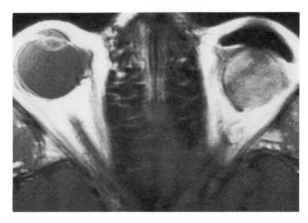

20–8A Axial T1W image. Note the curvilinear hypointense signal of the ophthalmic artery (*arrows*).

20–8B Axial Gd-DTPA–enhanced T1W image. The hydroxyapatite orbital implant demonstrates diffuse and heterogeneous enhancement.

FIGURE 20-9 *Hydroxyapatite Sphere Implanted in a 20-Year-Old Woman 6 Months Prior to MRI Studies*

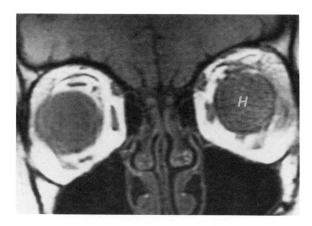

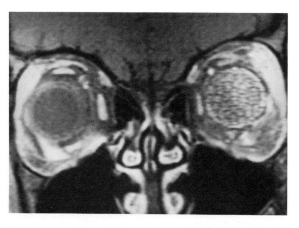

20-9A Coronal T1W image. The hydroxyapatite sphere (*H*) is seen to be well centered in the orbit.

20-9B Fat-suppressed coronal Gd-DTPA–enhanced T1W image. There is diffuse and homogeneous enhancement of the sphere, indicating total integration of the hydroxyapatite orbital implant.

MRI of the Eye and Orbit,
by Patrick De Potter, Jerry A. Shields, and Carol L. Shields.
J. B. Lippincott Company, Philadelphia © 1995.

21

Orbital Trauma

PATRICK DE POTTER

ROBERT A. ZIMMERMAN

Clinical and Pathological Features

Blunt or penetrating trauma to the orbital region can produce fractures, soft tissue injuries, localized or diffuse hemorrhage, and foreign bodies. Once the facial tissues and the globe are assessed, a careful orbital examination can be done. The motility of the eyelids, the position of the globe, and extraocular motility, with or without forced duction, must be evaluated. Palpation of the orbital rim may reveal a fracture site. Tissue emphysema and crepitus may suggest a paranasal fracture.

Direct fractures (involving the orbital rim) occur when force is applied to the bone. Indirect fractures (blowout or blowin) result from the force transmitted through the orbital soft tissues. The sites of least resistance are the orbital floor and the medial orbital wall. Motility disturbances, enophthalmos, infraorbital hypoesthesia, and pseudoproptosis may be seen. Medial blow-out fractures are usually minimal and may produce tissue emphysema.

Abrasions and avulsion of orbital tissues, such as the extraocular muscles and optic nerve, occur less commonly. Orbital hemorrhage can be classified according to the site of accumulated blood. Preseptal and/or postseptal hemorrhage, intraocular hemorrhage within the muscle cone, and subperiosteal hematoma or intracanalicular hemorrhage can occur.

Orbital foreign bodies are usually dormant and

well tolerated. Any laceration or puncture site should be explored for a foreign body.

Computed tomography (CT) remains the modality of choice for evaluating patients with a history of acute orbital trauma. CT studies can easily demonstrate bony defects or fragments in a blowout fracture, as well as the extent of soft tissue herniation. CT scans can also detect the presence of any type of intraorbital foreign body. However, CT has little value in detecting dry wood alone. Computer-reformatted CT scans produce an obvious loss of spatial resolution, and direct coronal scans may fail to demonstrate foreign bodies or lesions because of dental filling artifacts.

MR Features

Magnetic resonance imaging (MRI) is contraindicated if there is any suspicion of a ferromagnetic foreign body. The role of MRI is often complimentary to CT scanning in the evaluation of orbital trauma. Although bony fragments produce signal voids, orbital fractures can be diagnosed by the presence of hyperintense orbital fat that has prolapsed into the adjacent air-containing paranasal sinuses and by the interposition of tissue with increased signal intensity between fracture fragments (Figs. 21–1 and 21–2A). Kinking or entrapment of extraocular muscle and prolapse of the orbital fat (particularly on T1W images) in blow-out fractures will be best defined on a coronal plane or an oblique sagittal plane parallel to the axis of the inferior rectus muscle.

Intraorbital wood can be detected on MR studies. In such cases, a well-delineated, low-intensity, geometrically shaped intraorbital lesion suggestive of a retained foreign body is seen (Fig. 21–3B).

In acute orbital trauma, an increased linear and reticular pattern in the retro-orbital fat, along with vascular engorgement and edema, can be documented. The presence of a small orbital acute hemorrhage (deoxyhemoglobin) with low signal intensity on T1-(T1W) and T2-weighted (T2W) images may be difficult to detect (Fig. 21–4). In subacute hemorrhage, the hyperintense methemoglobin is easily identified on T1W images using fat-suppression techniques. The fat-suppressed images allow differentiation of the high signal intensity of the subacute hemorrhage from that of the orbital fat seen on standard T1W images (Fig. 21–2, A through D). Chronic hemorrhage with hemosiderin shows hyperintense to hypointense signals on both short time-to-repeat (TR) and time-to-echo (TE) studies. The presence of tissue fibrosis and globe or soft tissue distortion can be demonstrated in patients sustaining chronic orbital soft tissue trauma (Fig. 21–5). MR studies may also provide important information about the integrity of the intraocular tissues and may be helpful in ruling out luxation of the lens, retinal or choroidal detachment, rupture of the sclera, and vitreous hemorrhage (Figs. 21–1; 21–5, A and B; and 21–6).

BIBLIOGRAPHY

Bilaniuk LT, Zimmerman RA, Newton TH. Magnetic resonance imaging: Orbital pathology. In: Newton TH, Bilaniuk LT, eds. *Radiology of the Eye and Orbit.* New York: Raven Press; 1990, Chap 5.

Green BF, Kraft SP, Carter KD, Buncic JR, Nerad JA, Armstrong D. Intraorbital wood. Detection by magnetic resonance imaging. *Ophthalmology.* 1989; 97: 608–611.

Grove AS Jr. Computed tomography in the management of orbital trauma. *Ophthalmology.* 1982; 89:433–440.

Han JS, Benson JE, Bonstelle CT, Alfidi RJ, Kaufman B, Levine M. Magnetic resonance imaging of the orbit: A preliminary experience. *Radiology.* 1984; 150: 755–759.

McArdle CB, Amparo EG, Mirfakhraee M. MR imaging of blow-out fractures. *J Comput Assist Tomogr.* 1986; 10:116–119.

Rootman J, Neigel J. Trauma. In: Rootman J, ed. *Diseases of the Orbit.* Philadelphia: JB Lippincott; 1988: 504–523.

Tonami H, Nakagawa T, Ohguchi M, et al. Surface coil MR imaging of orbital blowout fractures: A comparison with reformatted CT. *AJNR.* 1987; 8:445–449.

Weisman RA, Savino PJ, Schut L, Schatz NJ. Computed tomography in penetrating wounds of the orbit with retained foreign bodies. *Arch Otolaryngol.* 1983; 109: 265–268.

Zimmerman RA, Bilaniuk LT, Hackney DB, Goldberg HI, Grossman RI. Paranasal sinus hemorrhage: Evaluation with MR imaging. *Radiology.* 1987; 162:499–503.

FIGURE 21-1 *Facial Trauma Producing a Left Orbital Blowout Fracture*
Coronal T1W image. The central vitreous in the left eye has a heterogeneous, hyperintense signal corresponding to blood in the methemoglobin state. Fractures of the medial orbital wall, as well as of the orbital floor, are evident and are associated with prolapse of the orbital fat through the bony defects (*arrows*).

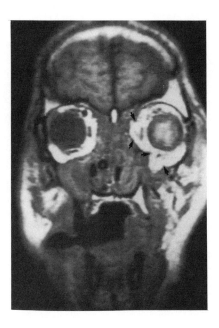

FIGURE 21-2 *Left Orbital Trauma*

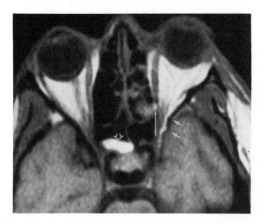

21-2A Axial T1W image. The irregular signal void in the cortical sphenoid wing suggests a bone fracture *(short arrows)*. Fracture of the left medial orbital wall has produced minimal herniation of orbital fat into the ethmoidal sinus *(long arrow)*. The intermediate, heterogeneous signal intensity in the left ethmoidal sinus most likely represents hemorrhage in the deoxyhemoglobin/methemoglobin state. The presence of methemoglobin is suggested by the high signal intensity in the posterior right sphenoid sinus *(open arrow)*. The left medial rectus muscle is slightly thickened by edema.

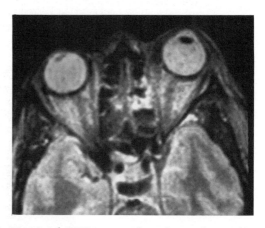

21-2B Axial T2W image. The subacute hemorrhage in the sphenoid sinus shows a hyperintense signal that is consistent with methemoglobin in an extracellular state.

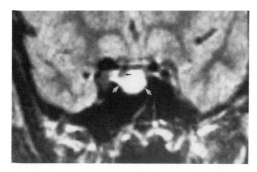

21-2C Coronal T2W image at the level of the sphenoid sinus. A hypointense linear signal represents a displaced bone fragment arising from the planum sphenoidale *(black arrow)* within the localized hemorrhage (methemoglobin state) *(white arrows)* in the sphenoid sinus.

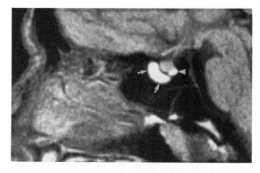

21-2D Parasagittal proton density-weighted image. Note the focal subacute hematoma *(arrows)* in the floor of the sellae. The normal posterior pituitary gland *(arrowhead)* has a hyperintense signal.

(continued)

FIGURE 21-2 *Left Orbital Trauma* (continued)

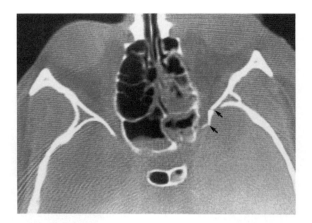

21-2E Axial nonenhanced CT scan (bone windows). Note the fractures (*arrows*) in the greater portion of the sphenoid wing.

FIGURE 21–3 *Intraorbital Wooden Foreign Body*

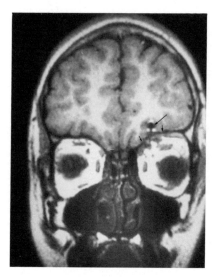

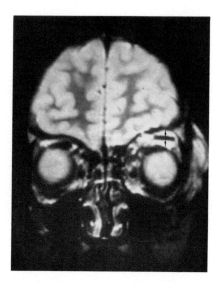

21–3A Coronal T1W image. The signal void in the left cortical frontal bone is irregular, suggesting a bony defect (*short arrows*). The rounded area of signal loss in the left frontal lobe represents an air bubble trapped within the gray matter (*long arrow*). The area of intermediate signal intensity adjacent to the orbital roof most likely represents tissue edema.

21–3B Coronal T2W image. The well-delineated rectangular signal void represents an intraorbital wooden foreign body (*arrows*). The surrounding area of high signal intensity represents tissue edema and/or hemorrhage (methemoglobin state).

FIGURE 21-4 *Bilateral Subperiosteal Hematomas Secondary to Facial Trauma*
Coronal T1W image. An isointense, lenticular fluid collection (*arrows*) is seen adjacent to the left orbital roof and overlying the superior rectus and levator palpebrae superioris muscles. The signal intensity is attributable to acute hemorrhage. Note the fracture of the roof of the right orbit with interposed tissue (*arrowhead*) between the two fracture fragments. A subperiosteal hematoma is present on this side as well (*arrow*).

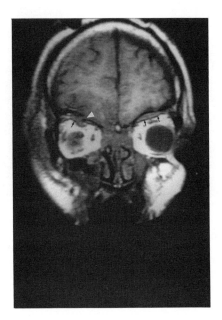

FIGURE 21-5 *Old Facial Trauma with Orbital and Intraocular Sequelae*

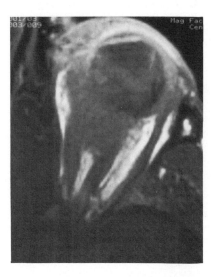

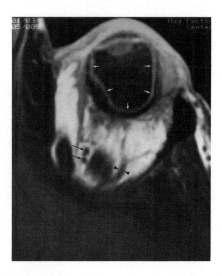

21-5A Axial T1W image. The ill-defined tissue of low signal intensity that lies adjacent to the globe and involves the left medial rectus muscle represents residual fibrotic tissue from orbital hemorrhage. The medial and lateral rectus muscles, as well as the optic nerve sheath complex, are involved.

21-5B Axial T1W image at a higher level than in *A*. The chronic post-traumatic choroidal effusion in the left eye has a crescent-shaped high signal intensity (*white arrows*). Note the ophthalmic artery (*black arrows*) and the superior ophthalmic vein (*arrowhead*).

FIGURE 21-6 *Traumatic Luxation of the Intraocular Lens*
Axial T2W image. The hypointense, ovoid area located at the posterior pole in the left eye corresponds to the luxated lens (*arrow*). Note the image degradation induced by motion artifact.

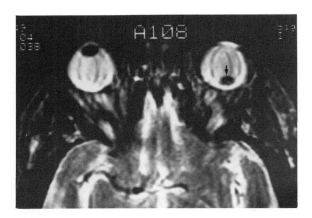

Index

Page numbers followed by *f* indicate a figure; *t* following a page number indicates tabular material.